Meet the editor

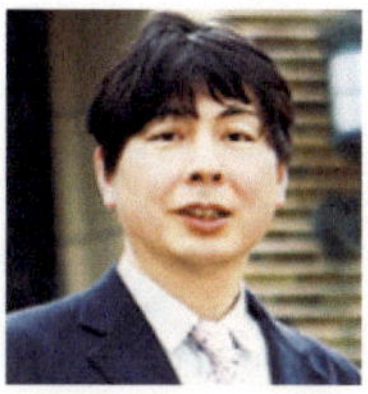

Dr. Naofumi Shiomi spent 15 years as a researcher at Kaneka's Industrial Technology Research Institute, researching recombinant yeast and its applications, until 1998. After receiving his Ph.D. in Engineering from Kyoto University, he taught applied microbiology, biotechnology, and life sciences for 27 years as a Professor at Kobe College's School of Human Sciences. At Kobe College, he specialized in bioremediation, and in recent years, his research has focused on preventing obesity and aging. He is currently affiliated with Kobe University, where he is developing new applications for microfibers in medicine and biotechnology.

Contents

Preface

The number of obese people worldwide is on the rise, and it is estimated that by 2030, the global obesity rate will reach 573 million. Due to changes in eating habits and working environments, metabolic syndrome is on the rise in both developed and developing countries, with the rate of increase being particularly rapid in developing countries compared to developed countries, and it is predicted that by 2030, approximately 80% of diabetes patients will be concentrated in developing countries. Furthermore, within Asia, South Asia has a high prevalence of obesity-related diseases, and in India, the number of adult type 2 diabetes patients is rapidly increasing. As such, obesity and metabolic syndrome are serious social issues that require solutions.

Obesity, resulting from an unbalanced diet and an irregular lifestyle, can lead to insulin resistance and chronic inflammation, resulting in a condition known as metabolic syndrome. Metabolic syndrome can progress to type 2 diabetes, heart disease, and hypertension. In 1998, the WHO established diagnostic criteria for metabolic syndrome. Over the 27 years since then, the mechanisms underlying metabolic syndrome have been elucidated, including the roles of paracrine factors such as adipokines and batokines secreted by tissues in insulin resistance and chronic inflammation, and the role of RNA in exosomes. It is also becoming clear that metabolic syndrome is involved in diseases initially thought to be unrelated to metabolic syndrome, such as non-alcoholic hepatitis, cancer, and dementia. Furthermore, numerous studies are underway to develop effective interventions for the prevention and treatment of metabolic syndrome.

Moreover, it is also important to note that obesity can lead to type 2 diabetes, not only causing insulin resistance and hyperglycemia but also hypoglycemia. In the case of diabetes, hypoglycemia can be caused by excessive administration of diabetes medication, and hypoglycemia can cause symptoms such as tremors, palpitations, cold sweats, headaches, and difficulty concentrating. Furthermore, there are also cases of hypoglycemia that are not related to diabetes. Therefore, in addition to treating hyperglycemia caused by diabetes, care must also be taken to prevent hypoglycemia.

This book covers the following topics related to metabolic syndrome and hypoglycemia. First, the authors discuss the relationship between obesity and metabolic syndrome, including the latest research on the role of exosomes in metabolic syndrome and its treatment, the relationship between lipedema and hormones, and factors contributing to the rise in obesity and diabetes in Southeast Asia. Next, the authors discuss the relationship between metabolic syndrome and other diseases, including factors affecting the development of heart disease, factors contributing to the development of pediatric chronic kidney disease, the relationship between endometriosis and metabolic syndrome, and the relationship between illicit opioids and metabolic syndrome. Finally, other authors discuss the causes and treatment of hypoglycemia, including characteristics of reactive hypoglycemia, hypoglycemia in diabetic patients, and hypoglycemic issues in non-diabetic patients. These expert reviews will provide readers with a broader understanding of metabolic syndrome and hypoglycemia. In addition, the related book, "Lifestyle-Related Diseases and Metabolic Syndrome," already published by IntechOpen, can also be used as reference material.

Finally, I would like to thank Ms. Mirna Papuga and the staff at IntechOpen Publishers for their generous support in writing and publishing this book.

Naofumi Shiomi
Research Center for Membrane and Film Technology,
Kobe University
Kobe, Japan

Chapter 1

The Role of Exosomes in Metabolic Syndrome and Cell Therapy

Naofumi Shiomi, Pengfei Zhang, Kazuo Kumagai and Hideto Matsuyama

Abstract

Metabolic syndrome (MetS) is a pathological condition in which diseases such as diabetes, dyslipidemia, and hypertension progress via a domino effect. Obesity induces adipose tissue hypertrophy and a chronic inflammatory state, leading to insulin resistance, glucose metabolism disorders, and MetS. Recent studies have revealed that not only adipokines secreted from white adipose tissue (WAT) and inflammatory cytokines secreted from immune cells, but also exosomes secreted from these cells transmit signals to various organs. The organs that receive the signals secrete hormones and exosomes in response to the next signal, thereby progressing the pathology. We focus here on the relationship between exosomes and MetS and explain their effects. Moreover, we discuss the trends in cell therapy using mesenchymal stem cells, beige fat cells, and brown fat cells, which are expected to be used as treatments for MetS.

Keywords: exosome, miRNA, mesenchymal stem cells, beige adipocyte, brown adipocyte

1. Introduction

Metabolic syndrome (MetS) is a cluster of interconnected metabolic disorders, including diabetes, dyslipidemia, and hypertension, which develop in a series of falling dominoes. Patients with MetS are 3–10 times more likely to develop cardiovascular disease, and those with 3–4 MetS risk factors have a 36-fold increased risk of heart disease [1]. MetS is also associated with metabolic disorders related to sugar and lipid abnormalities, as well as with the immune system and cancer [2, 3].

The diagnostic guidelines diagnose MetS when three of the following five conditions are met: Fasting plasma glucose ≥ 100 mg/dL (or type 2 diabetes mellitus receiving medical therapy for hypertension), hypertension ≥ 130/85 mmHg (or receiving medical therapy for hyperglycemia), triglycerides ≥ 150 mg/dL (or high plasma triglyceride levels), HDL-C < 40 mg/dL in men and < 50 mg/dL in women (or treatment for lowering HDL-C levels), and waist circumference ≥ 102 cm in men and ≥ 88 cm in women. The prevalence of MetS in adults is estimated at 20–25%, but it is widely accepted that age, lifestyle, and socioeconomic status also play a major role in its pathogenesis [4], and that its prevalence is increasing worldwide in both developed and developing countries [5]. For example, a study in the United States found that 39.8% of adults have obesity, and the proportion of those with diabetes or pre-diabetes was 34%, with an increased incidence in China. According to a survey conducted by the Japanese Ministry of Health, Labor, and Welfare, one in two men and one in five women are at risk of developing MetS. A recent report on the prevalence of MetS in China pointed out that several definitions of MetS lead to different prevalence rates [6], and it is important to establish a common definition in the future.

The onset of MetS is caused by insulin resistance and chronic inflammation associated with obesity; however, it is gradually becoming clear that the underlying mechanism is complex. In this review, we introduce the role of exosomes and miRNAs in the onset of MetS. We also discuss the current status of cell therapies for MetS using mesenchymal stem cells (MSCs), beige adipocytes, and brown adipocytes.

2. MetS development and adipokines

An overview of the association between MetS onset and obesity is shown in **Figure 1**. Pre-adipocytes and white adipocytes in white adipose tissue (WAT) act as hormone-secreting organs that secrete adipokines (or adipocytokines). Adipokines include more than 10 types of hormones, such as tumor necrosis factor (TNF)-α, plasminogen activator inhibitor (PAI)-1, leptin, adiponectin, and resistin, and are secreted from WAT, mainly loaded onto exosomes [7]. In a healthy state, WAT contains many pre-adipocytes and MSCs, and the adipokines and miRNAs secreted by these cells act on various organs and nerves to maintain normal blood glucose levels and lipid balance. However, when caloric intake continues and obesity occurs, most pre-adipocytes differentiate into white adipocytes and continue to accumulate fat, causing WAT hypertrophy. In hypertrophied WAT, the composition of

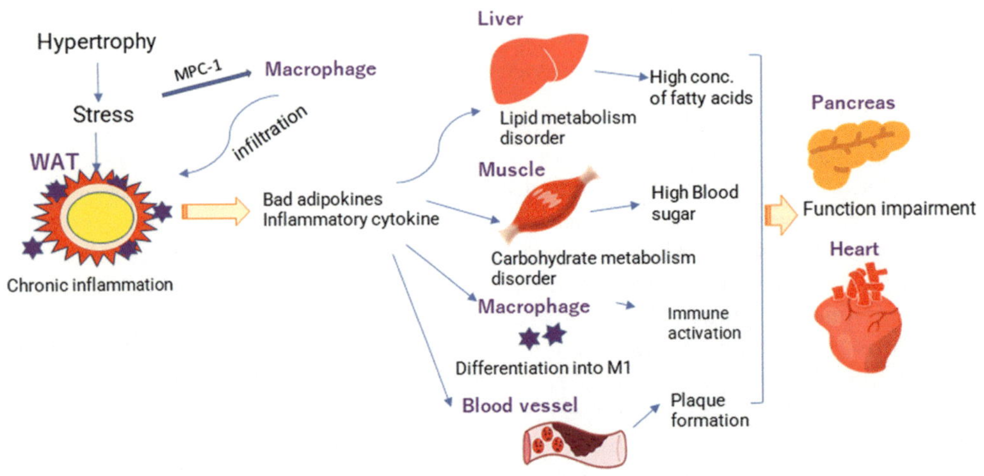

Figure 1.
MetS develops due to exosome information exchange. MetS, metabolic syndrome.

adipokines and miRNAs is altered [8], which suppresses the secretion of leptin and adiponectin. This promotes glucose metabolism and increases the secretion of TNFα, which promotes insulin resistance, and PAI-1, which increases blood pressure. Inflammatory adipokines such as TNFα activate inhibitory molecules such as SOCS and JNK, suppressing insulin receptor substrates (IRS)-1, thereby causing insulin resistance.

Furthermore, the mechanical stress caused by WAT hypertrophy induces stress in the endoplasmic reticulum and mitochondria, resulting in chronic inflammation [9–11]. This causes chemical mediators, such as monocyte chemo-attractant protein-1 (MCP-1), to be released from the inflammatory site, leading to the infiltration of inflammatory leukocytes, such as macrophages. In healthy individuals, macrophages make up 5–10% of all cells in adipose tissue; however, in hypertrophied adipose tissue, this number approaches 50% [10]. The infiltrated macrophages differentiate into M1 macrophages and become activated, and the inflammatory adipose tissue and macrophages produce inflammatory mediators such as TNF-α, interleukin (IL)-6, resistin, IL-1β, and monocyte chemotactic protein-1, which cooperate with adipokines from WAT to induce hyperglycemia and insulin resistance, while at the same time inhibiting the production of adiponectin and inducing leptin resistance, further worsening the MetS condition.

This leads to liver dysfunction, which increases lipolysis and free fatty acid and triglyceride levels in the blood. An increase in free fatty acids causes ectopic deposition in the liver and induces vascular plaque formation, leading to pancreatic and cardiac dysfunction [12]. These events activate pathways such as NF-κB, further accelerating inflammation and initiating a negative chain reaction. Thus, the increase and hypertrophy of WAT associated with obesity, the associated chronic inflammation, and changes in immunity are triggers for the progression of MetS.

Exosomes are small vesicles formed during endocytosis with a size of approximately 50–150 nm and are released by most cells. Exosomes can be detected in biological fluids such as serum, plasma, urine, saliva, and cerebrospinal fluid. More than 30 years ago, exosomes were thought to be used to release misfolded proteins and aggregated toxic proteins, such as amyloid beta and prions; however, subsequent research has revealed that exosomes are packages of signaling substances consisting of lipids, proteins, nucleic acids, mRNA, and miRNA, and play an important role in exchanging information with other tissues as paracrine signals [13–18]. It has become clear that adipokines contained in exosomes are responsible for the above-mentioned complex information exchange.

3. MetS development and miRNA

3.1 miRNAs and insulin resistance

In addition to adipokines, miRNAs, which are components of exosomes that play an important role in transporting and transmitting information to other tissues, have been found to be another major factor in causing MetS. MiRNAs are single-stranded RNA molecules of 21–25 bases that bind to complementary mRNAs to regulate gene expression [19]. WAT releases exosomes to control the function of various tissues, including the liver and macrophages. The number of exosomes in the plasma is increased in patients with T2DM [20], and the composition of miRNAs in exosomes

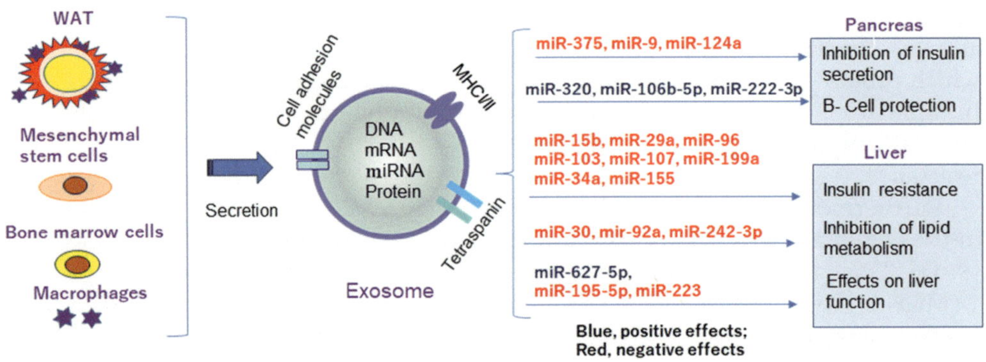

Figure 2.
Effects of miRNAs contained in exosomes secreted by various cells on the pancreas and liver.

differs between patients with T2DM and normal individuals [21]. These findings suggest a strong relationship between miRNAs and MetS onset. Primary miRNAs associated with MetS are shown in **Figure 2** and listed in **Table 1**.

miR-375 acts as a negative regulator, whereby increased expression of miR-375 reduces insulin secretion by decreasing the number of insulin-secreting beta cells and increasing glucagon-secreting alpha cells [22]. miR-9 and miR-124a also act as negative regulators that interfere with insulin endocytosis and decrease insulin secretion [23]. In contrast, miR-320 acts as a positive regulator of insulin, targeting the p85 kinase unit to increase the phosphorylation of serine/threonine kinase and GLUT-4, thereby improving insulin resistance [24]. miR-106b-5p and miR-222-3p, found in the exosomes of bone marrow cells, improve insulin levels by promoting beta cell proliferation after injury [25].

MetS, metabolic syndrome; WAT, white adipose tissue; MSCs, mesenchymal stem cells; UTR, untranslated regions; IRS, insulin receptor substrate; NAFLD, nonalcoholic fatty liver disease; NASH, nonalcoholic steatohepatitis.

miRNAs are also involved in the regulation of the insulin receptor (IR), IRS-1, and glucose transporter (GLUT)-4. miR-15b targets the untranslated region of the insulin receptor gene and suppresses its expression [26]. In the T2DM mouse model, overexpression of miR-15b in liver cells reduces the gene expression of IR. Decreased IRS-1 promotes insulin resistance in the skeletal muscle of patients with T2DM; miR-29a [27] and miR-96 [28] target downstream of IRS-1, and their overexpression reduces IRS-1 expression. Furthermore, miR-103 and miR-107 are overexpressed in the liver and adipocytes of obese mice, indirectly inhibiting IRS-1 expression [29]. miRNAs are also involved in GLUT4-mediated glucose uptake and lipid metabolism. miR-199a, when overexpressed in the serum of patients with T2DM, inhibits the expression of GLUT-4 in skeletal muscle and adipose tissue, resulting in insulin resistance [30]. Additionally, exosomal miRNAs suppress lipid synthesis in individuals with obesity. For example, miR-27a in adipocyte exosomes inhibits PPARγ to regulate lipid synthesis in the liver [31], and miR-30 and miR-92a in serum exosomes inhibit the lipid transporter ABCA1, thereby inhibiting lipid metabolism and cholesterol export [32]. miRNA-141-3p, secreted from adipose tissue to liver tissue, also significantly reduces insulin sensitivity [33].

Moreover, miRNAs are involved in chronic inflammation. In obesity, macrophages in adipose tissue increase, and exosomes derived from macrophages

miRNA	Source	Target	Effects of miRNA	Ref.
miR-375	Transformation	β cell decrease	Impaired blood sugar control	[22]
miR-124a	Pancreas	Mtpn ζ, Foxo2	Inhibition of glucose-induced insulin secretion	[23]
miR-320	Chemical synthesis	p85 subunit	Impairment of insulin resistance	[24]
miR-106b-5p/ miR-222	Pancreas	Growth of β cells	Induction improves hyperglycemia	[25]
miR-15b		Insurin receptor	Induction of insulin resistance	[26]
miR-96/miR-29		IRS-1 3'UTR	Glucose uptake via insulin receptor	[27, 28]
miR-103/miR-107		Caveolin-1	Regulates insulin sensitivity	[29]
miR-199a	Serum	GLUT4	Induction of abnormal sugar metabolism	[30]
miR-27		PPARγ	Induction and control of insulin resistance	[31]
miR-30/miR-92a	Serum	ABCA1	Negative correlation with cholesterol	[32]
miR-141-3p	WAT		Induction of hepatic insulin resistance	[33]
miR-34a	WAT	KLF4	Suppression of M2 differentiation	[35]
miR-155	WAT	PPARγ	Induction and control of insulin resistance	[34]
miR-29	β cells	TRAF3	Promoting inflammation and diabetes	[36]
miR-192-5p	Liver	Rictor/Akt/ FoxO1	Suppression of PCOSD development	[41]
miR-223	Macrophage		Attenuating progression to NASH and liver fibrosis	[42]
miR-627-5p	MSCs	Fat-related genes	Improvement of NAFLD and reduction of lipid deposition	[43]
miR-145	Serum	Secretion of renin, etc.	Control of high blood pressure	[47]

Table 1.
Effects of miRNAs on MetS.

affect insulin sensitivity [34]; exosomes released from the visceral adipose tissue of T2DM mice also induce insulin resistance and communicate with macrophages [35]. For example, miR-34a expression in the adipose tissue inhibits the polarization of M1 macrophages to M2 macrophages and promotes obesity-induced inflammation [36]. Furthermore, miR-155 is secreted from macrophages in adipocytes into hepatocytes, where it acts on PPARγ to reduce the activity of GLUT-4 [34]. Exosomal miR-29, secreted from β cells, induces inflammatory responses in macrophages and monocytes, promoting the progression of insulin resistance and T2DM [37].

Hormones also affect the amount and composition of secreted exosomes. Adiponectin stimulates exosome biogenesis in endothelial and skeletal muscle cells [38], ceramide influences exosome production [39], and vascular endothelial cells transmit several signals between distal organs and adipose tissue to control exosome production.

3.2 Relationship between non-alcoholic hepatitis, arteriosclerosis, and miRNA

A relationship between miRNAs and nonalcoholic fatty liver disease (NAFLD) has been identified [40]. For example, miR-192-5p from lipotoxic hepatocyte-derived exosomes plays a role in proinflammatory macrophage activation and is important in proinflammatory macrophage activation and disease progression in NAFLD [41]. In addition, the release of anti-fibrotic miR-223 from macrophages is promoted by IL-6 and attenuates the progression to nonalcoholic steatohepatitis (NASH) and liver fibrosis [42]. Human hepatic stem cell exosomes show anti-fibrotic and anti-inflammatory effects in a model of chronic liver disease and improve liver function [43]. Furthermore, UC-MSC exosomal miR-627-5p improves insulin resistance, liver injury, and glucose and lipid metabolism in NAFLD rats, reduces lipid deposition, and improves NAFLD [44].

In addition, a relationship between hypertension, arteriosclerosis (AS), and miRNAs has been reported [45]. Endothelial and immune cell exosomal miRNAs and proteins induce vascular smooth muscle cell proliferation and migration and are involved in vascular remodeling in hypertension [46], while circulating exosomes alter the expression of endothelial nitric oxide synthase, regulating vascular dilation and constriction, thereby contributing to blood pressure regulation. In addition, miR-34 and miR-21 affect renal tubular sodium reabsorption and maintain blood pressure homeostasis. Circulating exosomal miR-145 affects renin release, angiotensin II activation, and aldosterone secretion, thereby regulating hypertension [47]. Furthermore, human umbilical cord venous endothelial cell exosomes treated with oxidized lipids induced hyperlipidemia, inflammatory responses, and NETs release in a mouse model of AS [48]; macrophage-derived exosomal miR-223 promoted macrophage differentiation, inflammation, and disrupted lipid metabolism in adipose tissue [49], thereby promoting the progression of AS. Moreover, exosomes derived from visceral fat affect the formation and polarization of macrophage foam cells and the subsequent development of atherosclerosis [50].

As described above, miRNAs contained in exosomes play an important role in the complex crosstalk between organs. When this balance is disrupted by obesity, MetS progresses with a dominant effect involving many organs.

4. Cell therapy for MetS

4.1 Cell therapy using MSCs

Mesenchymal stem cells are expected to be effective against autoimmune and inflammatory diseases as well as in insulin resistance. For example, the main cause of type 1 diabetes mellitus (T1DM) is the destruction of β cells by autoimmunity, but MSCs suppress the destruction of pancreatic β cells by autoimmunity through their immunomodulatory effects, such as inhibiting the proliferation of T lymphocytes and B cells and blocking attacks by immune cells [51, 52]. In addition, M2 macrophages promote the resolution of inflammation and the repair of tissues, and MSCs differentiate and transition M1 macrophages to M2 macrophages, which have anti-inflammatory effects [51, 53]. Furthermore, the secretion of adipose tissue-derived MSCs (ATMSCs) increases GLUT-4 gene expression and suppresses PAI-1 and IL-6 gene expression, in addition to producing anti-inflammatory molecules

[54]. In light of this background, the use of MSCs in the treatment of MetS, especially diabetes, has attracted attention in recent years, and many research reports on this treatment method have been published [55–57]. Some of these reports are discussed below.

MSCs alleviate insulin resistance. For example, the administration of Wharton's jelly-derived MSCs (WJ-MSCs) to C57BL/6 db/db mice improved glucose and insulin tolerance [58]. In addition, the administration of placental mesenchymal stem cells (PMSCs) to rats improved insulin resistance by reconstituting the PI3K-Akt pathway and increasing GLUT-4 expression and glucose uptake in skeletal muscles [59]. The intravenous injection of amniotic membrane-derived MSCs (AMMSCs) or umbilical cord-derived MSCs (UCMSCs) into type 2 diabetic db/db mice improved insulin resistance and hepatic glycolipid metabolism [60].

MSCs also enhance insulin production. Co-transplantation of pancreatic islets and MSCs promotes immune tolerance to transplantation [61], and the secretion of cytokines by transplanted MSCs promotes β-cell engraftment, angiogenesis, and recovery of islet function [62, 63]. Furthermore, it has been shown that MSCs can differentiate into insulin-producing cells (IPCs). For example, Moriscot et al. induced human bone marrow-derived MSCs (BM-MSCs) to differentiate into IPCs and confirmed that the cells released insulin in a glucose-dependent manner [64]. Chandra also differentiated mouse adipose-derived stem cells (ASCs) into cells that secrete pancreatic hormones, encapsulated them in calcium alginate, and transplanted them intraperitoneally into streptozotocin-induced diabetic mice, restoring normal blood glucose levels within two weeks [65]. WJ-MSCs are most suitable for the differentiation of MSCs into IPCs and are easier to culture than UC-MSCs [66]. IPCs differentiated from WJ-MSCs exhibit β-cell function in vivo, and WJ-MSCs differentiate into IPCs when injected into NOD mice [67]. In addition, when undifferentiated human placenta-derived MSCs (PDMSCs) and cells differentiated into IPCs were microencapsulated and transplanted, normal blood glucose levels were restored, and the possibility of partial pancreatic regeneration was demonstrated [68]. Thus, MSCs may be an effective tool for cell replacement therapy in type-1 diabetes and cell therapy in T2DM.

On the other hand, exosomes secreted by MSCs (MSC–Exos) have also attracted attention. MSC–Exos can exert local and systemic effects, and because they have low antigenicity and low potential for tumor transformation due to their low expression of major histocompatibility class II (MHCII), they are expected to be an alternative treatment to current cell therapies [69, 70]. Notable effects of MSC–Exos on diabetes have been previously reported. For example, adipose-derived mesenchymal stem cell/mesenchymal stromal cell exosomes (ADMSC–Exos) improve hyperglycemic symptoms in T1DM mice by improving autoimmune and inflammatory responses and increasing the number of pancreatic islets [71]. MSC–Exos can attenuate the differentiation of Th1 and Th17 cells, prevent T-cell activation, enhance IL-10 production, and have therapeutic effects in the prevention of autoimmune diseases [72]. In addition, they protect β cells from hypoxia-induced apoptosis and improve the survival rate of pancreatic islets [73]. MSC–Exos are also expected to be useful in the treatment of T2DM. When exosomes derived from human UC–MSCs (UCMSC–Exos) were administered to T2DM rats, they increased insulin sensitivity via GLUT-4, suggesting that they could be a potential treatment for T2DM [74].

Recently, efforts have been made to develop exosomes that can selectively affect target cells, and exosomes with drug delivery properties have also been considered.

In rats with T1DM, selenium-loaded MSC-Exos induced pancreatic regeneration and anti-inflammatory effects [75]. The administration of artificial sEVs that overexpress apelin via gene transfer significantly reduced plasma glucose levels, promoted pancreatic β-cell proliferation, improved insulin and glucose tolerance, and regulated the inflammatory cytokine profile [76]. As described above, MSCs or MSC-Exos can control autoimmunity, improve insulin resistance, and may become an important treatment for diabetes in the future.

4.2 Cell therapy using beige and brown adipose tissue

Treatment of MetS using beige or brown adipocytes has attracted attention [77]. Brown adipocytes were discovered as fat-storing cells despite being brown like muscles, whereas beige adipocytes were discovered as cells that appear when WAT is exposed to cold and were named beige adipocytes because they are not as brown as brown adipocytes. Brown adipocytes develop from Myf5 +, Sca1 +, Pax7 + cells in the dermal muscle layer via pre-brown adipocytes, whereas beige adipocytes have been reported to be derived from pre-adipocytes or adipocytes, or from MyoD +, smooth muscle-like, or PDGFRα+ + neural precursor cells, suggesting the existence of multiple types [78–80]. Specific marker genes for beige adipocytes include Cd137 and Cited1, whereas specific marker genes for brown adipocytes include Zic1 and Lhx8, indicating that the two are different cells [81, 82].

The responses of beige and brown fat cells to cold stimulation are shown in **Figure 3**. Brown or beige adipocytes have excellent sugar and fat decomposition functions owing to the following mechanisms [83]: Brown and beige adipocytes have many mitochondria and express uncoupling protein 1 (UCP1) in the inner mitochondrial membrane. When UCP1 is activated by cold stimulation, the ion

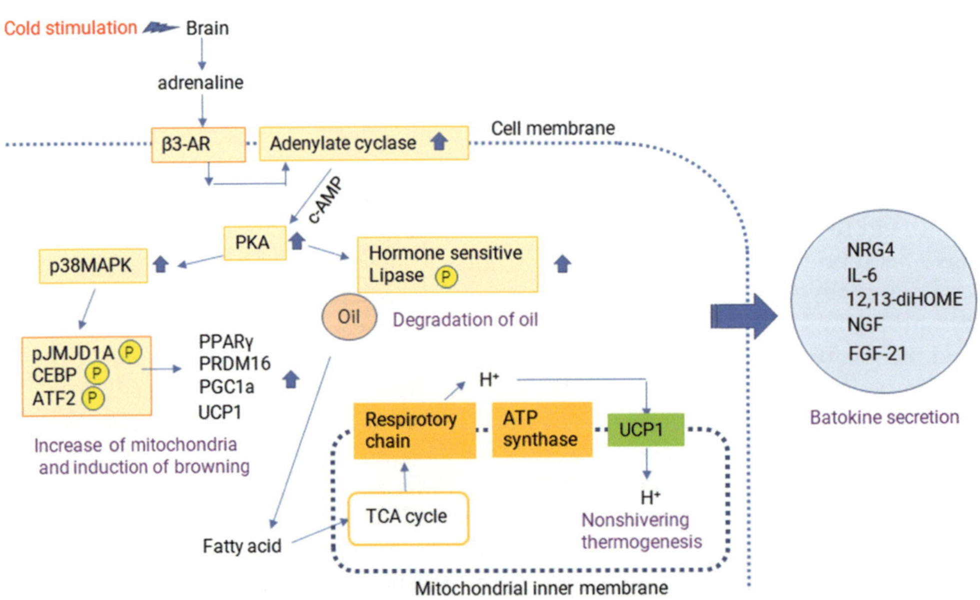

Figure 3.
Pathways of cold-induced non-shivering thermogenesis and browning in brown and beige adipocytes.

channel of UCP1 opens and couples with anions to take in H^+ ions present on the outside of the inner membrane, converting the potential energy lost in the process into heat energy and generating non-shivering heat. After that, β-oxidation is activated in the inner mitochondrial membrane, and as a result, sugar metabolism and fat decomposition are actively carried out to compensate for the lost energy.

Increases in UCP1 and browning occur via the following pathways: Adrenaline is secreted from the brain by cold stimulation, binds to β3-adrenergic receptors (β3-AR), and activates adrenaline cyclase. This signal activates PKA, which phosphorylates CEBP, ATF2, etc., via p38MAPK, and increases the expression of PPARγ and PRDM16, which induce browning, and PGC1a, which increases mitochondria. PRDM16, Zfp516, and IRF4 are the most important factors that induce browning [84, 85]; individuals with PRDM16 disruption are unable to maintain brown adipose tissue, whereas individuals with Zfp516 overexpression undergo browning. Furthermore, mice have a special auxiliary non-shivering heat production system that generates non-shivering heat through a UCP1-independent pathway (β3-AR-independent pathway) [86, 87]. However, the existence of this pathway in humans is not fully understood.

Recent studies have shown that brown adipose tissue (BAT) functions as a paracrine hormone-producing cell, similar to WAT. When activated by thermogenic activation or cold stimulation, BAT produces hormones called batokines, which play important roles in suppressing MetSs [88]. The removal of BAT in mice leads to systemic hypertension and heart disease; therefore, batokines act as cardiac signals. For example, 12,13-dihydroxy-9Z-octadecenoic acid (12,13-diHOME) increases calcium circulation and restores cardiac function [89, 90]. In addition, activation of BAT leads to the secretion of FGF21, which protects against the development of NAFLDs [91]. Batokines are also involved in the immune system; for example, CXCL14 and GDF-15, which are secreted in coordination with thermogenesis in BAT, reduce inflammatory activity [92, 93].

Thermogenesis by UCP1 and cytokine secretion is closely related to obesity and MetS, and increasing the number of brown or beige adipocytes may be an effective treatment for MetS [94, 95]. Although brown adipocytes are abundant in babies, their number and precursor cells decrease with age [96], making it difficult to increase brown adipocytes in adults. In contrast, beige adipocytes can be induced from adipocytes or their precursor cells; therefore, efficient induction of beige adipocytes in the body can improve MetS [97]. Cold stimulation is the most common method for inducing beige fat cells. BAT glucose uptake is eight times higher than that of skeletal muscle and is highly active [98], and cold exposure increases total energy expenditure [99]. Continuous cold exposure in humans increases basal metabolism by 22% [100]. In addition, although they do not have a dramatic effect on cold stimulation, foods such as capsaicin and resveratrol [101, 102] contain compounds that increase BAT, and a diet that includes long-term intake of these compounds can lead to the improvement and prevention of MetS.

In patients with chronic obesity or MetS, it has been pointed out that BAT function itself is impaired, and in such cases, drug or surgical treatment is effective. BAT is activated by the agonists of receptors related to BAT. For example, the β3-AR agonist mirabegron [103] and the PPARγ receptor agonist troglitazone [104] activate BAT and induce browning of WAT. However, these receptors are distributed throughout the body, so there are problems with side effects. BAT removal increases obesity and insulin resistance, whereas BAT transplantation into mice increases insulin sensitivity, enhances fat metabolism [100, 105], and improves the defense and motor functions of T2DM in mice [106]. Therefore, a suitable treatment method for BAT transplantation is required. For BAT transplantation, methods have been proposed to generate brown and beige adipocytes from human pluripotent stem cells [107, 108] and beige adipocytes from MSCs [109]. In addition, transplantation of the obtained beige and brown adipocytes was considered, and mice transplanted with ADSC-derived beige adipocytes showed increased glucose metabolism and thermogenic activity [110, 111].

However, there have been few studies on exosomes secreted by BAT. BAT exosomes contain components that promote glucose metabolism and high insulin resistance [112]; however, 12,13-diHOMO acts as an inflammatory mediator and promotes allergic inflammation in newborns [113], so there may be good and bad aspects. Therefore, further research is required on this aspect.

5. Conclusion

The term MetS has been used for more than 30 years. MetS was initially thought to be caused mainly by insulin resistance due to the abnormal secretion of adipokines by WAT; however, it has been found that chronic inflammation is also a factor. Furthermore, the characteristics of hormones and miRNAs contained in exosomes have been elucidated, and it has been found that each tissue exchanges information through exosomes. MetS is a more complex pathology in which changes in the composition of exosomes associated with obesity interact like an orchestra to transmit signals. Therefore, the treatment of MetS may not be straightforward. Currently, research is being conducted on treating MetS using mesenchymal stem cells (MSCs), beige fat cells, and their secreted exosomes. We hope that these treatments will be put to practical use in the future.

Conflict of Interest

The authors declare no competing interests.

Author details

Naofumi Shiomi*, Pengfei Zhang, Kazuo Kumagai and Hideto Matsuyama
Research Center for Membrane and Film Technology, Kobe University, Kobe, Japan

*Address all correspondence to: n-shiomi@people.kobe-u.ac.jp

References

[1] Cornier M-A, Dabelea D, Hernandez TL, Lindstrom RC, Steig AJ, Stob NR, et al. The metabolic syndrome. Endocrine Reviews. 2008;**29**:777–822

[2] Esposito K, Chiodini P, Colao A, Lenzi A, Giugliano D. Metabolic syndrome and risk of cancer a systematic review and meta-analysis. Diabetes Care. 2012;**35**:2402–2411. DOI: 10.2337/dc12-0336

[3] Andersen CJ, Murphy KE, Fernandez ML. Impact of obesity and metabolic syndrome on immunity. Advances in Nutrition. 2016;**7**:66–75. DOI: 10.3945/an.115.010207

[4] Nestel P, Lyu R, Low LP, Sheu W-H-H, Nitiyanant W, Saito I, Tan CE. Metabolic syndrome: Recent prevalence in East and Southeast Asian populations. Asia Pacific Journal of Clinical Nutrition. 2007;**16**:362–367

[5] Saklayen MG. The global epidemic of the metabolic syndrome. Current Hypertension Reports. 2018;**20**:12. DOI: 10.1007/s11906-018-0812-z

[6] MaKel K, Haiyang M, Guo L, Li J, Lei Y, Li X, et al. Comparison of metabolic syndrome prevalence and characteristics using five different definitions in China: A population-based retrospective study. Frontiers in Public Health. 2024;**12**:1333910. DOI: 10.3389/fpubh.2024.1333910

[7] Clemente-Suárez VJ, Redondo-Flórez L, Beltrán-Velasco AI, Martín-Rodríguez A, Navarro-Jiménez E, Laborde-Cárdenas CC. C, et al. The role of adipokines in health and disease. Biomedicines. 2023;**11**:1290

[8] Lee J-E, Moon P-G, Lee I-K, Baek M-C. Proteomic analysis of extracellular vesicles released by adipocytes of Otsuka Long-Evans Tokushima Fatty (OLETF) rats. The Protein Journal. 2015;**34**:220–235. DOI: 10.1007/s10930-015-9616-z

[9] Kraakman MJ, Murphy AJ, Jandeleit-Dahm K, Kammoun HL. Macrophage polarization in obesity and Type 2 diabetes: Weighing down our understanding of macrophage function? Frontiers in Immunology. 2014;**5**:470. DOI: 10.3389/fimmu.2014.00470

[10] Lumeng CN, Bodzin JL, Saltiel AR. Obesity induces a phenotypic switch in adipose tissue macrophage polarization. Journal of Clinical Investigation. 2007;**117**:175–184. DOI: 10.1172/JCI29881

[11] Weisberg SP, McCann D, Desai M, Rosenbaum M, Leibel RL, Ferrante Jr AW. Obesity is associated with macrophage accumulation in adipose tissue. Journal of Clinical Investigation. 2003;**112**:1796–1808. DOI: 10.1172/JCI19246

[12] Guilherme A, Virbasius JV, Puri V, Czech MP. Adipocyte dysfunctions linking obesity to insulin resistance and Type 2 diabetes. Nature Reviews Molecular Cell Biology. 2008;**9**:367–377. DOI: 10.1038/nrm2391

[13] Kalluri R, LeBleu VS. The biology, function, and biomedical applications of exosomes. Science. 2020;**367**:eaau6977. DOI: 10.1126/science.aau6977

[14] Pegtel DM, Gould SJ. Exosomes. Annual Review of Biochemistry.

2019;**88**:487–514. DOI: 10.1146/annurev-biochem-013118-111902

[15] Kita S, Maeda N, Shimomura I. Interorgan communication by exosomes, adipose tissue, and adiponectin in metabolic syndrome. Journal of Clinical Investigation. 2019;**129**:4041–4049. DOI: 10.1172/JCI129193

[16] Cione E, Cannataro R, Gallelli L, Sarro GD, Caroleo MC. Exosome microRNAs in metabolic syndrome as tools for the early monitoring of diabetes and possible therapeutic options. Pharmaceuticals (Basel). 2021;**14**:1257. DOI: 10.3390/ph14121257

[17] Wang N, Li J, Hu Z, Ngowi EE, Yan B, Qiao A. Exosomes: New insights into the pathogenesis of metabolic syndrome. Biology. 2023;**12**:1480. DOI: 10.3390/biology12121480

[18] Ali PSS, Ahmad MP, Parveen KMH. MicroRNAs in diabetes mellitus. Journal of Diabetes & Metabolic Disorders. 2025;**24**:77. DOI: 10.1007/s40200-025-01591-y

[19] Saliminejad K, Khorshid HRK, Fard SS, Ghaffari SH. An overview of microRNAs: Biology, functions, therapeutics, and analysis methods. Journal of Cellular Physiology. 2019;**234**:5451–5465. DOI: 10.1002/jcp.27486

[20] Diamant M, Nieuwland R, Pablo RF, Sturk A, Smit JW, Radder JK. Elevated numbers of tissue-factor exposing microparticles correlate with components of the Metabolic Syndrome in Uncomplicated Type 2 diabetes mellitus. Circulation. 2002;**106**: 2442–2447. DOI: 10.1161/01.cir.0000036596.59665.c6

[21] Santovito D, Nardis VD, Marcantonio P, Mandolini C, Paganelli C, Vitaleet E, et al. Plasma exosome microRNA profiling unravels a new potential modulator of adiponectin pathway in diabetes: Effect of glycemic control. The Journal of Clinical Endocrinology & Metabolism. 2014;**99**:E1681–5

[22] Latreille M, Herrmanns K, Renwick N, Tuschl T, Malecki MT, McCarthy MI, et al. miR-375 gene dosage in pancreatic β-cells: Implications for regulation of β-cell mass and biomarker development. Journal of Molecular Medicine. 2015;**93**:1159–1169

[23] Sebastiani G, Po A, Miele E, Ventriglia G, Ceccarelli E, Bugliani M, et al. MicroRNA-124a is hyperexpressed in type 2 diabetic human pancreatic Islets and negatively regulates insulin secretion. Acta Diabetologica. 2015;**52**: 523–530

[24] Ling HY, Ou HS, Feng SD, Zhang XY, Tuo QH, Chen LX, et al. Changes in MicroRNA (miR) profile and effects of miR-320 in insulin-resistant 3T3-L1 adipocytes. Clinical and Experimental Pharmacology and Physiology. 2009;**36**: e32–9

[25] Tsukita S, Yamada T, Takahashi K, Munakata Y, Hosaka S, Takahashi H, et al. MicroRNAs 106b and 222 improve hyperglycemia in a mouse model of insulin-deficient diabetes via pancreatic β-cell proliferation. EBioMedicine. 2017;**15**:163–172

[26] Li WD, Xia JR, Lian YS. MiR-15b can target insulin receptor to regulate hepatic insulin signaling in mice. Animal Cells and Systems. 2019;**23**

(2):82–89. DOI: 10.1080/19768354.2019.1583125

[27] Yang WM, Jeong HJ, Park SY, Lee W. Induction of miR-29a by saturated fatty acids impairs insulin signaling and glucose uptake through translational repression of IRS-1 in myocytes. FEBS Letters. 2014;**588**:2170–2176. DOI: 10.1016/j.febslet.2014.05.011

[28] Jeong HJ, Park SY, Yang WM, Lee W. The induction of miR-96 by mitochondrial dysfunction causes impaired glycogen synthesis through translational repression of IRS-1 in SK-Hep1 cells. Biochemical and Biophysical Research Communications. 2013;**434**(3):503–508. DOI: 10.1016/j.bbrc.2013.03.104

[29] Trajkovski M, Hausser J, Soutschek J, Bhat B, Akin A, Zavolan M, et al. MicroRNAs 103 and 107 regulate insulin sensitivity. Nature. 2011;**474**:649–653

[30] Yan ST, Li CL, Tian H, Li J, Pei Y, Liu Y, et al. MiR-199a is overexpressed in plasma of Type 2 diabetes patients which contributes to Type 2 diabetes by targeting GLUT4. Molecular and Cellular Biochemistry. 2014;**397**:45–51

[31] Lee JJ, Drakaki A, Iliopoulos D, Struhl K. MiR-27b targets PPARγ to inhibit growth, tumor progression and the inflammatory response in neuroblastoma cells. Oncogene. 2012;**31**:3818–3825. DOI: 10.1038/onc.2011.543

[32] Wang Z, Zhang J, Zhang S, Yan S, Wang Z, Wang C, et al. MiR–30e and miR–92a are related to atherosclerosis by targeting ABCA1. Molecular Medicine Reports. 2019;**19**:3298–3304

[33] Dang SY, Leng Y, Wang ZX, Xiao X, Zhang X, Wen T, et al. Exosomal transfer of obesity adipose tissue for decreased miR-141-3p mediate insulin resistance of hepatocytes. International Journal of Biological Sciences. 2019;**15**:351–368

[34] Ying W, Riopel M, Bandyopadhyay G, Dong Y, Birmingham A, Seo JB, et al. Adipose tissue macrophage-derived exosomal miRNAs can modulate in vivo and in vitro insulin sensitivity. Cell. 2017;**171**(372–84):e12. DOI: 10.1016/j.cell.2017.08.035

[35] Deng ZB, Poliakov A, Hardy RW, Clements R, Liu C, Liu Y, et al. Adipose tissue exosome-like vesicles mediate activation of macrophage-induced insulin resistance. Diabetes. 2009;**58**:2498–2505

[36] Pan Y, Hui X, Hoo RLC, Ye D, Chan CYC, Feng T, et al. Adipocyte-secreted exosomal microRNA-34a inhibits M2 macrophage polarization to promote obesity-induced adipose inflammation. Journal of Clinical Investigation. 2019;**129**:834–849

[37] Sun Y, Zhou Y, Shi Y, Zhang Y, Liu K, Liang R, et al. Expression of miRNA-29 in pancreatic β cells promotes inflammation and diabetes via TRAF3. Cell Reports. 2021;**34**:108576. DOI: 10.1016/j.celrep.2020.108576

[38] Obata Y, Kita S, Koyama Y, Fukuda S, Takeda H, Takahashi M, et al. Adiponectin/T-cadherin system enhances exosome biogenesis and decreases cellular ceramides by exosomal release. JCI Insight. 2018;**3**:e99680

[39] Elsherbini A, Bieberich E. Ceramide and exosomes: A novel target in cancer biology and therapy. Advances in Cancer Research. 2018;**140**:121–154. DOI: 10.1016/bs.acr.2018.05.004

[40] Tamimi A, Javid M, Sedighi-Pirsaraei N, Mirdamadi A. Exosome prospects in the diagnosis and treatment of non-alcoholic fatty liver disease. Frontiers in Medicine (Lausanne). 2024;**11**:1420281. DOI: 10.3389/fmed.2024.1420281

[41] Liu XL, Pan Q, Cao HX, Xin FZ, Zhao ZH, Yang RX, et al. Lipotoxic hepatocyte-derived exosomal microRNA 192-5p activates macrophages through rictor/Akt/forkhead box transcription factor O1 signaling in nonalcoholic fatty liver disease. Hepatology. 2020;**72**:454–469

[42] Hou X, Yin S, Ren R, Liu S, Yong L, Liu Y, et al. Myeloid-cell–specific IL-6 signaling promotes microRNA-223-enriched exosome production to attenuate NAFLD-associated fibrosis. Hepatology. 2021;**74**:116–132

[43] Bruno S, Pasquino C, Sanchez MBH, Tapparo M, Figliolini F, Grange C, et al. HLSC-derived extracellular vesicles attenuate liver fibrosis and inflammation in a murine model of non-alcoholic steatohepatitis. Molecular Therapy. 2020;**28**:479–489

[44] Cheng L, Yu P, Li F, Jiang X, Jiao X, Shen Y, et al. Human umbilical cord-derived mesenchymal stem cell-exosomal miR-627-5p ameliorates non-alcoholic fatty liver disease by repressing FTO expression. Human Cell. 2021;**34**:1697–1708

[45] Li Z, Zhao Y, Suguro S, Suguro R. MicroRNAs regulate function in atherosclerosis and clinical implications. Oxidative Medicine and Cellular Longevity. 2023;**2023**:1–12. DOI: 10.1155/2023/2561509. 2561509

[46] Arishe OO, Priviero F, Wilczynski SA, Webb RC. Exosomes as intercellular messengers in hypertension. International Journal of Molecular Sciences. 2021;**22**:11685. DOI: 10.3390/ijms222111685. 11685

[47] Ong SG, Lee WH, Huang M, Dey D, Kodo K, Sanchez-Freire V, et al. Cross talk of combined gene and cell therapy in ischemic heart disease: Role of exosomal microRNA transfer. Circulation. 2014;**130**:S60–9

[48] Gao H, Wang X, Lin C, An Z, Yu J, Cao H, et al. Exosomal MALAT1 derived from ox-LDL-treated endothelial cells induce neutrophil extracellular traps to aggravate atherosclerosis. Biological Chemistry. 2020;**401**:367–376

[49] Ismail N, Wang Y, Dakhlallah D, Moldovan L, Agarwal K, Batte K, et al. Macrophage microvesicles induce macrophage differentiation and miR-223 transfer. Blood. 2013;**121**:984–995

[50] Xie Z, Wang X, Liu X, Du H, Sun C, Shao X, et al. Adipose-derived exosomes exert proatherogenic effects by regulating macrophage foam cell formation and polarization. Journal of the American Heart Association. 2018;**7**:e007442

[51] Su W, Yin Y, Cheng Y, Yu S, Hu R, Zhang H, et al. The phenotype and related gene expressions of macrophages in adipose tissue of T2D mice following MSCs infusion. Immunobiology. 2024;**229**:152788. DOI: 10.1016/j.imbio.2024.152788

[52] Hematti P, Kim J, Stein AP, Kaufman D. Potential role of mesenchymal stromal cells in pancreatic islet transplantation. Transplantation Reviews. 2013;**27**:21–29. DOI: 10.1016/j.trre.2012.11.003

[53] Geng Y, Zhang L, Fu B, Zhang J, Hong Q, Hu J, et al. Mesenchymal stem cells ameliorate rhabdomyolysis-induced acute kidney injury via the activation of M2 macrophages. Stem Cell Research & Therapy. 2014;**5**:80

[54] Xie Z, Hao H, Tong C, Cheng Y, Liu J, Pang Y, et al. Human umbilical cord-derived mesenchymal stem cells elicit macrophages into an anti-inflammatory phenotype to alleviate insulin resistance in type 2 diabetic rats. Stem Cells. 2016;**34**: 627–639

[55] Zang L, Hao H, Liu J, Li Y, Han W, Mu Y. Mesenchymal stem cell therapy in type 2 diabetes mellitus. Diabetology & Metabolic Syndrome. 2017;**9**:36. DOI: 10.1186/s13098-017-0233-1

[56] Zeinhom A, Fadallah SA, Mahmoud M. Human mesenchymal stem/stromal cell based-therapy in diabetes mellitus: Experimental and clinical perspectives. Stem Cell Research & Therapy. 2024;**15**:384. DOI: 10.1186/s13287-024-03974-z

[57] Huang X, Liu Y, Li Z, Lerman LO. Mesenchymal stem/stromal cells therapy for Metabolic Syndrome: Potential clinical application? Stem Cells. 2023;**41**:893–906. DOI: 10.1093/stmcls/sxad052

[58] Ma Y, Wang L, Yang S, Liu D, Zeng Y, Lin L, et al. The tissue origin of human mesenchymal stem cells dictates their therapeutic efficacy on glucose and lipid metabolic disorders in Type II diabetic mice. Stem Cell Research & Therapy. 2021;**12**:385

[59] Kotikalapudi N, Sampath SJP, Sinha SN, Bhonde R, Mungamuri SK, Venkatesan V, et al. Human placental mesenchymal stromal cell therapy restores the cytokine efflux and insulin signaling in the skeletal muscle of obesity-induced Type 2 diabetes rat model. Human Cell. 2022;**35**:557–571

[60] Wang Z, Li H, Fang J, Wang X, Dai S, Cao W, et al. Comparative analysis of the therapeutic effects of amniotic membrane and umbilical cord derived mesenchymal stem Cells for the treatment of Type 2 diabetes. Stem Cell Reviews and Reports. 2022;**18**: 1193–1206

[61] Duprez IR, Johansson U, Nilsson B, Korsgren O, Magnusson PU. Preparatory studies of composite mesenchymal stem cell islets for application in intraportal islet transplantation. Upsala Journal of Medical Sciences. 2011;**116**:8–17. DOI: 10.9/03009734.2010.524320

[62] Gamble A, Pawlick R, Pepper AR, Bruni A, Adesida A, Senior PA, et al. Improved islet recovery and efficacy through co-culture and co-transplantation of islets with human adipose-derived mesenchymal stem cells. PLoS ONE. 2018;**13**:e0206449

[63] Kuppan P, Seeberger K, Kelly S, Rosko M, Adesida A, Pepper AR, et al. Co-transplantation of human adipose-derived mesenchymal stem cells with neonatal porcine islets within a prevascularized subcutaneous space augments the xenograft function. Xenotransplantation. 2020;**27**:e12581

[64] Moriscot C, de Fraipont F, Richard MJ, Marchand M, Savatier P,

Bosco D, et al. Human bone marrow mesenchymal stem cells can express insulin and key transcription factors of the endocrine pancreas developmental pathway upon genetic and/or microenvironmental manipulation in vitro. Stem Cells. 2005;**23**:594–603

[65] Chandra V, Swetha G, Phadnis S, Nair PD, Bhonde RR. Generation of pancreatic hormone-expressing islet-like cell aggregates from murine adipose tissue-derived stem cells. Stem Cells. 2009;**27**:1941–1953. DOI: 10.1002/stem.117

[66] Chao KC, Chao KF, Fu YS, Liu SH. Islet-like clusters derived from mesenchymal stem cells in Wharton's Jelly of the human umbilical cord for transplantation to control Type 1 diabetes. PLoS ONE. 2008;**3**:e1451. DOI: 10.1371/journal.pone.0001451

[67] Tsai PJ, Wang HS, Lin GJ, Chou SC, Chu TH, Chuan WT, et al. Undifferentiated Wharton's jelly mesenchymal stem cell transplantation induces insulin-producing cell differentiation and suppression of T-cell-mediated autoimmunity in nonobese diabetic mice. Cell Transplantation. 2015;**24**: 1555–1570

[68] Lee RH, Seo MJ, Reger RL, Spees JL, Pulin AA, Olson SD, et al. Multipotent stromal cells from human marrow home to and promote repair of pancreatic islets and renal glomeruli in diabetic NOD/SCID Mice. Proceedings of the National Academy of Sciences. 2006;**103**:17438–17443

[69] Jiao YR, Chen KX, Tang X, Tang YL, Yang HL, Yin YL, Li CJ. Exosomes derived from mesenchymal stem cells in diabetes and diabetic complications. Cell Death & Disease. 2024;**15**:271. DOI: 10.1038/s41419-024-06659-w

[70] Sun F, Sun Y, Wu F, Xu W, Qian H. Mesenchymal stem cell-derived extracellular vesicles: A potential therapy for diabetes Mellitus and Diabetic complications. Pharmaceutics. 2022;**14**:2208. DOI: 10.3390/pharmaceutics14102208

[71] Nojehdehi S, Soudi S, Hesampour A, Rasouli S, Soleimani M, Hashemi SM. Immunomodulatory effects of mesenchymal stem cell-derived exosomes on experimental type-1 autoimmune diabetes. Journal of Cellular Biochemistry. 2018;**119**: 9433–9443. DOI: 10.1002/jcb.27260

[72] Shigemoto-Kuroda T, Oh JY, Kim DK, Jeong HJ, Park SY, Lee HJ, et al. MSC-derived extracellular vesicles attenuate immune responses in two autoimmune murine models: Type 1 diabetes and uveoretinitis. Stem Cell Reports. 2017;**8**:1214–1225

[73] Chen J, Chen J, Cheng Y, Fu Y, Zhao H, Tang M, et al. Mesenchymal stem cell-derived exosomes protect beta cells against hypoxia-induced apoptosis via miR-21 by alleviating ER stress and inhibiting p38 MAPK phosphorylation. Stem Cell Research & Therapy. 2020;**11**:97

[74] Yap SK, Tan KL, Rahaman NYA, Hamid NFS, Ooi J, Tor YS, et al. Human umbilical cord mesenchymal stem cell-derived small extracellular vesicles ameliorated insulin resistance in type 2 diabetes mellitus rats. Pharmaceutics. 2022;**14**:649

[75] Khalil DY, Hussein RH, El-Kholy WM. Mesenchymal stem cell-derived exosomes loaded with selenium or Nano Selenium as a novel therapeutic

paradigm for Streptozotocin-Induced Type 1 diabetes in rats. Biology (Basel). 2024;**13**:253. DOI: 10.3390/biology 13040253

[76] Cui J, Wang M, Zhang W, Sun J, Zhang Y, Zhao L, et al. Enhancing insulin sensitivity in type 2 diabetes mellitus using apelin-loaded small extracellular vesicles from Wharton's jelly-derived mesenchymal stem cells: A novel therapeutic approach. Diabetology & Metabolic Syndrome. 2024;**16**:84

[77] Harms M, Seale P. Brown and beige fat: Development, function and therapeutic potential. Nature Medicine. 2013;**19**:1252–1263. DOI: 10.1038/nm.3361

[78] Lee YH, Petkova AP, Konkar AA, Granneman JG. Cellular origins of cold-induced brown adipocytes in adult mice. The FASEB Journal. 2015;**29**: 286–299. DOI: 10.1096/fj.14-263038

[79] Chen Y, Ikeda K, Yoneshiro T, Scaramozza A, Tajima K, Wang Q, et al. Thermal stress induces glycolytic beige fat formation via a myogenic state. Nature. 2019;**565**:180–185

[80] Long JZ, Svensson KJ, Tsai L, Zeng X, Roh HC, Kong X, et al. A smooth muscle-like origin for beige adipocytes. Cell Metabolism. 2014;**19**:810–820

[81] Garcia RA, Roemmich JN, Claycombe KJ. Evaluation of markers of beige adipocytes in white adipose tissue of the mouse. Nutrition & Metabolism. 2016;**13**:24. DOI: 10.1186/s12986-016-00 81-2

[82] Pilkington AC, Paz HA, Wankhade UD. Beige adipose tissue identification and marker specificity-overview. Frontiers in Endocrinology. 2021;**12**:599134. DOI: 10.3389/fendo.2021.599134

[83] Crichton PG, Lee Y, Kunji ERS. The molecular features of uncoupling protein 1 support a conventional mitochondrial carrier-like mechanism. Biochimie. 2017;**134**:35–50. DOI: 10.101 6/j.biochi.2016.12.016

[84] Harms MJ, Ishibashi J, Wang W, Lim HW, Goyama S, Sato T, et al. Prdm16 is required for the maintenance of brown adipocyte identity and function in adult mice. Cell Metabolism. 2014;**19**:593–604

[85] Dempersmier J, Sambeat A, Gulyaeva O, Paul SM, Hudak CSS, Raposo HF, et al. Cold-inducible Zfp516 activates UCP1 transcription to promote browning of white fat and development of brown fat. Molecular Cell. 2015;**57**: 235–246

[86] Pan R, Zhu X, Maretich P, Chen Y. Combating obesity with thermogenic fat: Current challenges and advancements. Frontiers in Endocrinology. 2020;**11**:185. eCollection 2020. DOI: 10.3389/fendo. 2020.00185

[87] Huo C, Song Z, Yin J, Zhu Y, Miao X, Qian H, et al. Effect of acute cold exposure on energy metabolism and activity of brown adipose tissue in humans: A systematic review and meta-analysis. Frontiers in Physiology. 2022;**13**:917084. DOI: 10.3389/fphys. 2022.917084

[88] Yang FT, Stanford KI. Batokines: Mediators of inter-tissue communication (a mini-review). Current Obesity Reports. 2022;**11**:1–9. DOI: 10.1007/s136 79-021-00465-7

[89] Cittadini A, Mantzoros CS, Hampton TG, Travers KE, Katz SE, Morgan JP, Flier JS, Douglas PS, et al. Cardiovascular abnormalities in transgenic mice with reduced brown fat: An animal model of human obesity. Circulation. 1999;**100**:2177–2183

[90] Pinckard KM, Shettigar VK, Wright KR, Abay E, Baer LA, Vidal P, et al. A novel endocrine role for the BAT-released lipokine 12,13-diHOME to mediate cardiac function. Circulation. 2021;**143**:145–159

[91] Zarei M, Pizarro-Delgado J, Barroso E, Palomer X, Vázquez-Carrera M. Targeting FGF21 for the treatment of nonalcoholic steatohepatitis. Trends in Pharmacological Sciences. 2020;**41**(3):199–208. DOI: 10.1016/j.tips.2019.12.005

[92] Cereijo R, Gavaldà-Navarro A, Cairó M, Quesada-López T, Villarroya J, Morón-Ros S, et al. CXCL14, a brown adipokine that mediates brown-fat-to-macrophage communication in thermogenic adaptation. Cell Metabolism. 2018;**28**:750–63.e6

[93] Campderrós L, Moure R, Cairó M, Gavaldà-Navarro A, Quesada-López T, Cereijo R, et al. Brown adipocytes secrete GDF15 in response to thermogenic activation. Obesity. 2019;**27**:1606–1616

[94] Brondani LA, Assmann TS, Duarte GCK, Gross JL, Canani LH, Crispim D. The role of the uncoupling protein 1 (UCP1) on the development of obesity and type 2 diabetes mellitus. Arq Bras Endocrinol Metabol. 2012;**56**:215–225. DOI: 10.1590/s0004-27302012000400001

[95] Kozak LP, Anunciado-Koza R. UCP1: Its involvement and utility in obesity. International Journal of Obesity. 2008;**32**(Suppl 7):S32–8. DOI: 10.1038/ijo.2008.236

[96] Cypess AM, Lehman S, Williams G, Tal I, Rodman D, Goldfine AB, et al. Identification and importance of brown adipose tissue in adult humans. New England Journal of Medicine. 2009;**360**:1509–1517

[97] Magro BS, Penteado D, Dias M. Brown and beige adipose tissue: New therapeutic targets for metabolic disorders. Health Science Review. 2024;**10**:100148. DOI: 10.1016/j.hsr.2024.100148

[98] Carpentier AC, Blondin DP, Virtanen KA, Richard D, Haman F, Turcotte ÉE ÉE. Brown adipose tissue energy metabolism in humans. Frontiers in Endocrinology. 2018;**9**:447. DOI: 10.3389/fendo.2018.00447

[99] Orava J, Nuutila P, Lidell ME, Oikonen V, Noponen T, Viljanen T, et al. Different metabolic responses of human brown adipose tissue to activation by cold and insulin. Cell Metabolism. 2011;**14**:272–279

[100] Stanford KI, Middelbeek RJW, Townsend KL, An D, Nygaard EB, Hitchcox KM, et al. Brown adipose tissue regulates glucose homeostasis and insulin sensitivity. Journal of Clinical Investigation. 2013;**123**:215–223

[101] Yoneshiro T, Aita S, Matsushita M, Kayahara T, Kameya T, Kawai Y, et al. Recruited brown adipose tissue as an antiobesity agent in humans. Journal of Clinical Investigation. 2013;**123**:3404–3408

[102] Wang S, Liang X, Yang Q, Fu X, Rogers CJ, Zhu M, et al. Resveratrol

induces brown-like adipocyte formation in white fat through activation of AMP-activated protein kinase (AMPK) α1. International Journal of Obesity. 2015;**39**:967–976

[103] Cypess AM, Weiner LS, Roberts-Toler C, Elía EF, Kessler SH, Kahn PA, et al. Activation of human brown adipose tissue by a β3-adrenergic receptor agonist. Cell Metabolism. 2015;**21**:33–38

[104] Ohno H, Shinoda K, Spiegelman BM, Kajimura S. PPARγ agonists induce a white-to-brown fat conversion through stabilization of PRDM16 protein. Cell Metabolism. 2012;**15**:395–404. DOI: 10.1016/j.cmet.2012.01.019

[105] Shankar K, Kumar D, Gupta S, Varshney S, Rajan S, Srivastava A, et al. Role of brown adipose tissue in modulating adipose tissue inflammation and insulin resistance in high-fat diet fed mice. European Journal of Pharmacology. 2019;**854**:354–364

[106] Brown AC. Brown adipocytes from induced pluripotent stem cells—how far have we come? Annals of the New York Academy of Sciences. 2019;**1463**:9–22. DOI: 10.1111/nyas.14257

[107] Guénantin AC, Briand N, Capel E, Dumont F, Morichon R, Provost C, et al. Functional human beige adipocytes from induced pluripotent stem cells. Diabetes. 2017;**66**:1470–1478

[108] Ahfeldt T, Schinzel RT, Lee YK, Hendrickson D, Kaplan A, Lum DH, et al. Programming human pluripotent stem cells into white and brown adipocytes. Nature Cell Biology. 2012;**14**:209–219

[109] Wang YL, Lin SP, Hsieh PC, Hung SC. Concomitant beige adipocyte differentiation upon induction of mesenchymal stem cells into brown adipocytes. Biochemical and Biophysical Research Communications. 2016;**478**:689–695. DOI: 10.1016/j.bbrc.2016.08.008

[110] Singh AM, Zhang L, Avery J, Yin A, Du Y, Wang H, et al. Human beige adipocytes for drug discovery and cell therapy in metabolic diseases. Nature Communications. 2020;**11**:2758

[111] Lu KY, Dass KTP, Lin SZ, Harn HJ, Liu SP. The application of stem cell therapy and brown adipose tissue transplantation in metabolic disorders. Cytotherapy. 2020;**22**:521–528. DOI: 10.1016/j.jcyt.2020.06.004

[112] Camino T, Lago-Baameiro N, Sueiro A, Bravo SB, Couto I, Santos FF, et al. Brown adipose tissue sheds extracellular vesicles that carry potential biomarkers of metabolic and thermogenesis activity which are affected by high fat diet intervention. International Journal of Molecular Sciences. 2022;**23**:10826. DOI: 10.3390/ijms231810826

[113] Levan SR, Stamnes KA, Lin DL, Panzer AR, Fukui E, McCauley K, et al. Elevated faecal 12,13-diHOME concentration in neonates at high risk for asthma is produced by gut bacteria and impedes immune tolerance. Nature Microbiology. 2019;**4**:1851–1861

Chapter 2

Lipedema as a Hormone-Driven Gynecological Disorder: The Estrogen Receptor Connection

Diogo Pinto da Costa Viana

Abstract

Lipedema is a chronic, progressive disorder of adipose tissue that predominantly affects women, characterized by symmetrical fat accumulation in the extremities, pain, and resistance to caloric restriction. Recent insights suggest that lipedema represents a hormone-driven gynecological fat disorder, in which estrogen receptor (ER) imbalance plays a central role. The predominance of ERβ activity and suppression of ERα signaling are hypothesized to drive adipose hypertrophy, fibrosis, and inflammation, particularly in the context of intracrine estradiol excess. This model aligns lipedema with other estrogen-sensitive conditions, such as endometriosis and uterine fibroids, and provides a novel framework for understanding its pathophysiology. Therapeutically, this reframing opens new perspectives for hormonal modulation using selective progestins (drospirenone, gestrinone) and metabolic adjuncts such as tirzepatide, beyond the current symptomatic or surgical approaches.

Keywords: lipedema, gynecological fat disorders, estrogen receptors, ERα/ERβ imbalance, aromatase, intracrine estrogen, estradiol, progesterone resistance, menopause, hormone-driven disorders

Key highlights:

- Lipedema is an estrogen receptor–driven gynecological disorder characterized by ERβ predominance and ERα suppression.

- Local intracrine estrogen production sustains disease activity even after menopause.

- Lipedema shares molecular mechanisms with endometriosis, fibroids, and adenomyosis, including progesterone resistance.

- Menopause exacerbates lipedema progression through metabolic deterioration and the loss of estrogenic protective pathways.

Hormonal modulation with selective progestins and metabolic therapies, like tirzepatide, represents a promising treatment approach.

1. Introduction

Lipedema is a chronic, progressive disorder of subcutaneous adipose tissue, almost exclusively affecting women. Clinically, it is characterized by a symmetrical and bilateral accumulation of subcutaneous fat predominantly in the lower extremities, sparing the hands and feet. This leads to a striking disproportion between the trunk and limbs, frequently associated with pain, easy bruising, tenderness on palpation, and resistance to weight loss, even under caloric restriction and exercise.

Despite being first described over 80 years ago [1], lipedema remains underdiagnosed and is often misclassified as obesity or lymphedema. Prevalence data suggest that it may affect up to 11% of women worldwide, although methodological variability in diagnosis likely leads to underestimation [2].

A key observation that differentiates lipedema from other fat disorders is its close association with hormonal transitions. The condition often emerges or worsens during life stages marked by significant hormonal shifts, including puberty, pregnancy, and menopause [3]. This clinical pattern suggests that lipedema may be a hormonally responsive disorder, with a pathogenesis deeply influenced by estrogen signaling.

Growing evidence supports the notion that lipedema shares mechanistic overlaps with classical estrogen-dependent gynecological diseases such as endometriosis, uterine fibroids, adenomyosis, and premenstrual dysphoric disorder (PMDD). These conditions are all characterized by local estrogen excess, resistance to progesterone, and alterations in estrogen receptor expression, particularly with a pathological shift toward ERβ dominance [3, 4].

This receptor imbalance is not just a molecular anomaly but a pivotal driver of the disease. It results in adipocyte dysfunction, impaired lipid metabolism, chronic low-grade inflammation, extracellular matrix remodeling, and lymphatic dysfunction. These processes combine to create the clinical and histological hallmarks of lipedema, including fibrotic and painful subcutaneous fat that is highly resistant to metabolic interventions [3].

Understanding lipedema through the lens of estrogen signaling provides a powerful framework for reframing it not merely as an adipose tissue disorder but as a hormone-driven gynecological disease. This chapter aims to explore the mechanistic underpinnings of estrogen signaling in adipose tissue, the pathological receptor shifts in lipedema, its association with other gynecological diseases, the exacerbating role of menopause, and the therapeutic opportunities that arise from this hormonal perspective.

This chapter presents a mechanistic model centered on ERβ predominance and ERα suppression as key drivers of lipedema progression. While this framework draws from robust molecular analogies with estrogen-sensitive disorders, it remains a working hypothesis due to limited direct human evidence. Future studies quantifying estrogen receptor expression in lipedema tissue at different stages are needed.

2. Estrogen and adipose tissue: Mechanisms of action

Adipose tissue is not merely an inert energy storage site but a dynamic endocrine organ profoundly influenced by sex steroid hormones, particularly estrogens [5].

The biological actions of estrogen are mediated through two main nuclear receptors – estrogen receptor alpha (ERα) and estrogen receptor beta (ERβ) – which often exert opposing effects on adipose tissue homeostasis.

ERα plays a crucial role in metabolic regulation, promoting lipid storage in subcutaneous depots, maintaining insulin sensitivity, supporting mitochondrial function, and facilitating adipose tissue expandability in a metabolically healthy manner [6]. Through ERα signaling, estradiol contributes to the gynoid pattern of fat distribution observed in premenopausal women, which is protective against cardiometabolic diseases [7].

Conversely, ERβ acts as a counter-regulatory receptor. It inhibits adipogenesis, suppresses lipogenesis, and exerts anti-proliferative, anti-inflammatory, and anti-fibrotic actions [3, 8]. While the balance between ERα and ERβ maintains adipose tissue homeostasis, a pathological shift favoring ERβ over ERα disrupts this balance and contributes to metabolic dysfunction, inflammation, and fibrosis.

An additional layer of complexity arises from the capacity of adipose tissue to function as an intracrine organ. It expresses enzymes such as aromatase and 17β-hydroxysteroid dehydrogenase isoforms (17β-HSD1 and 17β-HSD2), which regulate local estrogen biosynthesis independently of systemic hormone levels [4, 8]. Aromatase catalyzes the conversion of androgens to estradiol, while 17β-HSD1 increases estradiol production by converting estrone into estradiol. In contrast, 17β-HSD2 inactivates estradiol by converting it back into estrone.

In lipedema, as well as in other estrogen-dependent gynecological conditions, this enzymatic equilibrium is disrupted. There is upregulation of aromatase and 17β-HSD1, coupled with suppression of 17β-HSD2, resulting in localized estradiol excess within adipose tissue [8]. This local hyperestrogenism fosters adipocyte hypertrophy, extracellular matrix remodeling, and chronic inflammation. **(Figure 1)**

Compounding the effects of estrogen overproduction is the shift in estrogen receptor expression. The downregulation of ERα impairs mitochondrial function,

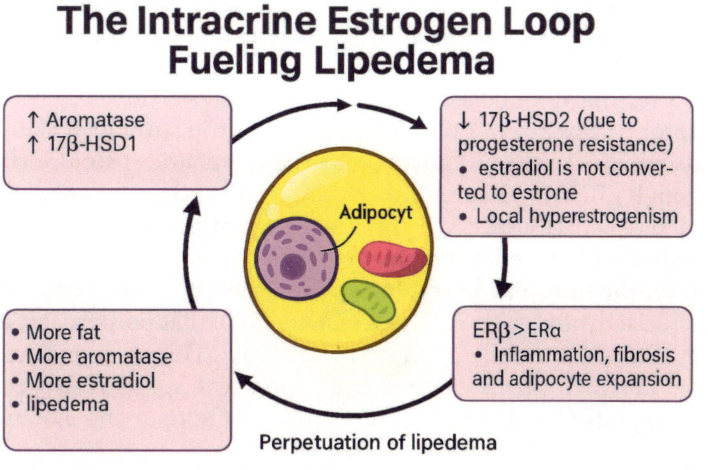

Figure 1.
The intracrine estrogen loop fueling lipedema. Upregulation of aromatase and 17β-HSD1, combined with downregulation of 17β-HSD2, sustains local estradiol excess. This hormonal microenvironment promotes ERβ predominance over ERα, driving inflammation, fibrosis, and adipocyte hypertrophy. The resulting adipose dysfunction perpetuates the pathological cycle characteristic of lipedema.

Author (Year)	Type of evidence	Methods	Main findings	Level of evidence
Tomada et al. [12]	Experimental study	Immunohistochemistry and qPCR on adipose tissue from lipedema patients vs. controls.	Increased ERβ and reduced ERα in lipedema tissue; ERβ correlated with fibrosis and inflammation.	High
Cione et al. [13]	Experimental study	Immunohistochemical staining and gene expression analysis of ERα and ERβ in subcutaneous fat.	Confirmed ERβ upregulation and ERα downregulation in advanced lipedema; associated with symptom severity.	High
Katzer et al. [3]	Narrative review	Literature-based theoretical model on ERβ dominance and ERα suppression.	Proposes ERβ predominance promotes adipogenesis, inflammation, and fibrotic resistance to weight loss.	Moderate
Al-Ghadban et al. [14]	Narrative review	Conceptual discussion based on previous literature linking estrogen and fat distribution.	Suggests that estrogen receptor imbalance may contribute to lipedema, but does not differentiate ERα/ERβ clearly.	Low
Viana et al. 2025 [8]	Narrative review	Narrative review based on mechanistic hypotheses.	ERβ predominance and ERα predominance drive fibrosis and inflammation.	Low

Table 1.
Summary of evidence supporting estrogen receptor dysregulation in lipedema. This table consolidates published findings on the expression of ERα and ERβ in lipedematous tissue, distinguishing between direct evidence from human studies and inferred mechanisms based on related gynecological or preclinical models. It highlights study types, methods used, and key molecular outcomes.

reduces oxidative metabolism, promotes insulin resistance, and facilitates adipocyte dysfunction [9, 10]. Meanwhile, ERβ dominance promotes a fibrotic and inflamed adipose microenvironment, characterized by increased collagen deposition, capillary fragility, and immune cell infiltration [3]. Although ERβ is typically associated with anti-fibrotic effects in healthy tissues, its role may differ in pathological contexts. In lipedema, aberrant ERβ activation in the presence of persistent estrogen signaling may paradoxically promote fibrotic remodeling through TGF-β1 upregulation, as suggested by preclinical models.

This receptor imbalance not only contributes to the pathological expansion of subcutaneous adipose tissue but also affects the lymphatic system. Estrogen signaling through ERα supports endothelial integrity and lymphangiogenesis, and its suppression likely contributes to the microvascular dysfunction and impaired lymphatic drainage observed in lipedema [11].

In summary, the interplay between estrogen biosynthesis, receptor imbalance, and mitochondrial dysfunction creates a vicious cycle that perpetuates adipose tissue hypertrophy, fibrosis, and inflammation in lipedema. This hormonal landscape is the foundation upon which the disease develops, progresses, and resists conventional metabolic treatments (see **Table 1** for a summary of supporting evidence).

3. Estrogen receptor imbalance in lipedema

The estrogen receptor landscape within adipose tissue is a critical determinant of metabolic homeostasis, structural integrity, and inflammatory balance. In lipedema, a pathological inversion of the physiological balance between estrogen receptor alpha (ERα) and estrogen receptor beta (ERβ) emerges as a central molecular signature that drives the disease process [3].

In healthy subcutaneous adipose tissue, ERα predominates over ERβ. This predominance is crucial for maintaining metabolic flexibility, mitochondrial function, and adipose tissue expandability in a non-pathological manner [6, 7]. ERα promotes lipid storage in the gluteofemoral region, supports insulin sensitivity, enhances mitochondrial biogenesis, and maintains extracellular matrix (ECM) homeostasis [15].

In contrast, ERβ serves a modulatory role. Its physiological function is to act as a counterbalance, suppressing excessive adipocyte proliferation, downregulating lipogenesis, and exerting anti-fibrotic and anti-inflammatory effects. However, when ERβ expression predominates, as occurs in lipedema, these effects become maladaptive [3, 8].

Histological and molecular analyses of lipedema-affected tissue consistently reveal a downregulation of ERα expression, coupled with a pathological overexpression of ERβ [3]. This shift disrupts estrogen signaling homeostasis and contributes to three key pathological processes: uncontrolled adipocyte hypertrophy, progressive extracellular matrix fibrosis, and chronic low-grade inflammation.

First, the loss of ERα signaling impairs mitochondrial function and oxidative metabolism within adipocytes. This shift promotes lipid accumulation, reduces fatty acid oxidation, and increases susceptibility to insulin resistance. Compromised mitochondrial function also leads to elevated oxidative stress, further driving tissue inflammation and dysfunction [9, 10].

Second, ERβ dominance profoundly influences ECM remodeling. It upregulates the expression of fibrogenic genes and promotes collagen deposition, leading to a stiff, fibrotic adipose tissue phenotype. This fibrotic transformation not only impairs adipose tissue plasticity but also exacerbates pain, tenderness, and mechanical dysfunction characteristic of lipedema [3, 16].

Third, the receptor imbalance perpetuates chronic inflammation. ERβ-driven signaling enhances the recruitment of immune cells, increases the expression of pro-inflammatory cytokines, and contributes to the maintenance of a pro-inflammatory microenvironment. This inflammatory state further damages the lymphatic and vascular systems, compounding edema and tissue hypoxia [17].

Notably, this receptor profile in lipedema mirrors that observed in other estrogen-dependent gynecological disorders, including endometriosis and adenomyosis, where ERβ dominance drives local estrogenic activity, fibrosis, and immune dysregulation [4, 14]. This convergence of receptor dynamics across distinct but related conditions reinforces the hypothesis that lipedema should be classified within the spectrum of hormone-driven gynecological diseases.

Additionally, the receptor imbalance explains a key clinical paradox: why lipedema progresses or worsens even in the postmenopausal period, when systemic estradiol levels decline. The combination of enhanced local estrogen production via upregulated aromatase and 17β-HSD1, together with ERβ predominance, sustains a microenvironment of estrogenic activity independent of systemic hormone levels [9].

In this context, ERα is not merely reduced – it is functionally silenced in favor of ERβ-driven pathways. This silencing eliminates estrogen's protective metabolic functions while unleashing fibrotic, inflammatory, and adipogenic processes that are characteristic of advanced lipedema.

The receptor imbalance is, therefore, not a downstream consequence of lipedema but a primary driver of its pathogenesis. This molecular signature shapes not only the metabolic and structural dysfunctions of adipose tissue but also its resistance to caloric restriction, exercise, and conventional metabolic therapies [18]. This concept is supported by findings in other metabolic conditions, such as obesity and Type 2 diabetes, where ERβ dominance similarly contributes to adipocyte dysfunction, inflammation, and therapeutic resistance [13].

To a broader estrogen-sensitive gynecological phenotype, recognizing ERβ predominance as a defining feature of lipedema provides a mechanistic framework for understanding its progression and refractoriness. It also underscores the potential for receptor-targeted interventions aimed at rebalancing estrogen signaling as a therapeutic strategy.

4. Lipedema and gynecological comorbidities

Lipedema does not occur in isolation but is part of a broader cluster of estrogen-sensitive gynecological disorders. Clinical and epidemiological observations consistently reveal an elevated prevalence of gynecological comorbidities in women with lipedema, including endometriosis, uterine fibroids, adenomyosis, and PMDD. This pattern strongly suggests a shared hormonal and molecular etiology rooted in dysregulated estrogen signaling (**Figure 2**).

Recent clinical analyses indicate that approximately 15% of women with lipedema are also diagnosed with uterine fibroids, 17% present with polycystic ovary syndrome (PCOS), and around 4% have endometriosis [19]. These rates are

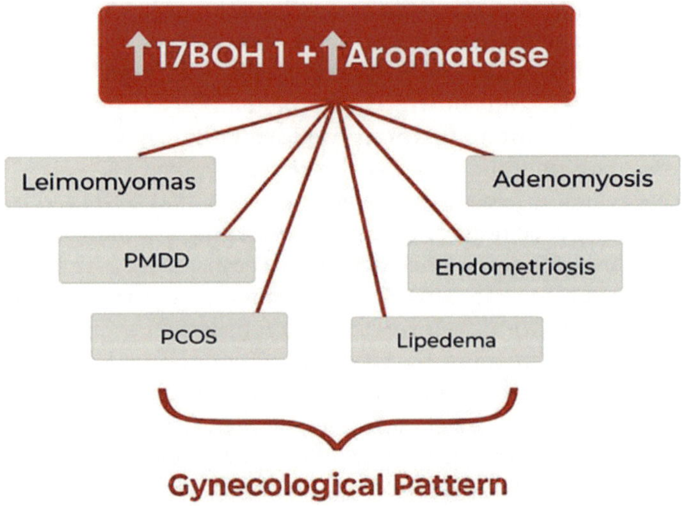

Figure 2.
Gynecological disease pattern shared by lipedema.
Lipedema shares molecular features with estrogen-sensitive disorders – endometriosis, adenomyosis, fibroids, and PMDD – including ERβ predominance, intracrine estrogen excess, fibrosis, inflammation, and progesterone resistance.

significantly higher than those observed in the general female population, reinforcing the hypothesis that lipedema is intrinsically linked to these conditions.

A common pathophysiological thread among these disorders is the dysregulation of local estrogen metabolism, coupled with a pathological shift in estrogen receptor expression. In particular, the predominance of ERβ over ERα is a molecular hallmark not only of lipedema but also of endometriosis, adenomyosis, and uterine fibroids [3, 4, 8].

This receptor imbalance drives a triad of pathological processes: chronic inflammation, extracellular matrix remodeling with progressive fibrosis, and progesterone resistance. These mechanisms form the biological substrate for the persistence, progression, and therapeutic resistance observed across these estrogen-dependent diseases [8].

In endometriosis, for instance, the overexpression of ERβ within ectopic endometrial lesions suppresses ERα-mediated anti-inflammatory signaling, leading to persistent inflammation, angiogenesis, and fibrogenesis [4]. A nearly identical receptor signature is observed in lipedema-affected adipose tissue, where ERβ dominance contributes to adipocyte dysfunction, fibrotic matrix expansion, and chronic low-grade inflammation [20].

Similarly, in uterine fibroids, enhanced local estrogen production through overactive aromatase and 17β-HSD1, combined with ERβ predominance, promotes smooth muscle proliferation and ECM deposition, resulting in fibroid growth and mechanical dysfunction [18]. This hormonal profile mirrors the adipose tissue environment in lipedema, where uncontrolled ECM remodeling leads to tissue stiffness, pain, and progressive loss of adipose tissue plasticity.

Another critical feature shared by lipedema and these gynecological disorders is progesterone resistance. Under physiological conditions, progesterone acts via PRβ to antagonize the proliferative and pro-inflammatory effects of estradiol. However, in lipedema – as in endometriosis and adenomyosis – PRβ expression is downregulated, impairing the anti-inflammatory and anti-fibrotic actions of progesterone [4, 8]. This resistance exacerbates the unchecked influence of estradiol signaling through ERβ, perpetuating disease progression.

Beyond endometriosis and fibroids, there is also emerging evidence linking lipedema with PMDD and mood disorders. This connection is likely mediated by the brain's sensitivity to fluctuations in sex steroids, particularly the imbalance between estradiol and progesterone. While not yet fully elucidated, the presence of estrogen receptor dysregulation in both central and peripheral tissues likely contributes to this association [21]. Collectively, these shared mechanisms suggest that lipedema is not merely an adipose tissue disorder but part of a systemic phenotype of estrogen-driven, progesterone-resistant gynecological diseases [8]. This conceptual framework has profound clinical implications, advocating for the inclusion of lipedema within the taxonomy of estrogen-sensitive gynecological disorders.

From a therapeutic perspective, recognizing this shared pathophysiology opens the door to hormonal strategies that have shown efficacy in conditions like endometriosis and fibroids. Modulating estrogen receptor dynamics, restoring PRβ function, and correcting intracrine estrogen excess represent promising targets not only for managing lipedema but also for improving outcomes across this spectrum of diseases [8]. This alignment reinforces the necessity for clinicians to screen women with lipedema for coexisting gynecological conditions and vice versa, as the presence of one disorder substantially increases the likelihood of others. Moreover, it underscores the importance of developing integrated therapeutic approaches that address the underlying hormonal and molecular dysfunction rather than treating each condition as an isolated entity. Important controversies remain unresolved. For instance, the phenotypic overlap with Dercum's disease complicates clinical differentiation, particularly in patients presenting with nodular fat deposits and chronic pain – features common to both conditions. Moreover, some reviews highlight inconsistencies in the literature regarding estrogen receptor dysregulation, with conflicting reports as to whether ERα or ERβ predominates in affected tissues. Independent research groups have further emphasized the methodological heterogeneity and the urgent need for standardized receptor quantification techniques, which currently hinder cross-study comparability and clinical applicability [22].

5. Menopause and clinical deterioration in lipedema

Menopause represents a critical inflection point in the natural history of lipedema. Clinically, many women report a marked worsening of symptoms after the onset of menopause, characterized by accelerated adipose tissue growth, increased pain, edema, and progression toward lipolymphedema. This observation stands in stark contrast to the conventional expectation that estrogen-dependent conditions improve with declining systemic estradiol levels, as is often seen with endometriosis or fibroids. Instead, in lipedema, menopause frequently marks a phase of clinical deterioration [12]. This paradox is explained by the unique endocrinological landscape of lipedema-affected adipose tissue. While systemic estradiol levels decline with ovarian failure during menopause, the local production of estradiol within adipose tissue remains active and, in many cases, is further upregulated. This phenomenon is driven by the overexpression of aromatase and 17β-HSD1, coupled with a deficiency of 17β-HSD2, which together sustain an intracrine hyperestrogenic microenvironment [4, 8].

Compounding this hormonal milieu is the persistent and perhaps worsening imbalance in estrogen receptor expression. As systemic estradiol declines, ERα expression is further suppressed, while ERβ predominance persists or becomes amplified [3]. This receptor dynamic removes the protective metabolic functions typically mediated by ERα – including mitochondrial biogenesis, oxidative metabolism, and insulin sensitivity – while enhancing ERβ-driven pathways that promote fibrosis, inflammation, and adipocyte dysfunction.

The result is a shift from a premenopausal state of hormonally modulated adipose dysfunction to a postmenopausal state dominated by metabolic derangement, immune dysregulation, and irreversible structural changes in the extracellular matrix. Mitochondrial dysfunction becomes a central feature, contributing to decreased fatty acid oxidation, impaired ATP production, increased reactive oxygen species (ROS) generation, and exacerbation of insulin resistance [9, 10]. Additionally, the loss of estradiol's vasoprotective effects, mediated through ERα, worsens endothelial dysfunction and lymphatic impairment. Estrogen deficiency contributes to capillary rarefaction, increased vascular permeability, and deterioration of lymphatic drainage, all of which accelerate the progression toward lipolymphedema [23].

From a metabolic standpoint, menopause further promotes a redistribution of fat toward visceral depots, while simultaneously amplifying the growth of lipedema-affected subcutaneous adipose tissue. This dual pattern of adiposity – visceral and gynoid – is associated with worsening insulin resistance, increased systemic inflammation, and higher cardiovascular risk [9]. Clinically, this is reflected in a dramatic decline in quality of life. Patients report increased pain, reduced mobility, worsening limb volume, and higher rates of depression and anxiety. The failure of conservative measures such as calorie restriction and exercise becomes even more pronounced in the postmenopausal period, reflecting the deepening of the underlying molecular dysfunction.

This menopausal exacerbation also reinforces the argument that lipedema is fundamentally distinct from obesity. While obesity may stabilize or even regress with weight management interventions, lipedema persists and progresses, particularly after menopause, due to its intrinsic hormonal pathophysiology, which is resistant to energy balance-based strategies [23].

Furthermore, the worsening of lipedema after menopause strongly validates its classification as a hormone-driven gynecological disorder. The parallels with the postmenopausal progression of other estrogen-dependent conditions – particularly those where local estrogen production and ERβ predominance play dominant roles, such as endometriosis persisting beyond menopause – are striking [4]. This understanding has profound therapeutic implications. It suggests that postmenopausal lipedema requires not only mechanical interventions like compression and physical therapy but also metabolic and hormonal modulation targeting the underlying receptor imbalance and intracrine estrogen excess. Without addressing these root causes, the disease will continue to progress despite conventional symptom-based management.

Menopause is not a neutral event in the trajectory of lipedema but a critical accelerator of its pathological processes. The hormonal shifts of this life stage amplify the receptor-driven, fibrotic, and inflammatory mechanisms already present, resulting in rapid clinical deterioration. Recognizing this pattern is essential for designing effective, targeted therapies that transcend superficial symptom control and aim for disease modification.

6. Hormonal and metabolic therapeutic strategies in lipedema

The recognition of lipedema as an estrogen receptor-driven gynecological disorder has profound therapeutic implications. Traditional management strategies for lipedema have focused on mechanical and supportive interventions, such as manual lymphatic drainage, compression therapy, exercise, and, in advanced cases, liposuction. While these strategies offer symptomatic relief, they do not address the underlying hormonal and molecular dysfunctions that drive the disease. A growing body of evidence suggests that targeted hormonal modulation represents a promising therapeutic avenue. Specifically, therapies that correct the pathological imbalance of estrogen receptor expression, reduce local estrogen biosynthesis, and restore progesterone receptor functionality hold significant potential for altering the disease course [8].

6.1. Progestins with selective profiles: Gestrinone and drospirenone

While selective progestins, such as drospirenone and gestrinone, show mechanistic promise in modulating ER imbalance, clinical validation through lipedema-specific trials remains lacking. Among the most promising hormonal agents are the selective progestins gestrinone and drospirenone. Both exhibit unique pharmacodynamic properties that directly counteract the hormonal abnormalities observed in lipedema.

Gestrinone exerts a multi-targeted hormonal action. It downregulates aromatase and 17β-HSD1, reducing local estradiol biosynthesis, while simultaneously upregulating 17β-HSD2, enhancing estradiol inactivation [24]. This enzymatic modulation shifts the intracrine balance away from hyperestrogenism. Furthermore, gestrinone binds to progesterone receptors, particularly PRβ, which is often downregulated in lipedema. By restoring PRβ activity, it counteracts the chronic inflammation, fibrosis, and proliferative signaling driven by unopposed ERβ activation [8]. Additionally, gestrinone has been shown to modulate estrogen receptor expression itself, contributing to the rebalancing of ERα and ERβ dynamics. This leads to improved adipocyte metabolism, reduction in extracellular matrix fibrosis, and mitigation of the pro-inflammatory adipose tissue microenvironment [8].

Drospirenone offers a complementary mechanism of action. As a synthetic progestin with potent anti-mineralocorticoid and anti-androgenic properties, drospirenone not only restores progesterone receptor signaling but also antagonizes aldosterone receptors. This dual action is particularly beneficial in lipedema, where aldosterone-mediated water retention exacerbates edema and tissue dysfunction [8, 25, 26]. Drospirenone is typically used at doses of 3 mg in combined oral contraceptives or 2–4 mg in postmenopausal hormone therapy formulations, often in combination with 1 mg of oral or transdermal estradiol.

Drospirenone's impact extends beyond fluid regulation. By restoring PRβ-mediated anti-fibrotic signaling and downregulating aromatase, it contribute to reductions in adipocyte hypertrophy, extracellular matrix remodeling, and chronic low-grade inflammation. Clinical studies in postmenopausal women further demonstrate its ability to improve body composition by reducing fat mass while preserving or increasing lean tissue – outcomes that are highly relevant to lipedema management [8, 25].

Gestrinone's androgenic profile, including potential effects on lipid metabolism, mood, and liver function, should be cautiously considered. Similarly, drospirenone's anti-mineralocorticoid activity may offer additional benefits but may not be suitable for patients with renal or adrenal compromise.

6.2. Tirzepatide: A metabolic adjunct in lipedema therapy

Tirzepatide has emerged as a promising metabolic agent for patients with coexisting lipedema and insulin resistance. However, its role in estrogen receptor modulation is indirect and remains exploratory. Beyond hormonal agents, recent evidence highlights the role of metabolic therapies, particularly GLP-1/GIP receptor agonists such as tirzepatide, as adjuncts in lipedema treatment [8]. While tirzepatide does not directly modulate estrogen signaling, it addresses the metabolic consequences of estrogen receptor dysfunction, particularly insulin resistance, visceral adiposity, and chronic inflammation.

Tirzepatide's dual agonism of GLP-1 and GIP receptors improves glycemic control, reduces visceral and subcutaneous fat mass, and exerts anti-inflammatory effects. Importantly, its impact on adipose tissue fibrosis and mitochondrial function offers benefits that align with the pathogenic mechanisms of lipedema [27].

Moreover, tirzepatide appears particularly beneficial in the postmenopausal context, where metabolic dysfunction accelerates lipedema progression. By improving mitochondrial efficiency and reducing systemic and tissue-specific inflammation, tirzepatide can mitigate some of the downstream consequences of estrogen receptor imbalance [27].

6.3. An integrated approach to hormonal and metabolic modulation

The emerging therapeutic model for lipedema requires a paradigm shift away from purely mechanical or cosmetic approaches toward one that incorporates hormonal and metabolic modulation. This integrated approach addresses the root hormonal drivers of the disease while simultaneously targeting the metabolic and inflammatory sequelae that sustain and exacerbate its clinical manifestations [8]. The combination of selective progestins like gestrinone or drospirenone with metabolic agents such as tirzepatide represents a rational, physiologically informed strategy. Together, they target both the hormonal imbalances (ERβ predominance, progesterone resistance, intracrine estrogen excess) and the metabolic dysfunction (insulin resistance, mitochondrial impairment, chronic inflammation) that underpin lipedema.

Importantly, this approach also holds the potential to alter the natural history of lipedema. By intervening in the molecular mechanisms that drive adipose tissue dysfunction and fibrosis, it may not only alleviate symptoms but also slow or even halt disease progression. Furthermore, hormonal treatment could enhance the outcomes of surgical interventions, such as liposuction. Patients with better-controlled inflammation, reduced fibrosis, and improved lymphatic function may experience superior surgical results, fewer complications, and more durable improvements in limb contour and function.

The therapeutic implications of recognizing lipedema as a hormone-driven gynecological disorder extend far beyond symptom management. They open the door to disease-modifying treatments grounded in the correction of estrogen receptor imbalance, intracrine steroidogenesis, and metabolic dysfunction. This represents a transformative shift in the clinical management of lipedema, with the potential to dramatically improve patient outcomes.

7. Future directions and research gaps

Despite the increasing body of evidence linking lipedema to a distinct hormonal and molecular signature – characterized by estrogen receptor imbalance, intracrine hyperestrogenism, and progesterone resistance – substantial gaps remain in both basic and clinical research. Addressing these gaps is critical to advancing the understanding, diagnosis, and treatment of lipedema as a hormone-driven gynecological disorder.

Although emerging evidence supports the role of ERβ dominance in lipedema, direct quantification studies remain limited. Future research should focus on validating receptor profiles in different disease stages and correlating them with clinical and histological markers.

7.1. Recognition of lipedema as a hormone-driven gynecological disorder

The first and most urgent priority is the formal recognition of lipedema within the framework of estrogen-sensitive gynecological diseases. Despite sharing pathophysiological hallmarks with well-established conditions like endometriosis, adenomyosis, and uterine fibroids – specifically the predominance of ERβ signaling, local estradiol excess, and progesterone resistance – lipedema remains largely classified as a disorder of fat metabolism rather than hormonal regulation [3, 4, 8].

This misclassification has significant consequences. It delays diagnosis, limits access to hormonally targeted therapies, and reinforces the erroneous perception of lipedema as a variant of obesity or lymphedema. A shift in the nosological framework is essential not only for improving clinical care but also for attracting research funding and driving policy changes that support patients.

7.2. Molecular and translational research on estrogen receptors

A major research gap lies in the detailed characterization of estrogen receptor dynamics within lipedema-affected adipose tissue. While current studies confirm ERβ predominance and ERα suppression, the precise molecular mechanisms driving this receptor shift remain unclear. Whether this imbalance is primarily genetically determined, epigenetically regulated, or induced by environmental factors such as endocrine-disrupting chemicals (EDCs) is not yet fully understood [8]. Furthermore, little is known about the downstream signaling pathways activated by ERβ in lipedema, particularly those involved in extracellular matrix remodeling, immune modulation, and mitochondrial dysfunction. Addressing these questions will require advanced molecular profiling techniques, including transcriptomics, proteomics, and epigenomic mapping of lipedema tissue compared to healthy controls.

7.3. Role of intracrine estrogen metabolism

Another critical avenue for research is the role of intracrine estrogen metabolism in lipedema pathogenesis. Current evidence demonstrates that lipedema tissue exhibits upregulated aromatase and 17β-HSD1 activity alongside reduced 17β-HSD2, resulting in persistent local estradiol production even in the postmenopausal state [8]. However, the regulation of these enzymes under different hormonal conditions and life stages remains poorly defined.

Additionally, the interactions between intracrine estrogen production and systemic hormonal environments, particularly during transitions such as menopause, have not been fully explored. Understanding these dynamics is crucial for developing timing-specific interventions that may prevent disease progression at vulnerable hormonal milestones.

7.4. Clinical trials for hormonal modulation

Despite the promising theoretical rationale for using selective progestins (gestrinone, drospirenone) and metabolic agents (tirzepatide) in lipedema, rigorous clinical trials are lacking. Most evidence to date is derived from observational studies, case series, and extrapolations from treatments for related gynecological conditions.

Randomized controlled trials are urgently needed to evaluate the efficacy, safety, and long-term outcomes of hormonal modulation in lipedema. These studies should also assess combination therapies that target both hormonal and metabolic pathways, as well as their impact on quality of life, limb volume reduction, pain, fibrosis, and prevention of lipolymphedema.

7.5. Development of diagnostic biomarkers

Current diagnostic approaches for lipedema are predominantly clinical and subjective, relying on physical examination and patient history. There is a pressing need for objective, molecular-based diagnostic tools. Potential biomarkers could include circulating indicators of estrogen receptor imbalance, aromatase activity, or extracellular matrix remodeling.

Advanced imaging modalities that capture tissue stiffness, lymphatic dysfunction, or ECM alterations may also enhance diagnostic accuracy and enable earlier intervention, particularly during subclinical or prodromal stages of lipedema [8].

7.6. Personalized medicine approaches

Finally, future research should prioritize the development of personalized treatment protocols. Not all women with lipedema exhibit the same degree of hormonal imbalance, metabolic dysfunction, or fibrosis. Stratifying patients based on their receptor profiles, metabolic status, and disease stage could enable more targeted, effective, and safer therapeutic strategies. Precision medicine approaches – integrating genomics, transcriptomics, and metabolomics – could help identify which patients are most likely to benefit from hormonal therapy, metabolic interventions, surgical approaches, or combinations thereof.

7.7. Limitations of the hormonal model

Although the hormonal model is central to the pathophysiology of lipedema – serving as the starting point for all clinical manifestations – it should not be interpreted in isolation. The immunological, vascular, lymphatic, and inflammatory responses characteristic of the disease ultimately stem from an imbalance between estradiol receptors α and β in subcutaneous adipose tissue, which triggers a dysfunctional intracrine environment. The occurrence of lipedema in male individuals, although extremely rare, is almost always associated with genetic syndromes involving X-chromosome abnormalities – such as Klinefelter syndrome – or with hypogonadal men with overlapping obesity, reinforcing the dependence of the condition on estrogenic dysfunction (citation). The clinical worsening observed during the climacteric phase is linked both to the pronounced hormonal fluctuations of the early menopausal transition (STRW–2) and to altered patterns of estradiol receptor expression, with reduced ERα and predominant ERβ, thereby perpetuating the core mechanisms of lipedema even after systemic estrogen levels decline.

8. Conclusion

Lipedema is best understood not as a simple disorder of fat accumulation but as a hormone-driven gynecological disease with a unique molecular signature centered around estrogen receptor dysregulation. The predominance of ERβ over

ERα in affected adipose tissue fundamentally alters the biological behavior of the tissue, promoting adipocyte hypertrophy, extracellular matrix remodeling, chronic inflammation, lymphatic dysfunction, and resistance to lipolysis. This receptor imbalance disrupts the protective metabolic, mitochondrial, and anti-inflammatory functions typically mediated by ERα, leaving ERβ-driven pathways unchecked.

Compounding this pathological receptor profile is a distinct intracrine hormonal environment characterized by upregulated aromatase and 17β-HSD1, and downregulated 17β-HSD2. This enzymatic dysregulation sustains local estradiol excess within the adipose tissue microenvironment, independent of systemic estrogen levels. As a result, lipedema persists – and often worsens – even after menopause, defying the expectations typically associated with other estrogen-dependent conditions.

Clinically, lipedema displays strong associations with other estrogen-sensitive gynecological disorders, such as endometriosis, adenomyosis, uterine fibroids, and PMDD. All of these conditions share common pathophysiological hallmarks: local hyperestrogenism, ERβ predominance, progesterone resistance, chronic inflammation, and tissue fibrosis. This striking overlap strengthens the argument for formally recognizing lipedema as part of the broader spectrum of hormone-driven gynecological diseases.

Menopause serves as a critical accelerant in the clinical course of lipedema. The loss of systemic estradiol exacerbates ERα suppression, further amplifying ERβ-driven pathways. This transition precipitates rapid clinical deterioration, characterized by increased fat accumulation, pain, edema, and progression toward lipolymphedema. The worsening of lipedema in the postmenopausal period underscores the centrality of local estrogen signaling in driving the disease.

From a therapeutic standpoint, the reframing of lipedema as a hormone-driven disorder opens avenues for targeted interventions. Selective progestins, such as gestrinone and drospirenone, demonstrate promise in modulating estrogen receptor balance, reducing local estradiol biosynthesis, and restoring progesterone receptor function. Additionally, metabolic agents like tirzepatide offer complementary benefits by addressing insulin resistance, mitochondrial dysfunction, and systemic inflammation.

This integrated therapeutic approach – combining hormonal modulation with metabolic correction – has the potential not only to alleviate symptoms but also to modify the underlying disease trajectory. Furthermore, it enhances the outcomes of adjunctive interventions such as physiotherapy and liposuction, offering patients a more comprehensive and effective treatment strategy.

Despite these advances, significant research gaps remain. Urgent priorities include formalizing the classification of lipedema within gynecological endocrinology, conducting clinical trials to evaluate hormonal and metabolic therapies, and developing molecular biomarkers to facilitate early diagnosis and personalized treatment.

Ultimately, the recognition of lipedema as a hormone-driven gynecological disorder represents a paradigm shift with the potential to transform clinical practice, improve patient outcomes, and advance scientific understanding of the complex interplay between estrogen signaling and adipose tissue biology. Far from being a mere cosmetic or mechanical problem, lipedema emerges as a sophisticated endocrine-metabolic disease that demands equally sophisticated solutions grounded in hormonal science, translational research, and integrative clinical care.

Conflicts of interest

The author declares no conflict of interest.

Funding

This research received no external funding.

Author details

Diogo Pinto da Costa Viana
President, Brazilian Society of Exercise and Sports Endocrinology and Metabolism (SBEMEE); Vice President, Brazilian Society of Obesity Medicine (SBEMO), Rio de Janeiro, Brazil

*Address all correspondence to: pinto.vianadiogo@gmail.com

References

[1] Wold LE, Hines EA, Allen EV. 1951. Lipedema of the legs; a syndrome characterized by fat legs and edema. Annals of Internal Medicine. **34**(5):1243–1250. DOI: 10.7326/0003-4819-34-5-1243

[2] Kruppa P, Georgiou I, Biermann N, Prantl L, Klein-Weigel P, Ghods M. 2020. Lipedema-pathogenesis, diagnosis, and treatment options.. Deutsches Arzteblatt International. **117**(22–23):396–403. DOI: 10.3238/arztebl.2020.0396

[3] Katzer K, Hill JL, McIver KB, Foster MT. 2021. Lipedema and the potential role of estrogen in excessive adipose tissue accumulation. International Journal of Molecular Sciences. **22**(21):11720. DOI: 10.3390/ijms222111720

[4] Bulun SE, Yildiz S, Adli M, Chakravarti D, Parker JB, Milad M, et al. Endometriosis and adenomyosis: Shared pathophysiology. Fertility & Sterility. 2023;**119**(5):746–750. DOI: 10.1016/j.fertnstert.2023.03.006.

[5] Richard AJ, White U, Elks CM, Stephens JM. Adipose tissue: Physiology to metabolic dysfunction. In Endotext [Internet]. South Dartmouth (MA): MDText.com; 2000. Available from: https://www.ncbi.nlm.nih.gov/books/NBK55560. [Accessed: 2025-July-15]

[6] Lizcano F, Guzmán G. Estrogen deficiency and the origin of obesity during menopause. BioMed Research International. 2014;**2014**:757461. 10.1155/2014/757461.

[7] Blüher M. 2013. Importance of estrogen receptors in adipose tissue function. Molecular Metabolism. **2**(3):130–132. DOI: 10.1016/j.molmet.2013.07.001

[8] Viana DPDC, Câmara LC. 2025. Hormonal links between lipedema and gynecological disorders: Therapeutic roles of Gestrinoneand Drospirenone. Journal of Advances in Medicine and Medical Research. **37**(2):175–188. DOI: 10.9734/jammr/2025/v37i25731

[9] Jeong HG, Park H. 2022. Metabolic disorders in menopause. Metabolites. **12**(10):954. DOI: 10.3390/metabo12100954

[10] Morfoisse F, Tatin F, Chaput B, Therville N, Vaysse C, Métivier R, et al. Lymphatic vasculature requires estrogen receptor-α signaling to protect from lymphedema. Arteriosclerosis, Thrombosis, and Vascular Biology. 2018;**38**(6):1346–1357. DOI: 10.1161/ATVBAHA.118.310997.

[11] DeBari MK, Abbott RD.Adipose tissue fibrosis: Mechanisms, models, and importance. International Journal of Molecular Sciences. 2020;**21**(17):6030

[12] Tomada I. 2025. Lipedema: From women's hormonal changes to nutritional intervention. Endocrines. **6**(2):24. DOI: 10.3390/endocrines6020024

[13] Cione E, Michelini S, Abrego-Guandique DM, Vaia N, Michelini S, Puleo V, et al. Identification of specific microRNAs in adipose tissue affected by lipedema. Curr. Issues Mol. Biol. 2024;**46**(11):11957–11974. DOI: 10.3390/cimb46110710.

[14] Al-Ghadban S, Teller ML, Bunnell BA. Estrogen as a contributing

factor to the development of lipedema. In Heshmati HM. Hot Topics in Endocrinology and Metabolism. Rijeka: IntechOpen; 2021. DOI: 10.5772.

[15] Foryst-Ludwig A, Kintscher U. Metabolic impact of estrogen signalling through ERalpha and ERbeta. The Journal of Steroid Biochemistry and Molecular Biology. 2010;**122**(1–3):74–81

[16] Heshmati HM, Organizador. Estrogen as a contributing factor to the development of lipedema. Em: Hot Topics in Endocrinology and Metabolism. Internet]. Rijeka: IntechOpen; 2021. Available from: https://www.intechopen.com/books/hot-topics-in-endocrinology-andmetabolism/estrogen-as-a-contributing-factor-to-the-development-oflipedema. [Accessed: 2025-July-15]

[17] Poojari A, Dev K, Rabiee A. 2022. Lipedema: Insights into morphology, pathophysiology, and challenges. Biomedicines. **10**(12):3081. DOI: 10.3390/biomedicines10123081

[18] Borahay MA, Asoglu MR, Mas A, Adam S, Kilic GS, Al-Hendy A. 2017. Estrogen receptors and signaling in fibroids: Role in pathobiology and therapeutic implications. Reproductive Sciences. **24**(9):1235–1244. DOI: 10.1177/1933719116678686

[19] Patton L, Ricolfi L, Bortolon M, Gabriele G, Zolesio P, Cione E, et al. Observational study on a large Italian population with lipedema: Biochemical and hormonal profile, anatomical and clinical evaluation, self-reported history. International Journal of Molecular Sciences. 2024;**25**(3):1599. DOI: 10.3390/ijms25031599.

[20] Kruppa P, Gohlke S, Łapiński K, Garcia-Carrizo F, Soultoukis GA, Infanger M, et al. Lipedema Stage Affects Adipocyte Hypertrophy, Subcutaneous Adipose Tissue Inflammation and Interstitial Fibrosis. Front Immunol [Internet]. 2023. Available from: https://www.frontiersin.org/articles/10.3389/fimmu.2023.1223264/full. [Accessed: 2025-July-15]

[21] Hantsoo L, Epperson CN. Premenstrual dysphoric disorder: Epidemiology and treatment. Current Psychiatry Reports. 2025;**17**(11). DOI: 10.1007/s11920-015-0628-3

[22] Al-Ghadban S, Isern SU, Herbst KL, Bunnell BA. The expression of adipogenic marker is significantly increased in estrogen-treated lipedema adipocytes differentiated from adipose stem cells in vitro. Biomedicines. 2024;**12**(5):1042. DOI: 10.3390/biomedicines12051042

[23] Fontaine C, Morfoisse F, Tatin F, Zamora A, Zahreddine R, Henrion D, et al. The impact of estrogen receptor in arterial and lymphatic vascular diseases. International Journal of Molecular Sciences. 2020;**21**(9):3244. DOI: 10.3390/ijms21093244.

[24] Canivilo L, Caseri L. Gestrinona: Ciência & Prática. São Paulo: Lura Editorial; 2023. p. 112

[25] Fedotcheva TA, Fedotcheva NI, Shimanovsky NL. Progesterone as an anti-inflammatory drug and immunomodulator: New aspects in hormonal regulation of the inflammation. Biomolecules. 2022;**12**(9):1299. DOI: 10.3390/biom12091299

[26] Karakus M, Gelisgen R, Topcuoglu A, Guralp O, Topcuoglu D,

Simsek G, et al. The effects of 17 β-estradiol plus drospirenone on anthropometric and biochemical measures of adiposity in menopausal women. Archives of Gynecology & Obstetrics. 2012;**286**(5):1233–1239. DOI: 10.1007/s00404-012-2437-9.

[27] Viana DP DC, Câmara LC. Metabolic therapy for lipedema: Can tirzepatide overcome the treatment gap? Journal of Pharmaceutical Research International. 2025;**37**(3):21–28. DOI: 1 0.9734/jpri/2025/v37i37664

Chapter 3

Women with Diabetes in South East Asia and Associated Risk Factors: A Review

Nalini Kumari, Vijay M. Motghare, Kalpana Dash and Sumana Sen

Abstract

The prevalence of diabetes is rising at an alarming rate in Southeast Asia (SEA). According to the International Diabetes Federation (IDF) atlas, approximately 10.5% of adults aged 20–79 years, equating to 537 million people, had diabetes globally in 2021, with this figure expected to reach 783 million by 2045. Of those with diabetes, three in four are living in low- and middle-income countries, whereas 44.7% of cases still remain undiagnosed. Diabetes is a significant contributor to non-communicable disease (NCD) mortality in SEA countries, causing 2% of all annual deaths and highlighting the substantial economic and healthcare burden. This review aims to examine the prevalence of diabetes and its associated risk factors using data from NFHS-4 and NFHS-5 from India; National Survey data of diabetes from Pakistan, Bangladesh, and Nepal were taken along with literature from PubMed, Google Scholar, Embase, the *Journal of Endocrine Society*, and the IDF Atlas. Statistical methods, including descriptive statistics and logistic regression, were applied to evaluate predictors of diabetes and its complications. Biomarker data included measurements of height, weight, hemoglobin levels, and waist-to-hip ratios for adults and children, as well as blood pressure and random blood glucose levels for adults aged 15 and above. Overweight, obesity, and high waist-to-hip ratios were more prevalent among urban women than rural women in Southeast Asia, and this indicates higher risks of diabetes and chronic disease complications in urban populations. All these addressing the risk factors, such as impaired glucose tolerance, is essential to mitigate diabetes-related complications.

Keywords: diabetes, Southeast Asia, women with diabetes, prevalence, biomarker, socioeconomic barriers

1. Introduction

'The occurrence, growth, and distribution of diabetes vary greatly by country and are increasing rapidly, as indicated by data from the International Diabetes Federation (IDF)'. The burden of diabetes is rising and predominantly affects middle-income nations such as India and Pakistan. Key factors contributing to this include economic growth, shifts in lifestyle, and dietary changes that result in high rates of obesity, unhealthy food behaviors, and a sedentary lifestyle. Diabetes is associated with almost all chronic diseases and can exacerbate existing health conditions, and over time, complications may lead to significant cardiovascular issues, damage to the eyes, kidneys, and nervous system, limb amputation, loss of vision, and early death. The worldwide prevalence of diabetes is approaching 463 million, with cases of impaired glucose tolerance (IGT) also on the rise. Projections suggest that by 2045, the number of individuals with diabetes will reach 700 million, while IGT cases may continue to increase to 548 million, according to the IDF [1, 2]. Reports from the World Health Organization (WHO) also indicate that non-communicable diseases (NCDs) are responsible for 74% of global fatalities, with diabetes alone contributing to nearly 1.6 million deaths and making it the ninth leading cause of death worldwide, as supported by data. With diabetes escalating to epidemic levels, it is estimated that by 2035, deaths attributed to diabetes could reach around 592 million. Type 2 diabetes, which represents about 90% of all diabetes cases, was once thought to be primarily prevalent in wealthy Western countries; however, it has now impacted middle-income populations and developing nations like India [3, 4].

South Asian individuals mainly include the Indian subcontinent, encompassing countries such as India, Pakistan, Sri Lanka, Nepal, Bangladesh, Bhutan, the Maldives, and Afghanistan. In 2021, global health expenditure on diabetes was approximately USD 966 billion and is projected to rise to USD 1028 billion by 2030. However, the current discussions are focused on India, Pakistan, Bangladesh and Nepal, and present statistics show it has now become a global issue and significantly contributes to disability and mortality, including among younger populations [5–9].

Diabetes has become a wide-spread issue in several developing countries including China, India, Pakistan, and other nations in Southeast Asia. 'According to the information provided by the IDF, one-third of the population resides in Southeast Asia, particularly in India'. Diabetes is linked with numerous risk factors, as various studies have demonstrated [1, 4]. The major contributors to diabetes are obesity and being overweight, both of which have seen a notable increase in the recent past, especially in the Southeast Asia region [3, 4]. As per IDF data from 2021, the prevalence of diabetes in the SEA was 8.5%, with around 90 million adults aged between 20 and 79 years affected. Additionally, the IDF predicts that the prevalence of diabetes in SEA will rise by 30%, reaching a rate of 13%, with undiagnosed cases accounting for 51.2% and hyperglycemia affecting pregnancies at a rate of 25.9% [1, 10–12].

The World Health Organization (WHO) in 2021 proposed the Global Diabetes Compact, a worldwide initiative aimed primarily at enhancing diabetes prevention and care, particularly for individuals in low and middle-income countries (LMICs) such as India. 'According to the ICMR-INDIAB study conducted across 15 states, the prevalence of pre-diabetes in India varies between 6 and 14.7%, with an average rate of 10.3%' [5, 6, 12–15]. Evidence from the National Family Health Survey-5 (2019–2021), conducted in Haryana, India, shows that diabetes rates among women aged 15 and older in urban areas stand at 13.5%, considerably higher than the national figure, both men and women are similarly impacted, although men exhibit a marginally higher prevalence at 10.8% compared to 10.2% in women based on the shared data [1, 5, 6, 12–15]. The increase in industrialization and urban growth has resulted in population increases, sedentary lifestyles, modifications in dietary patterns, mainly processed foods, and evolving eating habits, which play a crucial role in the diabetes epidemic [3, 4, 12, 16].

The prevalence of diabetes is rising, particularly among lower socioeconomic groups, with an increase in the likelihood of the condition in females as well. Due to insufficient and inconsistent data, we cannot determine whether diabetes is more common in men in countries such as India. Moreover, diabetes poses a considerable risk for mortality associated with cardiac complications [17–21]. Data from India's National Family Health Survey (NFHS-4) and (NFHS-5) indicate that 42% of individuals with diabetes are unaware of their diagnosis. The survey also reports that approximately 45% of the population has access to healthcare services, with significant regional variances among Indian states [5, 6, 12–15, 17–19]. In the Southeast Asia region, Pakistan covers an area of 796,095 km^2 and has a population of 207.7 million, ranking as the sixth most populous and the 36th largest country globally [2, 3]. Prior to 2018, a national diabetes survey was conducted in Pakistan in 1999, later published in 2007, which estimated the prevalence of type 2 diabetes to be 11% using the oral glucose tolerance test (OGTT) and the survey also reported specific regional prevalence rates for certain areas in Pakistan. 'In contrast, the IDF estimated a 6.8% prevalence rate among adults aged 20–79 in its 10th Atlas edition' [1–3]. However, local healthcare professionals believe this figure is underestimated, as represented by the IDF [17, 20, 21]. Subsequent studies have indicated that prevalence rates vary significantly across different regions, ranging from 7.2 to 19.21%. A diabetes prevalence study done in Pakistan, which was the first in the region to employ HbA1c testing as a biomarker, revealed a substantial population suffering from type 2 diabetes and prediabetes. The results show that the rates of type 2 diabetes and prediabetes in Pakistan are markedly higher than earlier estimates [22–24].

In the SEA region, Bangladesh is an emerging economy where the incidence of diabetes rose by 26% from 2011 to 2018, according to previous studies. The rate of diabetes among women in Bangladesh has notably increased, climbing from 11.25% in 2011 to 13.81% in 2018, and it may actually be higher than what the data indicates [1, 2]. Nepal is a neighboring country of India within the SEA region and also encompasses a diverse age range in its overall population. A nationally representative study conducted there showed a high rate of diabetes among participants, surpassing the IDF estimate of 4% prevalence for Nepal in 2017 [1, 25, 26].

The incidence of diabetes in Nepal rises with age, with participants aged 60 and older showing nearly five times the prevalence of those between 20 and 39 years old; additionally, male participants have a greater likelihood of developing diabetes compared to their female counterparts, while urban dwellers are about twice as likely to be affected as those in rural areas [26]. Factors associated with a higher prevalence include gender, marital status, educational attainment (none or secondary education), rural living, wealth status (middle to richest), obesity, unemployment, and hypertension [16, 26]. A national survey in Nepal has found that the absolute prevalence of diabetes is most pronounced among individuals living in urban settings and within the wealthiest segment, whereas the relative increase in prevalence is disproportionately greater among those in rural areas who belong to the poorest wealth groups and are of normal weight; approximately one-third of these individuals go undiagnosed [27]. The current evaluation of data encompasses findings from India, Pakistan, Bangladesh, and Nepal.

2. Methodology

A cross-sectional descriptive study was conducted on countries by the National Survey to gather information involving various demographics and biomarkers [13, 18, 19, 24–27].

In India, a descriptive cross-sectional investigation focusing on NCDs like diabetes data was taken from NFHS-4, 2015–2016 and NFHS-5, 2019–2021. NFHS-5 collected information from 636,699 households, encompassing 724,115 women and 101,839 men. The survey employed a multistage stratified sampling technique, which involved probability proportional to size and systematic sampling to select households for interviews across 707 districts, seven union territories, and 29 states. Women aged 15-49 years and men aged 15-54 years were involved conducting biomarker assessments by interviewing eligible participants. Data pertaining to women were gathered at the district level, whereas men's information was collected at the state level during the interviews. Trained field workers performed data collection through the interview process using the computer-assisted personal interviewing (CAPI) method [13, 18, 19, 27].

1. The NFHS used a structured questionnaire to collect information on age, gender, place of residence, ethnicity, and smoking habits. The household wealth was evaluated using a wealth index, which was established *via* principal component analysis. Each household was assigned scores based on the types and amounts of consumer goods they possessed. These scores were then attributed to household members, ranked, and distributed into five wealth quintiles (poorest, poorer, middle, richer, and most prosperous), each representing 20% of the population. The survey inquired whether participants were currently experiencing diabetes, capillary plasma glucose measurements and fasting blood sugar assessments [18, 19, 27].

2. In Pakistan, a nationwide cross-sectional study was done investigating the prevalence of diabetes, conducted from April to November 2017 by the Department of Diabetes, Endocrine, and Metabolic Diseases in Hayatabad, alongside the Department of Health, Government of Khyber Pakhtunkhwa. The research received technical support from the Institute of Public Health at Khyber Medical University in Peshawar, the University of Manchester in the United Kingdom, and the Pakistan Endocrine Society. Trained field teams, overseen by epidemiologists, gathered demographic information and blood samples from the participants chosen for the study [24].

3. Cross-sectional study data taken from the Bangladesh Demographic and Health Survey (BDHS), which was conducted in 2011 and 2017–2018, were utilized to estimate the prevalence of diagnosed diabetes among non-institutionalized individuals in Bangladesh aged 35 and older. Diabetes testing and corresponding questionnaires were only included in the surveys of 2011 and 2018 [25].

4. A population-based cross-sectional study was carried out across all seven provinces of Nepal between 2016 and 2018. The sample size was determined based on the 4% prevalence of elevated blood glucose reported in Nepal's 2013 NCDs Risk Factors STEPS Survey. This study involved 13,200 participants aged 20 and above who were selected by using a multistage cluster sampling method. Individuals who declined to participate in either the questionnaire or the physical and biochemical measurements were excluded from the relevant stages according to the consent provided [26].

2.1 Statistical analysis

Statistical evaluation was conducted to determine the prevalence from NFHS 4 to NFHS 5 in India, utilizing a binary logistic regression model that was adjusted for age and gender. In Pakistan, the research employed a stratified two-stage cluster design that encompassed all metropolitan areas and randomly chosen districts [24, 27].

Descriptive analyses for each outcome variable were performed using complex sample analysis that considered primary sampling units (PSUs), strata, and weights. Bivariate and multivariate analyses were done to explore the relationships between explanatory variables and the outcome variable in the surveys conducted in Pakistan, Bangladesh, and Nepal. Explanatory variables with a p-value <0.05 in the bivariate analysis were incorporated into the multivariate binary logistic regression model to evaluate their independent influence on the occurrence of diabetes across all studies. The strength of these associations was expressed using adjusted odds ratios (AOR) along with 95% confidence intervals (CI). A p-value of <0.05 signified statistical significance. The statistical analyses were performed using SPSS [28].

3. Results

3.1 Prevalence of diabetes in India

See **Tables 1–3.**

State/UT	Prevalence of diabetes (%)		Prevalence of pre-diabetes (%)	
	Urban	Rural	Overall	Urban
Andhra Pradesh	12.6	6.3	8.4	11.1
Arunachal Pradesh	5.8	4.9	5.1	14.2
Assam	12.4	4.4	5.5	13.6
Bihar	10.5	3.5	0.3	15.5
Chandigarh	14.2	8.3	13.6	14.5
Gujarat	9.5	5.1	7.1	8.4
Jharkhand	13.5	3	5.3	10.7
Karnataka	11.1	5.6	7.7	14.1
Maharashtra	10.9	6.5	8.4	15.2
Manipur	7.1	4.4	5.1	7.2
Meghalaya	8.9	3.5	4.5	7.4
Mizoram	7.9	3.6	5.8	6.2
Punjab	12	8.7	10	8.6
Tamil Nadu	13.7	7.8	10.4	9.8
Tripura	15.5	7.2	9.4	16.2

Above table denotes adjusted prevalence rates of Diabetes and pre-diabetes across 15 states and Union territories of India - the ICMR INDIAB Study [15].

Table 1.
Adjusted prevalence rates of diabetes and pre-diabetes across 15 states and Union territories of India – the ICMR-INDIAB study [Source Ref. [15]].

Category	NFHS-4 (per 100 persons, 95% CI)	NFHS-5 (per 100 persons, 95% CI)	RC (%)	Unadjusted OR (95% CI)	P-value	Adjusted OR* (95% CI)	P-value
Total Diabetes	3.50 (3.46–3.55)	3.99 (3.94–4.04)	14	1.14 (1.12–1.16)	<0.001	1.12 (1.10–1.14)	<0.001
Known Diabetes	2.08 (2.05–2.12)	2.35 (2.31–2.39)	17.9	1.13 (1.10–1.15)	<0.001	1.09 (1.07–1.12)	<0.001
Undiagnosed Diabetes	1.38 (1.35–1.41)	1.52 (1.49–1.56)	8.4	1.10 (1.07–1.14)	<0.001	1.09 (1.06–1.12)	<0.001
Gender							
Women	3.30 (3.25–3.35)	3.74 (3.69–3.79)	13.3	1.13 (1.11–1.16)	<0.001	1.10† (1.08–1.13)	<0.001
Men	4.70 (4.57–4.84)	5.70 (5.54–5.87)	21.2	1.22 (1.17–1.27)	<0.001	1.18† (1.13–1.24)	<0.001
Wealth Index							
Poorest	1.77 (1.69–1.85)	2.48 (2.38–2.57)	40.1	1.41 (1.32–1.49)	<0.001	1.40 (1.32–1.49)	<0.001
Poorer	2.24 (2.15–2.32)	3.00 (2.90–3.09)	33.9	1.35 (1.28–1.42)	<0.001	1.33 (1.27–1.40)	<0.001
Middle	3.03 (2.93–3.12)	3.88 (3.77–3.98)	28.1	1.29 (1.23–1.34)	<0.001	1.24 (1.19–1.29)	<0.001
Richer	4.53 (4.42–4.64)	4.89 (4.77–5.00)	7.9	1.08 (1.04–1.12)	<0.001	1.04 (1.01–1.08)	0.012
Richest	5.35 (5.23–5.46)	5.43 (5.31–5.55)	1.49	1.01 (0.98–1.05)	0.332	1.03 (0.96–1.03)	0.847
Age Group							
20–24	0.83 (0.77–0.87)	0.94 (0.88–0.99)	13.3	1.13 (1.04–1.23)	0.004	1.14‡ (1.05–1.24)	0.002
25–29	1.38 (1.31–1.44)	1.42 (1.35–1.48)	2.89	1.02 (0.95–1.10)	0.436	1.03‡ (0.96–1.10)	0.341
30–34	2.25 (2.16–2.34)	2.49 (2.39–2.58)	10.6	1.10 (1.04–1.17)	<0.001	1.11‡ (1.05–1.17)	<0.001
35–39	3.63 (3.51–3.74)	4.15 (4.02–4.26)	14.3	1.14 (1.09–1.20)	<0.001	1.15‡ (1.10–1.20)	<0.001
40–44	5.83 (5.67–5.99)	6.56 (6.39–6.72)	12.5	1.13 (1.09–1.17)	<0.001	1.13‡ (1.09–1.18)	<0.001
45–49	8.57 (8.38–8.76)	9.24 (9.05–9.43)	7.8	1.08 (1.05–1.12)	<0.001	1.09‡ (1.05–1.12)	<0.001
50–54	11.92 (11.24–12.63)	15.23 (14.46–16.03)	27.7	1.32 (1.21–1.45)	<0.001	1.32‡ (1.21–1.45)	<0.001
Residence							
Urban	4.95 (4.85–5.04)	5.26 (5.15–5.35)	6.3	1.06 (1.03–1.09)	<0.001	1.02 (1.00–1.05)	0.051
Rural	2.71 (2.66–2.76)	3.38 (3.32–3.43)	24.7	1.25 (1.22–1.28)	<0.001	1.23 (1.20–1.26)	<0.001

Category	NFHS-4 (per 100 persons, 95% CI)	NFHS-5 (per 100 persons, 95% CI)	RC (%)	Unadjusted OR (95% CI)	P-value	Adjusted OR* (95% CI)	P-value
BMI							
Underweight	1.26 (1.18–1.32)	1.39 (1.29–1.48)	10.3	1.10 (1.01–1.20)	0.029	1.12 (1.02–1.23)	0.007
Normal	1.87 (1.81–1.92)	2.16 (2.10–2.22)	15.5	1.16 (1.11–1.21)	<0.001	1.14 (1.09–1.19)	<0.001
Overweight	3.48 (3.35–3.61)	3.75 (3.62–3.88)	7.7	1.08 (1.02–1.13)	0.005	1.06 (1.00–1.12)	0.033
Obese	7.12 (6.97–7.25)	7.03 (6.90–7.15)	−1.2	0.98 (0.95–1.01)	0.362	0.98 (0.95–1.01)	0.384

Prevalence of Diabetes mellitus in India.
Adjusted for age and gender. RC: relative change.
†*Only available for females.*
‡*Adjusted for age; all variables entered simultaneously [27].*

Table 2.
National level prevalence of diabetes mellitus in India [Source Ref. [27]].

Category	NFHS-4 (per 100 persons) (95% CI)	NFHS-5 (per 100 persons) (95% CI)	Relative change (RC %)	Unadjusted OR (95% CI)	P-value	Adjusted OR (95% CI)	P-value
Undiagnosed Diabetes	1.38 (1.35–1.41)	1.52 (1.49–1.56)	10.1	1.10 (1.07–1.14)	<0.001	1.09 (1.06–1.12)	<0.001
Gender							
Women	1.25 (1.22–1.28)	1.41 (1.37–1.43)	11.7	1.12 (1.08–1.16)	<0.001	1.09 (1.06–1.13)	<0.001
Men	2.15 (2.05–2.25)	2.39 (2.28–2.49)	10.5	1.11 (1.04–1.18)	0.002	1.08 (1.01–1.15)	0.02
Age group							
20–24	0.38 (0.34–0.41)	0.37 (0.33–0.40)	−2.5	0.97 (0.85–1.11)	0.704	0.98 (0.86–1.12)	0.82
25–29	0.59 (0.54–0.63)	0.64 (0.59–0.68)	8.6	1.09 (0.98–1.20)	0.105	1.10 (0.99–1.22)	0.07
30–34	0.93 (0.87–0.99)	1.00 (0.94–1.06)	7.9	1.14 (1.01–1.29)	0.041	1.16 (1.02–1.31)	0.03
35–39	1.45 (1.36–1.55)	1.63 (1.54–1.71)	12.9	1.23 (1.12–1.35)	<0.001	1.27 (1.15–1.39)	<0.001
40–44	2.31 (2.21–2.41)	2.64 (2.52–2.74)	14.3	1.15 (1.07–1.24)	<0.001	1.15 (1.08–1.22)	<0.001
45–49	3.17 (3.05–3.29)	3.20 (3.10–3.32)	0.9	1.01 (0.96–1.07)	0.599	1.00 (0.95–1.08)	0.4
50–54	4.78 (4.32–5.25)	5.51 (5.00–6.05)	14.9	1.16 (1.01–1.34)	0.044	1.16 (1.01–1.34)	0.04
Wealth index							
Poorest	0.78 (0.72–0.83)	1.08 (1.01–1.13)	33.1	1.39 (1.27–1.52)	<0.001	1.38 (1.26–1.51)	<0.001

Category	NFHS-4 (per 100 persons) (95% CI)	NFHS-5 (per 100 persons) (95% CI)	Relative change (RC %)	Unadjusted OR (95% CI)	P-value	Adjusted OR (95% CI)	P-value
Poorer	1.04 (0.98–1.12)	1.28 (1.21–1.34)	20.4	1.22 (1.13–1.32)	<0.001	1.21 (1.12–1.30)	<0.001
Middle	1.38 (1.31–1.44)	1.56 (1.49–1.62)	12.8	1.12 (1.05–1.19)	<0.001	1.08 (1.01–1.15)	0.01
Richer	1.77 (1.69–1.84)	1.84 (1.76–1.91)	4.1	1.04 (0.99–1.10)	0.318	1.01 (0.96–1.08)	0.52
Richest	1.76 (1.69–1.83)	1.84 (1.74–1.89)	4.3	0.95 (0.91–0.99)	0.028	1.00 (0.95–1.05)	0.25
Residence							
Urban	1.78 (1.72–1.83)	1.85 (1.79–1.90)	3.9	1.04 (0.99–1.08)	0.091	1.04 (0.99–1.06)	0.46
Rural	1.17 (1.13–1.20)	1.38 (1.33–1.41)	17.9	1.20 (1.15–1.24)	<0.001	1.16 (1.12–1.21)	<0.001
BMI category							
Underweight	0.54 (0.49–0.58)	0.55 (0.50–0.59)	1.8	1.03 (0.93–1.15)	0.633	1.05 (0.92–1.21)	0.43
Normal	0.69 (0.65–0.72)	0.79 (0.75–0.84)	13.6	1.14 (1.07–1.22)	<0.001	1.13 (1.05–1.20)	<0.001
Overweight	1.30 (1.21–1.38)	1.33 (1.25–1.40)	2.3	1.02 (0.93–1.11)	0.629	1.00 (0.92–1.10)	0.85
Obese	2.82 (2.73–2.91)	2.84 (2.75–2.92)	0.7	1.00 (0.95–1.05)	0.854	1.00 (0.95–1.05)	0.86

**Adjusted for age and gender.*
†Adjusted for age.
‡Adjusted for gender, all variables entered simultaneously.
§Only available for females.
‖RC: relative change [27].

Table 3.
Prevalence of undiagnosed diabetes in India [Source Ref. [27]].

4. Prevalence of diabetes in Pakistan

See **Tables 4** and 5.

5. Prevalence of diabetes in Bangladesh

See **Tables 6** and 7.

6. Prevalence of diabetes in Nepal

See **Tables 8** and **9**.

Variables	Univariate OR (95% CI)	P-value	Multivariate OR (95% CI)	P-value
Age (years)				
20–30 (Ref)	1	—	1	—
31–40	2.21 (1.8 to 2.6)	<0.001	2.03 (1.7 to 2.4)	<0.001
41–50	3.93 (3.3 to 4.6)	<0.001	3.39 (2.9 to 4.0)	<0.001
51–60	5.97 (5.0 to 7.1)	<0.001	4.87 (4.1 to 5.8)	<0.001
61 and above	5.63 (4.7 to 6.7)	<0.001	4.93 (4.1 to 6.0)	<0.001
Gender				
Male (Ref)	1	—	1	—
Female	1.12 (1.0 to 1.2)	0.003	1.04 (0.9 to 1.1)	0.334
Education				
No formal education	2.02 (1.6 to 2.4)	<0.001	1.83 (1.5 to 2.3)	<0.001
Primary	1.85 (1.49 to 2.3)	<0.001	1.39 (1.1 to 1.8)	0.006
Secondary	1.89 (1.47 to 2.4)	<0.001	1.57 (1.2 to 2.0)	0.001
Graduation (Ref)	1	—	1	—
Area				
Urban (Ref)	1	—	1	—
Rural	1.26 (1.16 to 1.34)	<0.001	1.08 (0.9 to 1.2)	0.084
Family history				
Negative (Ref)	1	—	1	—
Positive	3.98 (3.6 to 4.3)	<0.001	3.94 (3.6 to 4.3)	<0.001
Smoking				
Never (Ref)	1	—	1	—
Ex-smoker	1.39 (1.1 to 1.8)	0.006	1.13 (0.9 to 1.5)	0.323
Current smoker	1.13 (0.9 to 1.3)	0.14	1.06 (0.9 to 1.3)	0.571
Systolic BP	1.02 (1.021 to 1.026)	<0.001	1.01 (1.01 to 1.02)	<0.001
Diastolic BP	1.01 (1.01 to 1.02)	<0.001	0.99 (0.9 to 1.0)	0.31
BMI (kg/m^2)				
Underweight (< 18.5)	0.64 (0.4 to 0.9)	0.001	0.71 (0.5 to 1.0)	0.077
Normal weight (Ref)	1	—	1	—
Overweight (25 to <30)	1.08 (0.9 to 1.2)	0.06	1.06 (0.9 to 1.1)	0.182
Class I obese (30 to <35)	1.57 (1.4 to 1.7)	<0.001	1.54 (1.3 to 1.7)	<0.001
Class II obese (35 to <40)	2.22 (1.8 to 2.6)	<0.001	2.13 (1.7 to 2.6)	<0.001
Class III obese ($\geq$ 40)	3.07 (2.2 to 4.2)	<0.001	2.44 (1.7 to 3.5)	<0.001
Waist circumference (WC)				
Normal weight (Ref)	1	—	1	—
Overweight	1.18 (1.04 to 1.34)	0.01	0.98 (0.8 to 1.1)	0.774
Obese	2.46 (2.19 to 2.77)	<0.001	1.86 (1.6 to 2.2)	<0.001

Variables	Univariate OR (95% CI)	P-value	Multivariate OR (95% CI)	P-value
Waist-hip ratio (WHR)				
Normal weight (Ref)	1	—	1	—
Overweight	1.02 (0.92 to 1.13)	0.4	0.8 (0.7 to 0.9)	<0.001
Obese	1.27 (1.07 to 1.51)	0.005	1.13 (0.9 to 1.4)	0.205

**n for WC and WHR is 12,865. The following variables were included in the multivariate regression: age, gender, education, residence area, family history of diabetes, smoking, systolic BP, diastolic BP, and BMI. BMI, body mass index; BP, blood pressure; DCCT, diabetes control and complication trial; HbA1c, glycated hemoglobin; WC, waist circumference; WHR, waist-to-hip ratio [24].*

Table 4.
Logistic regression analysis examining the participant linked to Diabetes (HbA1c ≥ 6.5% DCCT aligned/48 mmol/mol IFFC units) (n = 18,856) in Pakistan. [Source Ref. [24]].

Characteristics	Non-diabetic (N = 13,598)	Prediabetic (N = 2057)	Diabetic (N = 3201)	P-value
Age (years)				<0.001
20–30	2772 (20.37%)	218 (10.60%)	176 (5.52%)	
31–40	3503 (25.74%)	425 (20.66%)	511 (16.01%)	
41–50	3802 (27.94%)	654 (31.79%)	1033 (32.37%)	
51–60	1955 (14.37%)	412 (20.03%)	833 (26.10%)	
61 and above	1576 (11.58%)	348 (16.92%)	638 (19.99%)	
Gender				0.01
Male	7363 (54.15%)	1099 (53.43%)	1638 (51.17%)	
Female	6235 (45.85%)	958 (46.57%)	1563 (48.83%)	
Education				<0.001
No formal education	9853 (72.41%)	1516 (73.70%)	2439 (76.43%)	
Primary	1936 (14.23%)	354 (17.21%)	452 (14.16%)	
Secondary	818 (6.01%)	99 (4.81%)	184 (5.77%)	
Graduation	1001 (7.36%)	88 (4.28%)	116 (3.64%)	
Area				<0.001
Urban	9117 (67.00%)	1213 (58.97%)	1932 (60.55%)	
Rural	4491 (33.00%)	844 (41.03%)	1259 (39.45%)	
Family history				<0.001
Negative	10,325 (75.93%)	1210 (58.82%)	1320 (41.24%)	
Positive	3273 (24.07%)	847 (41.18%)	1881 (58.76%)	
Smoking				0.008
Never	12,682 (93.26%)	1893 (92.03%)	2937 (91.75%)	
Ex-smoker	275 (2.02%)	49 (2.38%)	91 (2.84%)	
Current smoker	641 (4.71%)	115 (5.59%)	173 (5.40%)	
Systolic BP (mean ± SD)	124.98	128.17	130.77	0.02

Characteristics	Non-diabetic (N = 13,598)	Prediabetic (N = 2057)	Diabetic (N = 3201)	P-value
Diastolic BP (mean ± SD)	82.75	84.13	84.84	0.006
BMI (kg/m^2)				<0.001
Underweight (<18.5)	279 (2.05%)	31 (1.51%)	35 (1.09%)	
Normal weight (18.5 to <25)	5137 (37.78%)	668 (32.47%)	1019 (31.83%)	
Overweight (25 to <30)	5884 (43.27%)	850 (41.32%)	1288 (40.24%)	
Class I obese (30 to <35)	1844 (13.56%)	396 (19.25%)	621 (19.40%)	
Class II obese (35 to <40)	372 (2.74%)	83 (4.04%)	178 (5.56%)	
Class III obese (≥40)	82 (0.60%)	29 (1.41%)	60 (1.87%)	
Waist circumference				<0.001
Normal weight	6787 (70.88%)	645 (51.68%)	1142 (55.93%)	
Overweight	1676 (17.50%)	285 (22.84%)	357 (17.48%)	
Obese	1113 (11.62%)	318 (25.48%)	543 (26.59%)	
Waist-to-hip ratio				0.002
Normal weight	3219 (33.62%)	394 (31.57%)	658 (32.22%)	
Overweight	5528 (57.73%)	768 (61.54%)	1171 (57.35%)	
Obese	828 (8.65%)	86 (6.89%)	213 (10.43%)	

**n for waist circumference and waist-to-hip ratio is 12,865. BP, blood pressure [24].*

Table 5.
Participant characteristics categorized by diabetes (n = 18,856) in Pakistan [Source Ref. [24]].

Variables	Distribution (%)	2011 BDHS diabetes prevalence (%) (SE)	2018 BDHS diabetes prevalence (%) (SE)	P-value	2011 vs. 2018 ratio
All adults aged 35 +	100	10.95 (0.0048)	13.75 (0.0056)	<0.001	1.26
Age group					
35–44	35.99	8.82 (0.0065)	11.21 (0.0078)	0.081	1.27
45–54	27.43	10.86 (0.0079)	14.82 (0.01)	0.008	1.36
55–64	18.65	14.69 (0.012)	15.78 (0.0115)	0.629	1.07
65–74	11.26	11.60 (0.0128)	15.97 (0.016)	0.112	1.38
75+	6.68	12.11 (0.0174)	13.43 (0.0189)	0.793	1.11
Sex					
Male	48.98	10.65 (0.0061)	13.69 (0.0072)	0.091	1.29
Female	51.02	11.25 (0.006)	13.81 (0.0072)	0.003	1.23
Marital status					
Not married	15.88	12.13 (0.0112)	12.54 (0.0111)	0.953	1.03
Married	84.12	10.73 (0.0049)	13.98 (0.006)	<0.001	1.3

Variables	Distribution (%)	2011 BDHS diabetes prevalence (%) (SE)	2018 BDHS diabetes prevalence (%) (SE)	P-value	2011 vs. 2018 ratio
Educational level					
No education	44.8	8.39 (0.0058)	10.64 (0.0072)	0.021	1.27
Primary	29.07	11.10 (0.0078)	13.59 (0.009)	0.141	1.22
Secondary	18.15	13.03 (0.0108)	17.80 (0.0121)	0.015	1.37
Higher	7.98	21.79 (0.018)	20.27 (0.0185)	0.209	0.93
Place of residence					
Urban	23.91	16.08 (0.0106)	18.95 (0.0106)	0.129	1.18
Rural	76.09	9.39 (0.0051)	12.06 (0.0065)	0.003	1.28

BDHS, Bangladesh demographic and health survey [25].

Table 6.
Prevalence of diabetes among adults aged 35 years and older in Bangladesh 2011–2018 [Source Ref. [25]].

Variables	2011 BDHS (OR, 95% CI)	P-value	2017–18 BDHS (OR, 95% CI)	P-value
Age groups				
35–44 (Ref)	Ref	—	Ref	—
45–54	1.36 (1.07 to 1.72)	0.012	1.41 (1.13 to 1.76)	0.002
55–64	2.11 (1.58 to 2.83)	<0.001	1.58 (1.24 to 2.03)	<0.001
65–74	1.60 (1.13 to 2.27)	0.008	1.67 (1.21 to 2.30)	0.002
75+	1.77 (1.14 to 2.74)	0.011	1.32 (0.86 to 2.01)	0.202
Sex				
Male (Ref)	Ref	—	Ref	—
Female	0.78 (0.58 to 1.05)	0.104	0.92 (0.75 to 1.13)	0.435
Marital status				
Not married (Ref)	Ref	—	Ref	—
Married	0.93 (0.72 to 1.20)	0.572	1.28 (0.99 to 1.64)	0.057
Educational level				
No education (Ref)	Ref	—	Ref	—
Primary	1.31 (1.05 to 1.64)	0.017	1.23 (0.99 to 1.53)	0.059
Secondary	1.32 (1.01 to 1.73)	0.045	1.23 (0.96 to 1.57)	0.108
Higher	1.87 (1.35 to 2.60)	<0.001	1.15 (0.83 to 1.60)	0.397
Place of residence				
Urban	1.08 (0.87 to 1.33)	0.7	0.96 (0.79 to 1.16)	0.678
Rural (Ref)	Ref	—	Ref	—
Geographical region				
Barisal	1.43 (1.04 to 1.96)	0.027	0.75 (0.54 to 1.06)	0.103
Chittagong	1.44 (1.09 to 1.89)	0.01	0.88 (0.67 to 1.16)	0.369
Dhaka (Ref)	Ref	—	Ref	—

Variables	2011 BDHS (OR, 95% CI)	P-value	2017–18 BDHS (OR, 95% CI)	P-value
Khulna	0.66 (0.50 to 0.89)	0.007	0.60 (0.46 to 0.79)	<0.001
Rajshahi	1.17 (0.87 to 1.57)	0.309	0.74 (0.55 to 1.00)	0.054
Rangpur	1.00 (0.69 to 1.45)	0.986	0.56 (0.41 to 0.76)	<0.001
Sylhet	1.22 (0.91 to 1.63)	0.183	0.75 (0.53 to 1.06)	0.101
Wealth index				
Poorest (Ref)	Ref	—	Ref	—
Poorer	0.89 (0.62 to 1.27)	0.514	0.99 (0.70 to 1.40)	0.957
Middle	0.86 (0.62 to 1.19)	0.365	1.33 (0.94 to 1.88)	0.103
Richer	1.18 (0.84 to 1.65)	0.345	1.84 (1.29 to 2.61)	0.001
Richest	1.96 (1.40 to 2.76)	<0.001	3.09 (2.18 to 4.38)	<0.001
Body mass index				
Underweight	0.82 (0.61 to 1.10)	0.177	0.77 (0.58 to 1.01)	0.055
Normal weight (Ref)	Ref	—	Ref	—
Overweight	1.54 (1.20 to 1.97)	0.001	1.22 (1.00 to 1.50)	0.052
Obese	1.51 (1.16 to 1.97)	0.003	1.44 (1.13 to 1.84)	0.003
Currently working				
No (Ref)	Ref	—	Ref	—
Yes	0.77 (0.59 to 1.01)	0.056	0.80 (0.65 to 0.99)	0.039
Hypertension				
No (Ref)	Ref	—	Ref	—
Yes	1.51 (1.26 to 1.81)	<0.001	1.57 (1.32 to 1.87)	<0.001

BDHS, Bangladesh demographic and health survey [25].

Table 7.
Modified odds ratios (ORs) for variables influencing Diabetes in adults aged 35 and above (BDHS 2011–2018) survey in Bangladesh [source Ref. [25]].

Variable	Characteristics	N	% (95% CI)
Smoking habit	Smokers	3955	31.9 (30.3 to 33.5)
	Non-smokers	8602	68.1 (66.5 to 69.7)
Users of smokeless tobacco	Users	3087	25.4 (24.1 to 26.8)
	Non-users	9470	74.6 (73.3 to 75.9)
Users of either smoke or smokeless tobacco	Users	1609	13.1 (12.2 to 14.1)
	Non-users	10,948	86.9 (86.0 to 87.8)
Alcohol consumption	Yes	3115	24.6 (22.98 to 26.3)
	No	9442	75.4 (73.7 to 77.02)
Blood pressure	Raised	4504	36.9 (35.4 to 38.5)
	Normal	8053	63.1 (61.6 to 64.6)
Body mass index	Underweight	1534	12.3 (11.3 to 13.4)
	Normal	7156	57.0 (55.6 to 58.5)

Variable	Characteristics	N	% (95% CI)
	Overweight and obese	3866	30.7 (28.9 to 32.5)
Increased waist-hip ratio	Increased	6896	55.3 (53.9 to 56.7)
	Normal	5101	44.7 (43.4 to 46.1)
Total cholesterol	Raised	3120	28.8 (27.3 to 30.4)
	Normal	7741	71.2 (69.6 to 72.7)
Triglycerides	Raised	3862	35.7 (34.2 to 37.2)
	Normal	7124	64.3 (62.8 to 65.9)

Above table shows behavioural and biological characteristics of the participant [26].

Table 8.
Behavioral and biological characteristics of the participant in Nepal [Source Ref. [26]].

Variables and characteristics	No. of participants	Proportion with DM (%)	Odds of having DM	COR (95% CI)	AOR (95% CI)
Age					
20–39	4046	3	1	—	—
40–59	4723	10.4	3.7	(2.9 to 4.9)***	3.1 (2.3 to 4.2)***
60+	2508	13.3	4.9	(3.7 to 6.5)***	4.7 (3.3 to 6.6)***
Sex					
Female	6952	6.7	1	—	—
Male	4325	11	1.7	(1.5 to 2.0)***	1.3 (1.1 to 1.6)**
Ethnicity					
Disadvantaged Janajatis	1130	6.6	1	—	—
Dalits	2369	6.7	1	(0.7 to 1.4)	1.3 (0.8 to 1.9)
Disadvantaged Non-Dalit Terai caste groups	1690	8.4	1.3	(1.0 to 1.7)	1.5 (1.1 to 2.1)*
Religious Minorities	285	17.5	2.9	(1.7 to 5.0)***	2.4 (1.2 to 4.7)*
Relatively advantaged Janajatis	1884	11.9	1.9	(1.4 to 2.5)***	1.2 (0.9 to 1.6)
Upper caste groups	3919	7.8	1.2	(0.9 to 1.5)	1.0 (0.7 to 1.3)
Education					
Illiterate/no formal schooling	6128	8.4	1	—	—
Below secondary (<10 years)	2548	7.9	1	(0.8 to 1.2)	1.1 (0.8 to 1.4)
Secondary and above (≥10 years)	2601	10.1	1.3	(1.1 to 1.6)**	1.4 (1.1 to 1.8)*

Variables and characteristics	No. of participants	Proportion with DM (%)	Odds of having DM	COR (95% CI)	AOR (95% CI)
Province					
Karnali Province	565	3.2	1	—	—
Province 1	1909	7.7	2.5	(1.2 to 5.2)*	2.2 (1.1 to 4.4)*
Province 2	1845	8.5	2.8	(1.3 to 5.8)**	1.8 (0.9 to 3.7)
Bagmati Province	2820	11.5	3.9	(1.9 to 8.0)***	1.8 (0.9 to 3.5)
Gandaki Province	1249	6.7	2.2	(1.0 to 4.6)*	1.1 (0.6 to 2.3)
Lumbini Province	1905	9.6	3.2	(1.5 to 6.6)**	1.9 (0.9 to 3.8)
Sudurpaschim Province	984	5.2	1.6	(0.7 to 3.8)	1.5 (0.7 to 3.5)
Place of residence					
Rural	5663	5.5	1	—	—
Urban	5614	11.3	2.2	(1.8 to 2.7)***	1.7 (1.4 to 2.2)***

$^{*}P < 0.05$, $^{***}p < 0.001$. AOR, adjusted OR; COR, crude OR. Association of socio-demographic factors with diabetes mellitus (DM) [26].

Table 9.
Association of socio-demographic factors with diabetes mellitus (DM) in Nepal [Source Ref. [26]].

7. Discussion

7.1 Diabetes in South East Asia

Diabetes presents a major challenge within the South Asian population as individuals from this different ethnic background are four times more likely to develop the disease compared to other groups based on global statistics [14]. Furthermore, South Asians with diabetes have an increased risk of heart disease, kidney issues, and a higher rate of mortality related to diabetes compared to the general population [15, 16, 29]. The prevalence of diabetes among women has sharply risen in women of Asian descent, and they are particularly at high risk for gestational diabetes, which raises the chances of their children developing type 2 diabetes in the future [14, 15]. Although data regarding diabetes prevalence is scarce in many areas, research indicates that the condition affects women in both affluent and low-income countries. Nevertheless, there is a significant shortage of data in sex difference on the wider effects of diabetes [14, 15, 27, 29–32]. This review concentrated on India, Pakistan, Bangladesh, and Nepal.

7.2 Diabetes in India

In India, the burden of diabetes-related illness has been quantified using the DALY (Disability-Adjusted Life Years) metric, which saw a fourfold increase by 2016, as per data suggested. The prevalence of diabetes has markedly increased among the top contributors

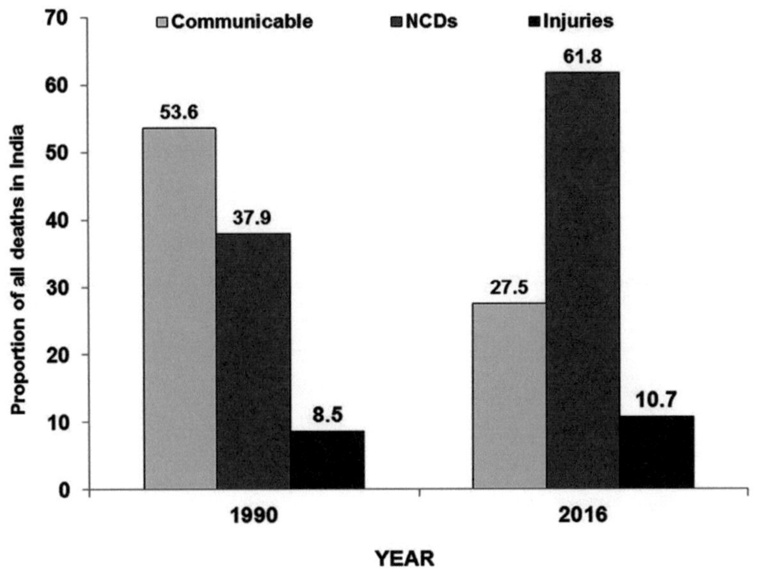

Figure 1.
Reasons for overall mortality in India, 1990 and 2016 (communicable diseases compared to non-communicable diseases and injuries [Refs. [34, 35]].

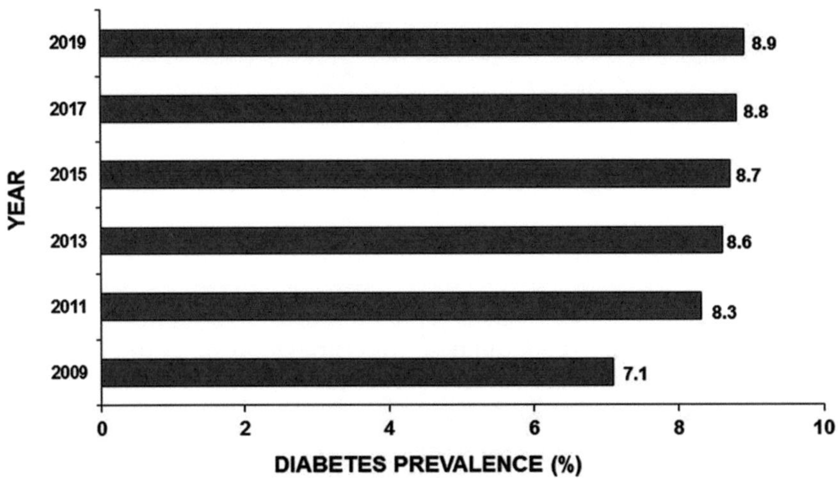

Figure 2.
Diabetes prevalence trends in India over the last 10 years [Source: Refs. [1, 35–40]].

to DALYs [33]. India moved up from the 35th position in 1990 to the 13th position in 2016, indicating a notable increase in its effect in comparison to other NCDs, which have also experienced a rise in ranking during the same time frame (**Figures 1** and **2**) [33, 34, 41].

The Centre for Cardio-metabolic Risk Reduction in South Asia (CARRS) Study was a population-based study. The results were found that 6 in 10 adults in South Asian cities have either diabetes or pre-diabetes [35, 42]. One study showed that diabetes prevalence was reported at 22.8% in Chennai and 25.2% in Delhi, while Karachi, Pakistan, showed a lower prevalence of 16.3% [4, 35]. The study also revealed that the lifetime risk of diabetes for 20-year-olds was 55.5% in men and 64.6% in women, rising significantly for obese individuals to 86.9% in men and 86.0% in women [32]. However, the lifetime risk decreased associated with diabetes, with age dropping to 37.7% for women and 27.5% for men at 60 years of age [35, 42–44].

In India, there is a lack of longitudinal studies examining the incidence of diabetes and pre-diabetes conditions. The Chennai Urban Population Study has documented incidence rates of 20.2 and 13.1 cases per 1000 person-years for diabetes and pre-diabetes state, respectively [45]. In a similar study, the Chennai Urban Rural Epidemiology Study (CURES) identified incidence rates of 22.2 for diabetes, 29.5 for pre-diabetes, and 51.7 for any form of dysglycemia per 1000 person-years [45] and among individuals with pre-diabetes, the rate at which they progressed to diabetes was 58.9%, with an incidence of 78.9 cases per 1000 person-years; however, for those with normal glucose tolerance, the conversion rate was 19.4% (**Figures 3** and **4**) [15, 17, 45–47].

India is a developing country and has a growing economy, which may have an impact on changes in lifestyle and food habits [46]. Previously, diabetes was a disease of the higher-income group, but now the lower-income group experienced a significantly higher increase in diabetes prevalence (135%) compared to the middle-income group (24%) from the studies suggest [46, 47].

7.3 Diabetes in Pakistan

In Pakistan, the prevalence of diabetes is between 7.6 and 11%, with differences influenced by many factors such as age, sex, location, and degree of urbanization [22]. Gestational diabetes impacts 3.2 to 3.5% of women, which is similar to rates found in Western populations; however, it is associated with greater maternal and fetal complications due to inadequate glycemic control, unawareness and lack of treatment, as highlighted in previous studies also [22, 24]. A cross-sectional survey conducted in Pakistan revealed that 6.8% of urban women were newly diagnosed

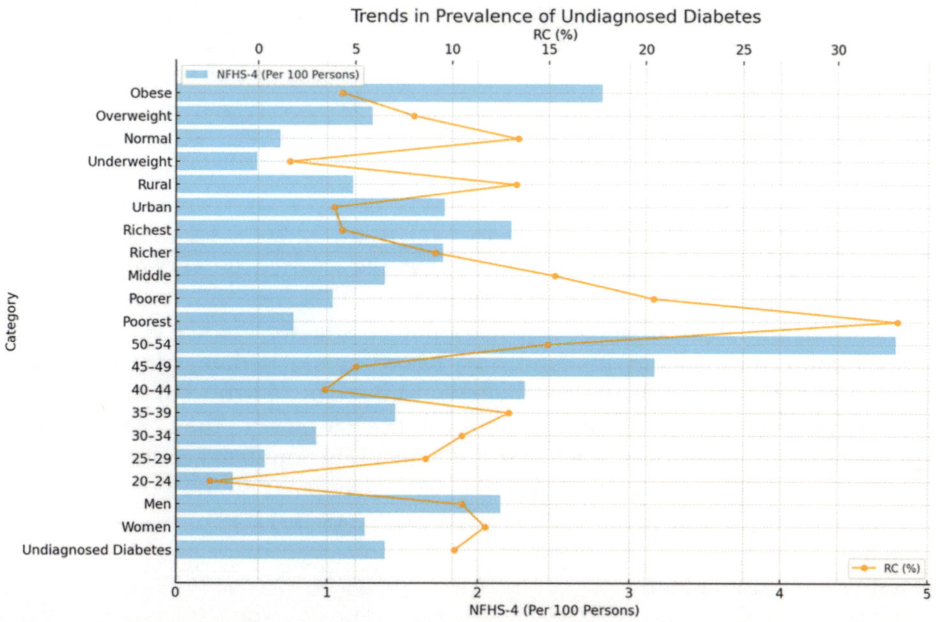

Figure 3.
Trends in the prevalence of undiagnosed diabetes in India [Ref. [13]].

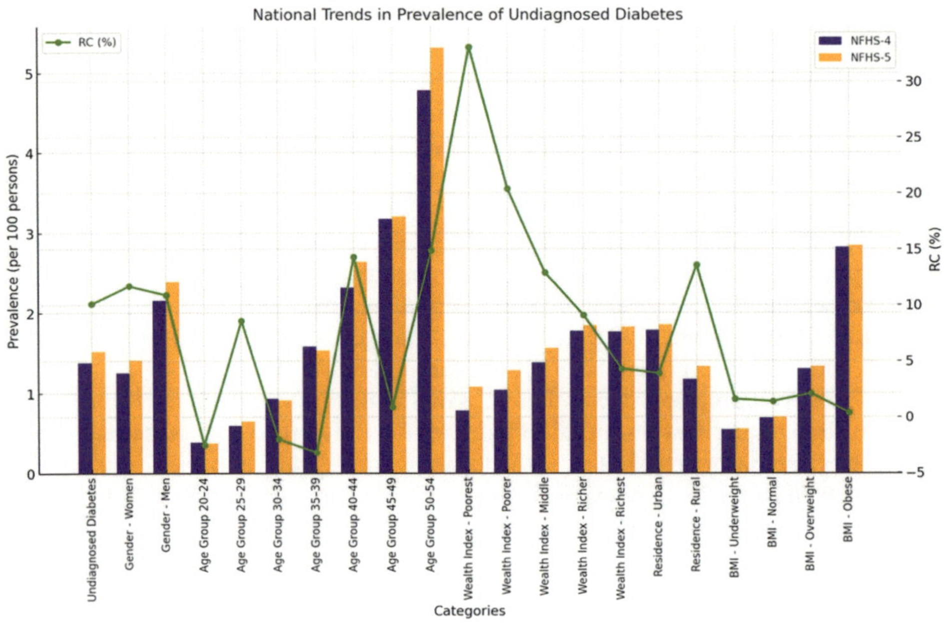

Figure 4.
National patterns in the occurrence of undiagnosed diabetes in the NFSH -4 and NFSH -5 Surveys of India [Ref. [27]].

with diabetes as compared to 5.1% of men, while the incidence of IGT was notably higher in women and has been recorded at 14.2% against 6.3% in urban settings and 10.9% against 6.9% in rural regions of Pakistan [24, 48, 49].

Obesity is considered a risk factor for diabetes. A study conducted by Aamir AH et al. [24] found that among the participants, 345 individuals (1.83%) were categorized as underweight, 6839 (36.20%) maintained a normal weight, 8038 (42.55%) were classified as overweight, 2864 (15.16%) fell into the class I obesity category, 633 (3.35%) were identified as class II obese, and 172 (0.91%) were marked as class III obese, based on WHO criteria. When Waist circumference (WC) was used as a biomarker (n = 12,865), 8574 individuals (66.64%) were found to have normal weight, 2318 (18.02%) were identified as overweight, and 1974 (15.34%) were classified as obese. Using the cut-offs for central obesity (WHR, n = 12,865), 4271 individuals (33.20%) had a normal weight, 7467 (58.04%) were classified as overweight, and 1127 (8.76%) were categorized as obese [48, 49].

Pakistan has the highest rate of diabetes among adults worldwide, with 26.7% of its population suffering from this condition, according to IDF data, which translates to around 33 million individuals with diabetes. More than one-third of these individuals remain undiagnosed, positioning Pakistan as the nation with the fourth-highest number of undiagnosed cases in the world. As a densely populated country without implementing any preventive strategies, the diabetic population in Pakistan is expected to nearly double to 62 million by the year 2045 [1, 17, 49].

7.4 Diabetes in Bangladesh

Bangladesh is among the seven nations in the IDF SEA region and diabetes prevalence based on the socio-demographic traits of participants indicate that most individuals fell within the 35–44 age bracket that represents 35.77% in the 2011 survey conducted and 36.03% in the 2018 survey reports. In both years, the prevalence rate was almost evenly divided between men and women with each group making up around 50% [25, 49].

The research indicated a consistent downward trend in education levels, and additionally, urbanization contributed to the rising incidence of diabetes nationwide and participants from urban areas surpassed those from rural areas in both years [4]. Weight is used as a biomarker, as obesity is a known risk factor for diabetes. The smallest percentage of individuals identified as overweight in 2011 was 12.97%, while in 2018, the lowest percentage was for those identified as obese at 13.36% [17, 25]. The overall diabetes prevalence among adults aged 35 and older increased from 10.95% in 2011 to 13.75% in 2018. The most significant relative growth (38%) was noted in the 65–74 age bracket, followed closely by a 36% rise in the 45–54 age group [1, 2, 25].

In addition, the study revealed that the rate of diabetes among women grew markedly from 11.25% in 2011 to 13.81% in 2018, whereas the rise for men was not considered statistically significant [1, 25]. Countries with low- and middle-income levels have experienced a faster rise in diabetes prevalence compared to those with high-income, with over two-thirds of their populations affected by the illness [46, 47]. Bangladesh is undergoing a transition from infectious diseases to chronic diseases, influenced by better socioeconomic conditions and rapid, unplanned urbanization, much like many other nations [4, 44, 45]. Elevated BMI was identified as a significant risk factor for diabetes in both 2011 and 2018. In 2011, overweight and obese individuals faced a 54% and 51% higher likelihood of developing diabetes, respectively, while in 2018, those figures changed to a 22 and 44% greater likelihood compared to individuals with normal weight [44, 45]. Changes in dietary habits and a sedentary lifestyle contributing to overweight and obesity are risk factors for the rising incidence of diabetes and are consistent with trends in other Southeast Asian countries [2, 32].

7.5 Diabetes in Nepal

A nationwide survey conducted in Nepal has revealed a significant correlation between age and diabetes, with those aged 60 and over displaying a greater likelihood of developing the disease. The WHO Stepwise approach to NCD risk factor monitoring identified weight, age, waist-hip ratio, and IGT as risk factors and biomarkers for evaluation. The findings indicate that older age is a crucial predictor of DM, which is consistent with results from various studies [50, 51]. In Nepal, life expectancy increased from 58 years in 1990 to 71 years in 2019, and the share of the elderly population continues to rise. This pattern is anticipated to continue to rise and possibly lead to a further escalation in the prevalence of diabetes [52].

In a semi-urban area of Nepal, the rate of diabetes among women was found to be 7.9%, while impaired glucose tolerance (IGT) was recorded at 15.4%. For women aged between 21 and 40 years, the rates for diabetes and IGT stood at 2.9 and 12.8%, respectively. In the age group of 41 to 60 years, the prevalence rates were 9.7% for diabetes and 13.8% for IGT, and among those aged over 60 years, these figures rose to 15.4% for diabetes and 27.7% for IGT [26, 53, 54]. Individuals living in urban areas are more susceptible to diabetes compared to their rural counterparts. Nepal is experiencing swift urbanization [26, 34, 41], leading to alterations in dietary patterns, a rise in sedentary behavior, and decreased physical activity. These aspects may have played a significant role in the increased prevalence of diabetes among urban dwellers [55]. The occurrence of overweight and obesity is escalating in Nepal, especially among women across all age groups. Considering that obesity is a critical risk factor for diabetes, implementing strategies to manage obesity could aid in mitigating the rising rates of Diabetes Mellitus in the nation [56].

8. Risk factor and problem statement of diabetes

The causes of diabetes are viewed as multifactorial, and several non-modifiable individual-level risk factors—such as genetics, age, ethnicity, and family history—have been prospectively associated with type 2 diabetes in prior research [44, 46, 47]. The increasing prevalence observed in numerous populations is likely influenced by modifiable risk factors, which include sedentary behavior, insufficient physical activity, rising rates of overweight and obesity, and poor dietary habits marked by a high intake of refined grains, fats, sugars, sweetened drinks, along with low consumption of fruits and vegetables [32]. Additionally, other contributing factors encompass smoking, alcohol consumption, exposure to environmental toxins, changed intrauterine conditions, mental health issues such as stress and depression, inadequate sleep duration, and characteristics of the built environment that contribute to the heightened incidence of diabetes [32, 46, 47, 57]. Many similar studies focusing on women indicate a higher proportion of individuals classified as high risk for diabetes. The study by Bala et al. [58] reported that 38% of high-risk subjects were women, with 57.4% of them falling within the 30–35 years' age group. Similarly, Sankar et al. [59] have identified 48.7% of high-risk individuals, of whom 64% were women under the age of 35 years, and these studies have been focused on women. These findings underscore the urgent need for early screening to assess diabetes risk among women under 35 years of age; lack of exercise or physical activity is a well-established risk factor for developing diabetes, and evaluation of the physical activity parameter using the IDRS showed that a significant proportion (67%) of women did not adhere to any exercise routine and led a predominantly sedentary lifestyle [46, 60]. Comparable findings were also reported by Brahmbhatt et al. [61] where 50.5% of women were observed to follow a sedentary lifestyle. Suri and Kapur [62] have reported that 63% of the subjects do not exercise, and Bala et al. [58] support the common findings from previous studies.

The transition from conventional diets to fast-food options and a lack of physical activity are contributing to the increase of NCDs, such as Diabetes in Bangladesh, Pakistan and Nepal, threatening a potential diabetes crisis [32, 46]. Overweight and obesity elevate the likelihood of diabetes and impaired glucose tolerance in women; numerous studies back this assertion. Additional factors, including low literacy rates, insufficient awareness, societal customs that restrict mobility (such as needing someone to accompany them to medical facilities) and extensive household responsibilities severely hinder women's access to healthcare services [31, 32, 63]. The prevalence of diabetes has escalated more rapidly among lower-income populations compared to those with middle incomes, raising concerns due to its impact on both the societal and governmental economic burden. Although the absolute prevalence rates differ among studies because of various methodologies, they consistently demonstrate an increasing trend [62, 63]. This rise is particularly affecting impoverished, normal weight individuals residing in rural areas, as well as those in lower- and middle-income brackets. A similar upward trajectory is noted in many research findings across the SEA region [63, 64].

9. Conclusion

Diabetes impacts women more severely due to their unique biological, cultural, and socioeconomic circumstances. Gender inequality continues to hinder the health and well-being of many rural women. Social, economic, and political barriers often limit access to high-quality care for women with diabetes. Factors such as illiteracy, lack of awareness, restrictive social customs (e.g., requiring accompaniment to medical facilities), and the heavy burden of household responsibilities further constrain their access to healthcare services. The lower-income group experienced a significantly higher increase in diabetes prevalence compared to the middle-income group. Although the absolute prevalence of diabetes varies across studies, all consistently reveal an upward trend in the prevalence of diabetes, and this increase disproportionately affects poor, normal weight individuals living in rural areas and lower and middle-income groups.

Conflict of interest

Nil

Author details

Nalini Kumari[1*], Vijay M. Motghare[2], Kalpana Dash[3] and Sumana Sen[4]

1 Department of Pharmacology, Apollo Institute of Medical Sciences, Hyderabad, India

2 Department of Pharmacology, Govt. Medical College, Nagpur, Maharashtra, India

3 Apollo Sugar Clinics, Raipur, India

4 Department of Pharmacology, Apollo Institute of Medical Sciences and Research, Hyderabad, India

*Address all correspondence to: dr.npuran@gmail.com

References

[1] Federation ID. IDF, Diabetes Atlas 10th ed. 2021. Available from: www.diabetesatlas.org [Preprint]

[2] Saeedi P, Petersohn I, Salpea P, Malanda B, Karuranga S, Unwin N, et al. Global and regional diabetes prevalence estimates for 2019 and projections for 2030 and 2045: Results from the international diabetes federation diabetes atlas, 9th edition. Diabetes Research and Clinical Practice (Elsevier B.V.). 2019;**157**:107843. DOI: 10.1016/j.diabres.2019.107843. Epub 2019 Sep 10.PMID: 31518657. 0168-8227/2019

[3] Ong KL et al. Global, regional, and national burden of diabetes from 1990 to 2021, with projections of prevalence to 2050: A systematic analysis for the global burden of disease study 2021. The Lancet. 2023;**402**(10397):203-234. DOI: 10.1016/S0140-6736(23)01301-6

[4] Rajendra P, Viswanathan M. Epidemiology of type 2 diabetes in India. Indian Journal of Ophthalmology. 2021;**69**(11):2932-2938. DOI: 10.4103/ijo.IJO_1627_21

[5] Collaborators, N. C. 2030. NCD countdown 2030: Pathways to achieving sustainable development goal target 3.4. Lancet. 2020;**396**:918-934

[6] Collaborators, N. C. 2030. NCD countdown 2030: Worldwide trends in non-communicable disease mortality and progress towards sustainable development goal target 3.4. Lancet. 2018;**392**:1072-1088

[7] Hunt D, Hemmingsen B, Matzke A, Varghese C, et al. The WHO global diabetes compact: A new initiative to support people living with diabetes. The Lancet Diabetes and Endocrinology. 2021;**9**(6):325-327. DOI: 10.1016/S2213-8587(21)00111-X. Epub April 13, 2021

[8] Hanif W, Ali SN, Bellary S, Patel V, Farooqi A, Karamat MA, et al. Pharmacological management of south Asians with type 2 diabetes: Consensus recommendations from the South Asian Health Foundation. Diabetic Medicine. 2021;**38**(4):e14497. DOI: 10.1111/dme.14497. Epub February 11, 2021

[9] Moody A, Cowley G, Fat LN, Mindell JS. Social inequalities in the prevalence of diagnosed and undiagnosed diabetes and impaired glucose regulation in participants in the health surveys for England series. BMJ Open. 2016;**6**:e010155

[10] Pradeepa R, Mohan V. Prevalence of type 2 diabetes and its complications in India and economic costs to the nation. European Journal of Clinical Nutrition. 2017;**71**:816-824

[11] Hills AP, Arena R, Khunti K, et al. Epidemiology and determinants of type 2 diabetes in South Asia. The Lancet Diabetes and Endocrinology. 2018;**6**:966-968

[12] Richards SE, Wijeweera C, Wijeweera A. Lifestyle and socioeconomic determinants of diabetes: Evidence from country-level data. PLoS One. 2022;**17**(7):e0270476. DOI: 10.1371/journal.pone.0270476

[13] Maiti S, Akhtar S, Upadhyay AK, et al. Socioeconomic inequality in awareness, treatment and control of diabetes among adults in India: Evidence from National Family Health Survey of India (NFHS), 2019-2021. Scientific Reports. 2023;**13**:2971. DOI: 10.1038/s41598-023-29978-y

[14] Hodgson S, Williamson A, Bigossi M, et al. Genetic basis of early onset and progression of type 2 diabetes in south Asians. Nature Medicine. 2025;**31**:323-331. DOI: 10.1038/s41591-024-03317-8

[15] Anjana RM, Deepa M, Pradeepa R, Mahanta J, Narain K, Das HK, et al. ICMR-INDIAB Collaborative Study Group. Prevalence of diabetes and pre-diabetes in 15 states of India: Results from the ICMR-INDIAB population-based cross-sectional study. The Lancet Diabetes and Endocrinology. 2017;**5**:585-596. Available from: https://www.sciencedirect.com/science/article/pii/S2213858717301742,elseivier

[16] Kumar GS, Kulkarni M, Rathi N. Evolving food choices among the urban Indian middle-class: A qualitative study. Frontiers in Nutrition. 2022;**9**:844413. DOI: 10.3389/fnut.2022.844413

[17] International Diabetes Federation. IDF 2019, Diabetes Atlas. 10th ed. 2021. Available from: https://idf.org/aboutdiabetes/what-is-diabetes/facts-figures.html [Accessed: March 11, 2022]

[18] Ministry of Health and Family Welfare. National Family Health Survey (NFHS-5), 2019-2021, India Report. Deonar, Mumbai, India: International Institute for Population Science. NFHS-5. Available from: http://rchiips.org/nfhs/, https://www.iipsindia.ac.in or https://main.mohfw.gov.in

[19] Ministry of Health and Family Welfare. National Family Health Survey (NFHS-4), 2015-2016, India Report. Deonar, Mumbai, India: International Institute for Population Sciences. NFHS-5. Available from: http://rchiips.org/nfhs/, https://www.iipsindia.ac.in or https://main.mohfw.gov.in

[20] Meo SA, Zia I, Bukhari IA, et al. Type 2 diabetes mellitus in Pakistan: Current prevalence and future forecast. The Journal of the Pakistan Medical Association. 2016;**66**:1637-1642

[21] Shera AS, Rafique G, Khwaja IA, et al. Pakistan National Diabetes Survey: Prevalence of glucose intolerance and associated factors in North West Frontier Province (NWFP) of Pakistan. The Journal of the Pakistan Medical Association. 1999;**49**:206-211

[22] Hasan SU, Siddiqui MAR. Epidemiology of diabetes mellitus in Pakistan: A systematic review protocol. BMJ Open. 2024;**14**(3):e079513. DOI: 10.1136/bmjopen-2023-079513

[23] Cho NH, Shaw JE, Karuranga S, Huang Y, da Rocha Fernandes JD, Ohlrogge AW, et al. IDF diabetes atlas: Global estimates of diabetes prevalence for 2017 and projections for 2045. Diabetes Research and Clinical Practice. 2018;**138**:271-281. DOI: 10.1016/j.diabres.2018.02.023. Epub 2018 Feb 26

[24] Aamir AH, Ul-Haq Z, Mahar SA, et al. Diabetes prevalence survey of Pakistan (DPS-PAK): Prevalence of type 2 diabetes mellitus and prediabetes using HbA1c: A population-based survey from Pakistan. BMJ Open. 2019;**9**:e025300. DOI: 10.1136/bmjopen-2018-025300

[25] Chowdhury MAB, Islam M, Rahman J, Uddin MJ, Haque MR. Diabetes among adults in Bangladesh: Changes in prevalence and risk factors between two cross-sectional surveys. BMJ Open. 2022;**12**(8):e055044. DOI: 10.1136/bmjopen-2021-055044

[26] Shrestha N, Karki K, Poudyal A, Aryal KK, Mahato NK, Gautam N, et al. Prevalence of diabetes mellitus and associated risk factors in Nepal: Findings from a nationwide population-based survey. BMJ Open. 2022;**12**(2):e060750. DOI: 10.1136/bmjopen-2022-060750

[27] Gupta R, Upadhyay A, Kohli S, Khadgwat R. Evolving landscape of diabetes epidemic in Southeast Asia: Insights from National Family Health Survey. Indian Journal of Endocrinology and Metabolism. 2023;**27**:492-500

[28] Martínez-Mesa J, González-Chica DA, Duquia RP, Bonamigo RR, Bastos JL. Sampling: How to select participants in my research study? Anais Brasileiros de Dermatologia. 2016;**91**(3):326-330. DOI: 10.1590/abd1806-4841.20165254

[29] Sohal PS. Prevention and management of diabetes in south Asians. Canadian Journal of Diabetes. 2008;**32**:206-210

[30] Dreyer G, Hull S, Aitken Z, Chesser A, Yaqoob MM. The effect of ethnicity on the prevalence of diabetes and associated chronic kidney disease. QJM. 2009;**102**:261-269

[31] Osman A, Curzio J. South Asian cultural concepts in diabetes. Nursing Times. 2012;**108**(28):30-32

[32] Ghosh S. India: Nutrition intake and economic growth, a causality analysis. Development Studies Research. 2018;**5**(1):69-82. DOI: 10.1080/21665095.2018.1468791

[33] Indian Council of Medical Research, Public Health Foundation of India, and Institute for Health Metrics and Evaluation. India: Health of the Nation's States - the India State-Level Disease Burden Initiative. New Delhi: ICMR, PHFI, and IHME; 2017

[34] Tandon N et al. The increasing burden of diabetes and variations among the states of India: The global burden of disease study 1990-2016. The Lancet Global Health. 2018;**6**(12):e1352-e1362

[35] Indian Council of Medical Research, Public Health Foundation of India, and Institute for Health Metrics and Evaluation. India: Health of the Nation's States - The India State-Level Disease Burden Initiative. New Delhi: ICMR, PHFI, and IHME; 2017. Public Health Foundation of India ©2025 All rights reserved

[36] Global Burden of Disease Collaborative Network. Global Burden of Disease Study 2021. Results. Institute for Health Metrics and Evaluation; 2024. Available from: https://vizhub.healthdata.org/gbd-results/

[37] International Diabetes Federation. IDF Diabetes Atlas. 5th ed. Brussels, Belgium: International Diabetes Federation; 2011

[38] International Diabetes Federation. IDF Diabetes Atlas. 6th ed. Brussels, Belgium: International Diabetes Federation; 2013

[39] International Diabetes Federation. IDF Diabetes Atlas. 7th ed. Brussels, Belgium: International Diabetes Federation; 2015

[40] International Diabetes Federation. IDF Diabetes Atlas. 8th ed. Brussels, Belgium: International Diabetes Federation; 2017

[41] Dandona L, Dandona R, Kumar GA, Shukla DK, Vinod KP, et al. Nations within a nation: Variations in epidemiological transition across the states of India, 1990-2016 in the global burden of disease study. The Lancet. 2017;**390**(10111):2437-2460. DOI: 10.1016/S0140-6736(17)32804-0. Available from: https://www.sciencedirect.com/science/article/pii/S0140673617328040. ISSN 0140-6736

[42] Kondal D, Patel SA, Ali MK, Mohan D, Rautela G, Gujral UP,

et al. Cohort profile: The Center for cArdiometabolic risk reduction in South Asia (CARRS). International Journal of Epidemiology. 2022;**51**(6):e358-e371. DOI: 10.1093/ije/dyac014

[43] Luhar S, Kondal D, Jones R, Anjana RM, Patel SA, Kinra S, et al. The lifetime risk of diabetes in metropolitan cities in India. Diabetologia. 2021;**64**:521-529

[44] Anjana RM, Deepa M, Subashini R, Patel SA, Kondal D, Unnikrishnan R, et al. Temporal changes in diabetes prevalence and achievement of care goals in urban South Asia from 2010 to 2016 - The Center for Cardio-metabolic Risk Reduction in South Asia Study. Diabetic Medicine. 2021;**38**(2):e14424. DOI: 10.1111/dme.14424. Epub November 2, 2020

[45] Anjana RM, Shanthi Rani CS, Deepa M, Pradeepa R, Sudha V, Divya Nair H, et al. Incidence of diabetes and prediabetes and predictors of progression among Asian Indians: 10-year follow-up of the Chennai urban rural epidemiology study (CURES). Diabetes Care. 2015;**38**(8):1441-1448. DOI: 10.2337/dc14-2814. Epub 2015 Apr 23

[46] Hill-Briggs F, Adler NE, Berkowitz SA, Chin MH, Gary-Webb TL, Navas-Acien A, et al. Social determinants of health and diabetes: A scientific review. Diabetes Care. 2020;**44**:258-279. DOI: 10.2337/dci20-0053

[47] Deepa M, Anjana RM, Manjula D, Narayan KMV, Mohan V. Convergence of prevalence rates of diabetes and cardiometabolic risk factors in middle and low-income groups in urban India: 10-year follow-up of the Chennai urban population study. Journal of Diabetes Science and Technology. 2011;**5**:918-927

[48] Azeem S, Khan U, Liaquat A. The increasing rate of diabetes in Pakistan: A silent killer. Annals of Medicine and Surgery. (London). 2022;**79**:103901. DOI: 10.1016/j.amsu.2022.103901

[49] Dagenais GR, Gerstein HC, Zhang X, et al. Variations in diabetes prevalence in low-, middle-, and high-income countries: Results from the prospective urban and rural epidemiological study. Diabetes Care. 2016;**39**:780-787

[50] Gyawali P, Bhandari S, Shrestha J. Horti-tourism; an approach for strengthening farmers' economy in the post-covid situation. Journal of Agriculture and Food Research. 2022;**7**:100278. DOI: 10.1016/j.jafr.2022.100278. Available from: https://www.sciencedirect.com/science/article/pii/S2666154322000114

[51] O'Neill A. Share of the urban population in Nepal from 2013 to 2023. Available from: https://www.statista.com/statistics/761126/share-of-urban-population-nepal/

[52] Dhungana RR, Pandey AR, Shrestha N. Trends in the prevalence, awareness, treatment, and control of hypertension in Nepal between 2000 and 2025: A systematic review and meta-analysis. International Journal of Hypertension. 2021;**2021**:6610649

[53] Population-aged-65-years-and-above, National statistics office, Thapathali, Kathmandu. Available from: https://censusnepal.cbs.gov.np/results/files/result-folder/Final_Population_compostion_12_2.pdf

[54] Ono K, Limbu YR, Rai SK, Kurokawa M, Yanagida J, Rai G, et al. The prevalence of type 2 diabetes mellitus and impaired fasting glucose in the semi-urban population of Nepal.

Nepal Medical College Journal. 2007, 2019;**9**:154-156

[55] WHO. Diabetes. 2019. Available from: http://www.searo.who.int/india/topics/diabetes_mellitus/en

[56] Rana K, Ghimire P, Chimoriya R, Chimoriya R. Trends in the prevalence of overweight and obesity and associated socioeconomic and household environmental factors among women in Nepal: Findings from the Nepal demographic and health surveys. Obesities. 2021;**1**(2):113-135. DOI: 10.3390/Obesities1020011

[57] Galicia-Garcia U, Benito-Vicente A, Jebari S, Larrea-Sebal A, Siddiqi H, Uribe KB, et al. Pathophysiology of type 2 diabetes mellitus. International Journal of Molecular Sciences. 2020;**21**(17):6275. DOI: 10.3390/ijms21176275

[58] Bala S, Pandve H, Kamala K, Dhanalakshmi A, Sarikonda H. Performance of Indian diabetic risk score as a screening tool of diabetes among women of the industrial urban area. Journal of Family Medicine and Primary Care. 2019;**8**:3569. DOI: 10.4103/jumps.jfmpc_799_19

[59] Sankar P, Ahmed WN, Mariam Koshy V, Jacob R, Sasidharan S. Effects of COVID-19 lockdown on type 2 diabetes, lifestyle and psychosocial health: A hospital-based cross-sectional survey from South India. Diabetes and Metabolic Syndrome: Clinical Research and Reviews. 2020;**14**:1815-1819

[60] Guilbert JJ. The world health report 2002 - reducing risks, promoting healthylife. Education for Health (Abingdon, England). 2003;**16**(2):230. DOI: 10.1080/1357628031000116808. PMID: 14741909

[61] Brahmbhatt K, Chakraborty T, Gopal C, Shwethashree M, Madappady S, Sowndarya TA, et al. Assessment of risk of type 2 diabetes using simplified Indian diabetes risk score-community-based cross-sectional study. International Journal of Medical Science and Public Health. 2016;**5**:2522. DOI: 10.5455/ijmsph.2016.16052016517

[62] Suri M, Kapur D. Putting knowledge into practice: Where are we going wrong in managing type 2 diabetes? A cross-sectional study on urban population in the millennium city of North India. Journal of Diabetology. 2022;**13**:56. DOI: 10.4103/jod.jod_81_21

[63] Okunogbe A, Nugent R, Spencer G, Powis J, Ralston J, Wilding J. Economic impacts of overweight and obesity: Current and future estimates for 161 countries. BMJ Global Health. 2022;**7**:e009773

[64] World Diabetes Foundation. Global Alliance for Women's Health. Diabetes, Women, and Development: meeting summary, expert recommendations for policy action, conclusions, and follow-up actions. International Journal of Gynaecology and Obstetrics. 2009;**104**(Suppl 1):S46-S50. DOI: 10.1016/j.ijgo.2008.11.014. Epub 2009 Jan 20. PMID: 19159877

Chapter 4

Adipose Tissue Metabolic Inflammation: A Key Driver of Cardiovascular Disease Pathogenesis and Underlying Mechanisms

Jiafu Ouyang, Wen Lu, Yubing Fan, Zhishan Jiang, Qian Du and Donghui Liu

Abstract

Obesity is a chronic metabolic disorder driven by dysregulated energy homeostasis, characterized by excessive adipose tissue accumulation and/or pathological redistribution. Beyond its primary role as an energy reservoir, adipose tissue functions as a dynamic endocrine organ that orchestrates adipokine secretion, immune cell crosstalk, and inflammatory signaling cascades. A hallmark of obesity is the induction of systemic insulin resistance and metabolic dysregulation, which significantly elevates cardiovascular disease (CVD) risk. Central to this pathophysiology is metabolic inflammation – a chronic low-grade inflammatory state initiated by caloric surplus and adipocyte dysfunction. Adipose tissue drives this inflammatory cascade through increased pro-inflammatory cytokine (e.g., TNF-α, IL-6) secretion and immune cell (e.g., macrophages, T cells) infiltration. This persistent low-grade inflammation acts as a critical mediator of metabolic dysfunction and cardiovascular complications, including atherosclerosis, hypertension, heart failure, and atrial fibrillation. Through a synthesis of adipose tissue-derived inflammatory responses in CVD pathogenesis, this review elucidates the mechanistic interconnections between metabolic inflammation and cardiac pathophysiology, while highlighting targeted therapeutic strategies for obesity-related CVD.

Keywords: adipose tissue, obesity, metabolic inflammation, cardiovascular diseases, atherosclerosis, hypertension, heart failure, atrial fibrillation

1. Introduction

Obesity stands as one of the most profound challenges to global public health. According to 2016 World Health Organization (WHO) estimates, approximately 1.9 billion adults were overweight, including 650 million with obesity (defined as

BMI ≥30 kg/m^2). These figures translate to 39% of adults aged ≥18 years being overweight and 13% living with obesity [1]. By 2021, about 1 billion adult males and 1.11 billion adult females were affected by overweight or obesity. Under current trajectories, this number is projected to reach nearly 3.8 billion adults globally by 2050, surpassing 50% of the world's adult population [2].

Obesity primarily arises from chronic excess energy intake, causing adipose tissue lipid overload [3]. Adipose tissue exhibits remarkable plasticity, dynamically adjusting its volume through lipid uptake (expansion) or mobilization (contraction) in response to metabolic demands [4]. Under physiological conditions, adipocytes hydrolyze triglycerides and release free fatty acids (FFAs) into the blood for peripheral energy supply [5]. However, sustained energy excess triggers adipose expansion via adipocyte hypertrophy (cell enlargement) and hyperplasia (cell proliferation) to buffer lipid overload [6]. Initially, adipocyte hypertrophy serves as an adaptive mechanism, sequestering excess lipids within adipocytes to prevent systemic lipotoxicity and maintain homeostasis during early weight gain [7]. Beyond critical thresholds, overwhelmed adipocytes exhibit impaired lipid metabolism and chronic low-grade inflammation [7].

Accumulating evidence indicates that elevated abdominal obesity and intermuscular adipose tissue (IMAT) are linked to heightened cardiovascular disease (CVD) risk and adverse outcomes [8, 9]. Notably, increased epicardial adipose tissue (EAT) correlates strongly with hypertension, heart failure, atrial fibrillation (AF), acute coronary syndrome (ACS), and major adverse cardiovascular events [10–12]. Visceral adipose tissue (VAT) in obesity exhibits upregulated NLR family pyrin domain-containing 3 (NLRP3) inflammasome activity alongside elevated monocyte chemoattractant protein-1 (MCP-1), interleukin (IL)-1β, IL-6, and tumor necrosis factor-α (TNF-α) levels compared to lean individuals [13, 14].

Given the critical roles of adipose tissue in CVD etiopathogenesis, this review primarily focuses on elucidating the mechanisms by which adipose tissue drives inflammation and its contributions to CVD, aiming to clarify the interplay between obesity-mediated metabolic inflammation and CVD development.

2. Adipose tissue as a modulator of metabolic inflammation

2.1 Adipocyte-driven inflammatory cascades

In individuals with obesity, vascular rarefaction within adipose tissue and the separation of hypertrophic adipocytes from the capillary network lead to insufficient blood perfusion and the occurrence of hypoxia in adipose depots [15]. Hypoxia activates hypoxia-inducible factor-1α (HIF-1α) signaling, which upregulates pro-inflammatory cytokine (e.g., IL-6, TNF-α) expression while suppressing anti-inflammatory adiponectin biosynthesis [16, 17]. Concurrently, hypertrophic adipocytes enhance basal lipolysis, promoting FFA overflow that triggers uncoupled respiration by activating adenine nucleotide translocase 2 (ANT2) [18, 19]. This metabolic shift elevates oxygen consumption, exacerbating adipocyte hypoxia and amplifying HIF-1α-driven inflammatory cascades. HIF-1α ablation attenuates adipose inflammation, manifesting as reduced pro-inflammatory cytokine expression, diminished macrophage infiltration, and enhanced insulin sensitivity [19]. Furthermore, lipid accumulation in adipocytes disrupts mitochondrial function, increases reactive oxygen species (ROS) production, and induces endoplasmic reticulum (ER) stress, which drives chronic adipose inflammation (**Figure 2**) [20]. ER stress mitigation reduces chronic adipose inflammation and ameliorates weight gain in high-fat diet (HFD)-fed mice [21]. Annexin A1 (ANXA1), an anti-inflammatory mediator, inhibits adipogenesis and pro-inflammatory cytokine secretion through competitively binding PDZ and LIM domain 7 (PDLIM7) and displacing its interaction with MYC-binding protein 2 (MYCBP2) [22].

Adipocyte apoptosis acts as a key driver of metabolic inflammation (**Figure 2**) [23]. Caspase-8 deficiency reduces adipocyte apoptosis and adipose inflammation, attenuates macrophage infiltration and MCP-1 expression, and prevents HFD-induced obesity and glucose intolerance in mice [24]. Necroptosis components also regulate metabolic inflammation. Receptor-interacting protein kinase 1 (RIPK1) inhibition attenuates HFD-induced weight gain and metabolic inflammation [25]. MLKL suppression reduces adipose inflammation and metabolic dysregulation in obese mice [26]. The precise mechanisms linking necroptosis to metabolic inflammation remain unclear.

2.2 Pro-inflammatory signaling in macrophages

Although adipocytes can produce pro-inflammatory mediators, macrophages represent the predominant source of inflammatory factors in adipose tissue [27]. BMI (19.4–60.1 kg/m^2) positively correlates with adipose tissue macrophage (ATM) marker CD68 expression in subcutaneous adipose tissue (SAT) [28]. In obesity, hypoxia, ER stress, and lipotoxicity synergistically induce adipose chemokine production, driving monocyte recruitment [29].

Obese mice exhibit elevated MCP-1 levels compared to lean controls, driving monocyte infiltration into adipose tissue [30]. Bariatric surgery reduces adipose macrophage content and MCP-1 expression [31]. MCP-1 deletion prevents macrophage infiltration in HFD-fed mice, whereas adipocyte-specific MCP-1 overexpression exacerbates macrophage accumulation and TNF-α/IL-6 levels [32, 33]. Leukotriene B4 (LTB4) can mediate monocyte migration. In HFD-fed mice, hypertrophic adipocytes release more LTB4, and circulating CD11b$^+$ monocytes also upregulate BLT1 receptor expression [34, 35]. This chemotactic response is abolished in adipose tissue in BLT1 knockout mice, indicating the critical role of the LTB4/BLT1 axis in metabolic inflammation [35]. Notably, MCP-1 and LTB4 establish a reciprocal activation loop. The elevated expression of MCP-1 is mediated by LTB4 in a BLT1-dependent manner. MCP-1 enhances LTB4 biosynthesis, perpetuating adipose inflammation [36]. Hypertrophic adipocytes release long-chain saturated fatty acids (LCFAs), suppressing proliferator-activated receptor gamma coactivator-1β (PGC-1β) in macrophages. Reduced PGC-1β promotes transforming growth factor-β-activated kinase 1 (TAK1)-TAK1 binding protein 1 (TAB1) complex formation, activating nuclear factor-κB (NF-κB)/JNK pathways to upregulate IL-1β, TNF-α, and MCP-1 [7, 37]. Additionally, LCFAs bind fetuin-A to activate Toll-like receptor 4 (TLR4)-mediated pro-inflammatory signaling (**Figure 1**) [38, 39].

ATMs predominantly exhibit the M2 phenotype in lean individuals, maintaining tissue homeostasis through IL-10 secretion [40, 41]. Hypoxia-induced ROS triggers adipocyte death in hypertrophic adipose tissue, which releases damage-associated molecular patterns (DAMPs) such as ATP and DNA, driving macrophage polarization

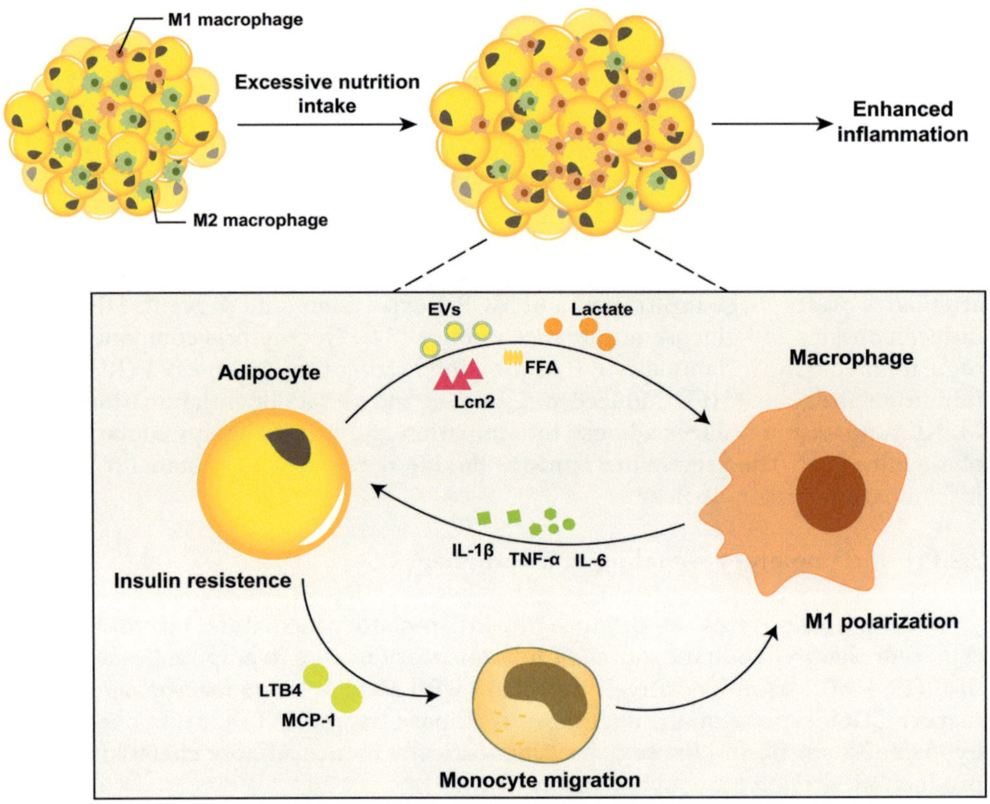

Figure 1.
Adipocyte-macrophage crosstalk drives obesity-associated inflammation through bidirectional metabolic dysregulation. Adipose tissue hypertrophy during obesity enhances the secretion of FFAs, lactate, Lcn2, and microRNA-containing EVs by hypertrophic adipocytes. These adipocyte-derived factors promote M1 macrophage polarization via NF-κB activation, driving the release of pro-inflammatory cytokines (IL-1β, IL-6, TNF-α). Insulin-resistant adipocytes, in turn, exacerbate FFA efflux through impaired insulin signaling, perpetuating macrophage activation and chronic inflammation. Hypertrophic adipocytes further amplify macrophage infiltration by secreting LTB4 and MCP-1, thereby establishing a self-sustaining inflammatory loop.

from the M2 to the M1 phenotype [42, 43]. M1 macrophages secrete pro-inflammatory cytokines (IL-1β, IL-6, TNF-α), exacerbating adipose inflammation and metabolic dysfunction [43]. Inositol-requiring enzyme 1α (IRE1α) regulates the M2–to–M1 macrophage transition in obesity, and macrophage-specific IRE1α deletion inhibits M1 polarization and attenuates HFD-induced weight gain [44].

In obese adipose tissue, over 90% of ATMs surround apoptotic and necrotic adipocytes, forming crown-like structures (CLS), a pathological hallmark of adipose inflammation [45]. Notably, CLS abundance correlates positively with TNF-α levels and adipocyte hypertrophy in SAT/VAT [46]. Expanded adipocytes exceed macrophage efferocytosis capacity (~25 μm) by about five-fold, impeding necrotic adipocyte clearance [47]. These uncleared necrotic cell debris accumulate within adipose tissue, persistently activating pro-inflammatory signaling cascades in obesity [15, 47].

Gut-derived lipopolysaccharide (LPS), translocating from the intestinal lumen into circulation, represents a key contributor to obesity-associated metabolic

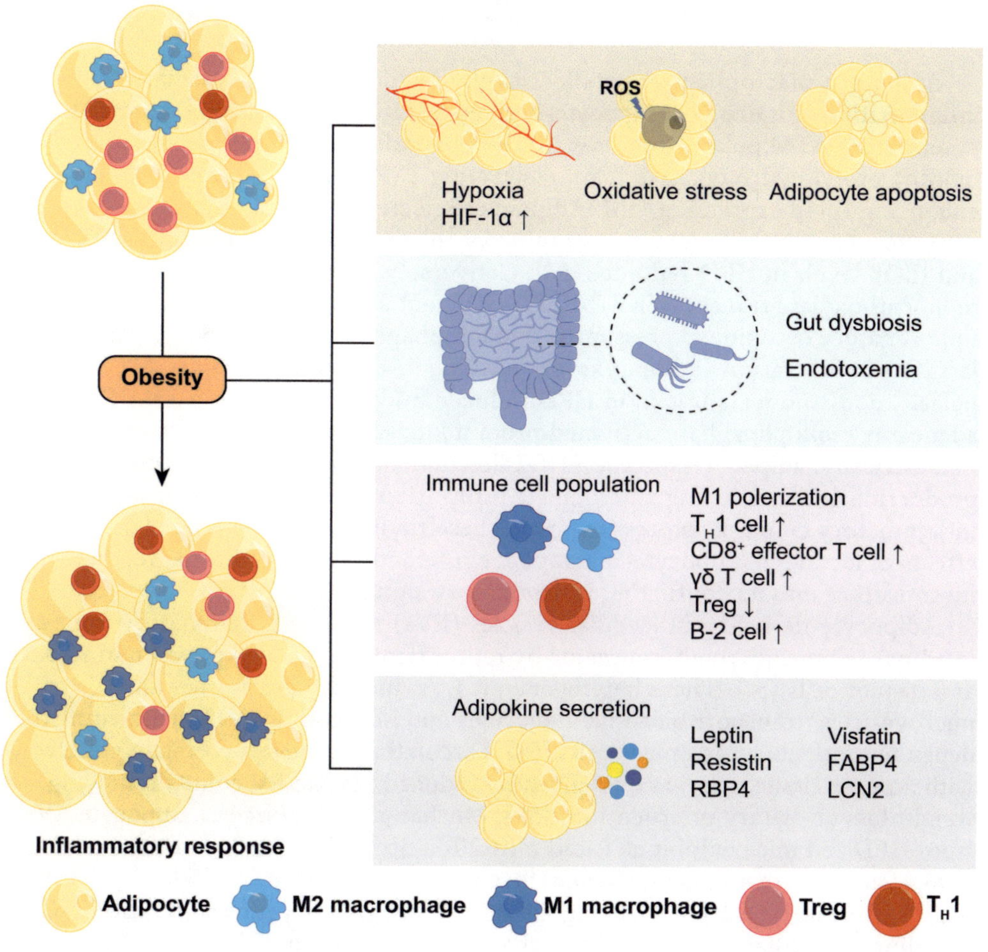

Figure 2.
Cytokines drive metabolic inflammation in obesity. Hypoxia in obese adipose tissue upregulates HIF-1α, driving the release of inflammatory mediators. Concurrently, lipid overload induces mitochondrial dysfunction and oxidative stress, exacerbating adipose inflammation. Adipocyte apoptosis in hypertrophic adipose tissue promotes macrophage recruitment and insulin resistance. Dysbiosis in the gut microbiota, exacerbated by a HFD, disrupts intestinal barrier integrity and facilitates LPS translocation into circulation, triggering systemic and adipose inflammation. Obesity induces adipose immune remodeling characterized by the expansion of M1 macrophages, TH1 cells, $CD8^+$ T cells, γδ T cells, and B cells, alongside the depletion of M2 macrophages and Tregs. Pro-inflammatory adipokines (e.g., leptin, resistin) sustain inflammation via cytokine upregulation and the activation of monocyte adhesion molecules.

inflammation (**Figure 2**) [48]. Obesity-induced gut dysbiosis alters microbial ethanolamine metabolism, and accumulated ethanolamine disrupts intestinal barrier integrity via zonula occludens-1 (ZO-1) degradation, thereby facilitating LPS leakage into the bloodstream and promoting ATM infiltration and M1 polarization [49, 50]. Mono-colonization of germ-free mice with LPS-producing *E. coli* recapitulates adipose inflammation and M1 macrophage activation, whereas immunologically inert *E. coli* MLK1067 fails to induce these responses [51]. Notably, germ-free mice resist HFD-induced adipose inflammation and insulin resistance, underscoring the critical role of LPS in metabolic dysregulation [52].

2.3 Intercellular crosstalk between adipocytes and macrophages

Adipocyte-macrophage crosstalk critically regulates obesity-associated metabolic inflammation (**Figure 1**). Adipocyte-derived lactate acts as a paracrine signal, potentiating ATM polarization toward the pro-inflammatory M1 phenotype by binding prolyl hydroxylase domain-containing 2 (PHD2), stabilizing HIF-1α, and enhancing IL-1β expression [53]. Adipocyte-selective deletion of lactate dehydrogenase A (LDHA) improves glucose tolerance and reduces ATM infiltration and IL-1β levels in HFD-fed mice [53]. Conversely, lactate retention in monocarboxylate transporter 1 (MCT1)-deficient adipocytes exacerbates pro-inflammatory cytokine expression and macrophage chemotaxis [54]. Moderate lactate administration (800 mg/kg/day) attenuates insulin resistance, M1 polarization, and weight gain in HFD-induced mice via protein kinase A (PKA)-adenosine monophosphate-activated protein kinase α1 (AMPKα1) activation [55]. Paradoxically, adipocyte-specific PHD2 deletion enhances glycolysis and lactate production while reducing macrophage infiltration without altering pro-inflammatory cytokine expression [56]. These findings highlight the pleiotropic effects of lactate in adipocyte-macrophage interactions, necessitating further investigation into its conflicting inflammatory signaling pathways.

Adipocyte-derived extracellular vesicles (EVs) regulate inflammatory processes in adipose tissue microenvironments by reprogramming gene expression in adjacent and distant cells [57]. These heterogeneous EVs, including exosomes and microvesicles, transport bioactive molecules and non-coding RNAs with context-dependent effects on recipient cells [58]. Circulating EV levels correlate positively with adipose tissue mass, as evidenced by reduced plasma EV counts following weight loss or dietary interventions [59]. Mechanistically, visceral adipocyte EVs from HFD-fed mice exhibit elevated miR-200a-3p/miR-200b-3p content, driving lipid accumulation and pro-inflammatory cytokine (IL-1β, IL-6, TNF-α) production in 3T3-L1 adipocytes [60]. Blocking the signaling regulatory protein α (SIRPα)-CD47 signaling axis enhances macrophage phagocytosis of adipose-derived EVs, ameliorating HFD-induced adipose inflammation and metabolic dysregulation [60]. Hypertrophic adipocytes release EVs containing miR-155 and miR-34a, which promote M1 macrophage polarization [61, 62].

Monocyte-derived macrophages adopt a pro-inflammatory M1 phenotype upon adipose infiltration, engaging in paracrine crosstalk with adipocytes [63]. Activated ATMs secrete pro-inflammatory cytokines (e.g., TNF-α, IL-1β), disrupting adipocyte insulin signaling and exacerbating insulin resistance in obesity. This creates a vicious cycle in which insulin-resistant adipocytes release more FFAs, further activating ATMs [64]. TNF-α-induced lipocalin 2 (Lcn2) in adipocytes activates macrophage NLRP3 inflammasomes through secondary signaling, and this bidirectional signaling further amplifies cytokine production (TNF-α, IL-1β), forming a self-sustaining adipose inflammation [65, 66]. Such paracrine interactions between adipocytes and macrophages lock adipose tissue in a chronic inflammatory state through chemokine-receptor crosstalk [40].

2.4 Adaptive immune cells in metabolic inflammation

Adipose lymphocytes critically drive metabolic inflammation alongside adipocytes and macrophages (**Figure 2**). $CD4^+$ T cells are broadly categorized into pro-inflammatory (TH1/TH17) and anti-inflammatory (TH2/regulatory T cells (Treg)) subsets. Obesity induces a pronounced immunological shift in adipose tissue, characterized by elevated TH1/TH2 ratios and depleted Treg populations [67, 68]. This Treg loss amplifies macrophage and effector T cell recruitment. Pro-inflammatory changes predominantly occur in VAT, fostering a localized inflammatory microenvironment and systemic metabolic dysregulation [68]. $CD8^+$ effector T cells expand in obese adipose tissue, directly inducing macrophage polarization and migration through paracrine signaling, thereby perpetuating adipose inflammation [67, 69]. $CD8^+$ T cell depletion attenuates adipose inflammation and improves insulin resistance, highlighting their central role in obesity-associated adipose pathology [69]. Additionally, γδ T cell infiltration increases in adipose depots, promoting IL-17-mediated metabolic inflammation in obese mice, and γδ T cell ablation reduces circulating IL-6 levels and ameliorates metabolic dysfunction [70, 71].

Obesity also drives B cell infiltration into VAT, while B cell deficiency attenuates adipocyte hypertrophy and macrophage recruitment [72]. This pro-inflammatory activity requires T cell collaboration. Adoptive transfer of B cells from HFD-conditioned mice into RAG1 deficiency recipients fails to induce glucose intolerance, establishing a T-cell-dependent pathway for B cell-mediated metabolic dysregulation [73].

2.5 Adipokine-induced pathogenesis of metabolic inflammation

Adipose-derived adipokines regulate metabolic inflammation by modulating immune responses and metabolic pathways, driving obesity-associated metabolic dysfunction and CVD development (**Figure 2**) [27]. Leptin shows elevated plasma levels during obesity. Inhibition of leptin signaling prevents weight gain in murine obesity models, underscoring its role in early pathogenesis [74, 75]. In preadipocytes, leptin enhances adipogenesis via upregulation of peroxisome proliferator-activated receptor γ (PPARγ) and sterol regulatory element-binding protein-1 (SREBP1c), while simultaneously stimulating pro-inflammatory cytokine (IL-1β, IL-6, TNF-α) production, establishing dual roles in adipose remodeling and inflammatory activation [76].

Visfatin, another adipokine implicated in metabolic inflammation, exhibits increased plasma levels in obesity [77, 78]. Bariatric surgery-induced weight loss reduces visfatin expression in SAT [79]. Mechanistically, visfatin activates NF-κB and p38 mitogen-activated protein kinase (MAPK) pathways to promote TNF-α, IL-1β, and IL-6 synthesis, exacerbating adipose inflammation [80].

Resistin, upregulated in the plasma of HFD-fed mice, enhances intercellular adhesion molecule-1 (ICAM-1) and vascular cell adhesion molecule-1 (VCAM-1) expression in vascular endothelium, promoting monocyte-endothelial interactions and atherosclerosis in apolipoprotein E (ApoE) knockout mice [81, 82].

Additional adipokines, including chemerin, fatty acid-binding protein 4 (FABP4), retinol-binding protein 4 (RBP4), and LCN2, further amplify metabolic inflammation by upregulating adhesion molecule expression and monocyte recruitment [83]. Collectively, these adipokines bridge adipose dysfunction and systemic metabolic inflammation.

3. Adipose-metabolic inflammation and CVD

3.1 Atherosclerosis

It has been reported that adipose tissue inflammation induces the development of CVD like atherosclerosis, hypertension, heart failure and atrial fibrillation (**Figure 3**).

Adipose tissue dysfunction drives atherosclerosis through inflammatory dysregulation. EAT exhibits volume-dependent inflammatory activity, where expanded EAT mass is correlated with local cytokine overexpression (TNF-α, IL-6) and coronary plaque burden in patients with atherosclerotic cardiovascular disease (ASCVD) [84]. Perivascular adipose tissue (PVAT) transplantation reveals that obese-derived PVAT grafts into low-density lipoprotein receptor (LDLR) knockout mice exacerbate atherosclerosis via MCP-1/TNF-α upregulation and adiponectin suppression [85]. MCP-1-deficient PVAT fails to induce neointimal hyperplasia in LDLR knockout mice, confirming its chemokine dependency [86]. Senescent VAT transplantation accelerates carotid plaque progression with local macrophage infiltration in young LDLR-deficient mice [87]. Mechanistically, aged adipocyte-derived TNF-α, C–X–C motif chemokine ligand 2 (CXCL2), and MCP-1 synergistically recruit monocytes to perivascular niches, amplifying vascular inflammation, and neutralizing these chemokines effectively attenuates atherogenesis [87].

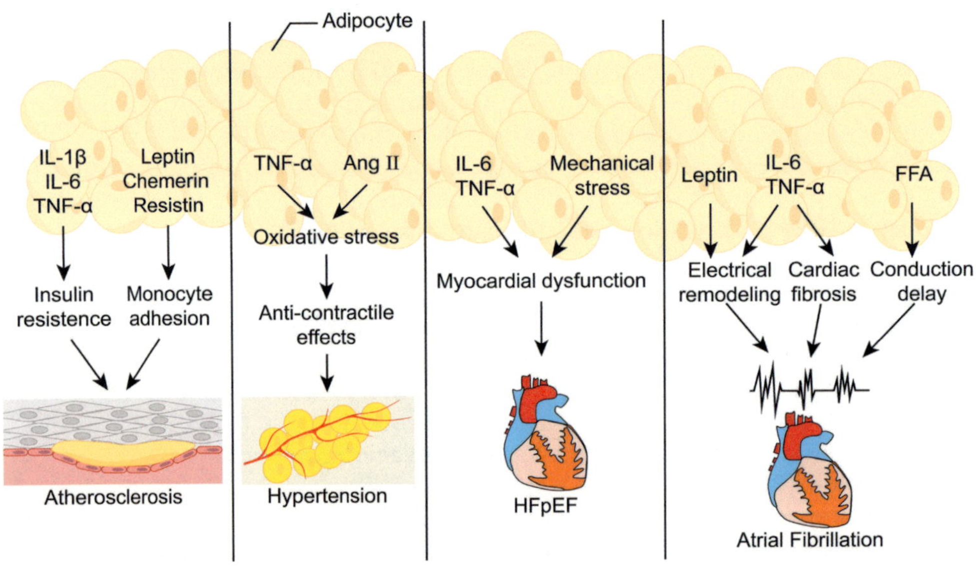

Figure 3.
Adipose tissue dysfunction plays a crucial role in the pathogenesis of cardiovascular disease (CVD). Adipose tissue dysfunction in obesity promotes CVD pathogenesis through pro-inflammatory cytokine secretion and metabolic dysregulation. Cytokine-driven monocyte adhesion and insulin resistance further accelerate atherogenesis. TNF-α and Ang II from adipose tissue exacerbate oxidative stress, impair vasodilation, and promote hypertension. Mechanical adipose expansion and IL-6/TNF-α synergistically induce myocardial dysfunction, contributing to HFpEF pathogenesis. EAT-derived IL-6/TNF-α triggers fibrosis and electrical remodeling in AF, while FFAs disrupt conduction. Leptin further alters cardiac ion dynamics, exacerbating arrhythmogenesis.

Cytokines critically accelerate atherosclerosis by inducing vascular dysfunction. TNF-α activates NF-κB and PPARγ signaling pathways in ApoE knockout mice, upregulating endothelial transcytosis proteins (e.g., caveolin-1) to enhance LDL retention and atherogenesis [88]. This process is exacerbated by TNF-α-mediated overexpression of ICAM-1 and VCAM-1, which promotes monocyte adhesion and upregulates pro-inflammatory interleukins and NADPH oxidase (NOX), forming coordinated effects for early atherogenesis [89]. IL-1β-driven insulin resistance contributes to collagen synthesis, LDL retention, and inflammatory cascades, accelerating atherosclerotic plaque progression [90, 91]. Canakinumab trials validate IL-1β as a therapeutic target for ASCVD [92]. IL-1β production relies on NLRP3 inflammasome activation, and its inhibition reduces pro-inflammatory gene expression, plaque macrophage infiltration, and necrotic core size in ApoE knockout mice [93]. Similarly, IL-6 exacerbates endothelial dysfunction and via mitochondrial dysfunction and ROS overproduction [94]. Ziltivekimab trials demonstrate that IL-6 blockade effectively lowers inflammatory biomarkers, highlighting its therapeutic potential for atherosclerosis [95].

In addition, pro-inflammatory adipokines (e.g., leptin, chemerin, FABP4, and resistin) also amplify atherogenesis by upregulating MCP-1 and adhesion molecule expression, as well as facilitating monocyte-endothelial interactions [83].

3.2 Hypertension

Obesity-induced metabolic inflammation disrupts vascular homeostasis through adipose tissue-derived cytokine dysregulation. Adipose tissue expansion correlates with progressive vascular dysfunction, characterized by impaired vasodilation and the development of hypertension. Administration of TNF-α and IL-6 to PVAT induces vasoconstriction in healthy vessels, while TNF-α blockade reverses obesity-associated ROS accumulation and restores PVAT-dependent vasodilation in HFD-induced mice [96, 97]. Mechanistically, TNF-α enhances ROS generation via NOX activation and reduces nitric oxide (NO) production through endothelial NO synthase (eNOS) inhibition in obese rat aortas [98]. Beyond oxidative stress, adipose immune cell remodeling also emerges as a key contributor to hypertension pathogenesis. In Dahl salt-sensitive rats with HFD, PVAT displays early macrophage and $CD4^+$ memory T cell infiltration prior to the onset of hypertension [99].

PVAT synthesizes key angiotensin components, including angiotensinogen, angiotensin II (Ang II), and angiotensin 1–7, which coordinately regulate vascular tone [100, 101]. Obesity causes dysregulation of these components. Angiotensinogen expression is consistently upregulated in adipose tissue in both obese humans and murine models [102]. HFD-induced transcriptional activation of angiotensinogen is reversed following weight loss [103]. Ang II exacerbates endothelial dysfunction through angiotensin type 1 receptor (AT1R)-mediated ROS overproduction, eNOS suppression, and NO reduction [104]. Concurrently, Ang II stimulates vasoconstrictor production, such as endothelin-1 (ET-1) and cyclooxygenase-1 (COX-1)-derived prostanoids, amplifying oxidative stress and vascular remodeling [105].

3.3 Heart failure

SAT serves as the primary lipid reservoir under physiological conditions, storing excess lipids to prevent ectopic lipid deposition in metabolically active peripheral organs such as the liver, heart, and skeletal muscle [106]. However, when SAT storage capacity is overwhelmed, excess lipids redistribute to ectopic depots, driving pathological outcomes [107]. Emerging evidence demonstrates that ectopic adiposity, particularly in heart failure with preserved ejection fraction (HFpEF), exacerbates myocardial dysfunction via lipotoxicity, inflammatory cytokine secretion, and fibrotic remodeling, ultimately contributing to adverse clinical outcomes [108, 109].

EAT anatomically resides between the myocardium and visceral pericardium, establishing bidirectional crosstalk with the heart through mechanical interactions and paracrine signaling to modulate cardiac structure and function [110]. EAT expansion directly compresses biventricular chambers, increasing cardiac workload and inducing left ventricular hypertrophy [111]. Compounded by the low-compliant pericardium, this mechanical constraint exacerbates myocardial stiffness and diastolic dysfunction, leading to elevated ventricular filling pressures and hemodynamic alterations mimicking constrictive pericarditis [112]. Elevated right atrial pressure (a surrogate for pericardial pressure) in patients with obesity and HFpEF further supports pericardial restraint mechanisms [113]. Notably, the square root sign in right ventricular pressure waveforms, a marker of pericardial constraint, correlates with both EAT volume and mean right atrial pressure in HFpEF, establishing a clinical nexus between epicardial adiposity and pericardial dysfunction [114]. In obesity, the shared coronary microcirculation and absence of fascial separation between EAT and myocardium facilitate lipid infiltration from expanded EAT depots into cardiac tissue, driving cardiomyocyte disorganization, functional impairment, and apoptosis [84, 115]. Clinical evidence further demonstrates that increased EAT volume independently associates with myocardial lipid accumulation, interstitial fibrosis, and contractile dysfunction in healthy populations [116].

Pathologically expanded EAT in obesity exhibits a pro-inflammatory phenotype, characterized by the upregulation of inflammatory mediators (e.g., TNF-α, IL-6), which induce myocardial disarray, fibrosis, and stiffness [10, 117, 118]. TNF-α and IL-6 synergistically impair cardiomyocyte calcium handling, contributing to diastolic dysfunction [119]. TNF-α drives cardiomyocyte apoptosis through dual TNFR1/TNFR2 receptor signaling [120, 121]. IL-6 promotes fibrotic remodeling via the upregulation of fibronectin and type I collagen in cardiac fibroblasts [122]. Chronic cytokine exposure activates endothelial NOX, triggering ROS-mediated NO depletion [123]. NO deficiency disrupts the cyclic guanosine monophosphate (cGMP)-protein kinase G (PKG) pathway, exacerbating maladaptive cardiomyocyte hypertrophy in HFpEF patients [118, 124].

3.4 Atrial fibrillation

Obesity independently increases AF risk, with BMI, waist circumference, and total fat mass correlating with 10-year AF incidence [125, 126]. AF patients exhibit elevated EAT cytokine secretion (e.g., TNF-α, IL-6) compared to non-AF controls [127]. 18-fluorodeoxyglucose-positron emission tomography/computerized tomography (18 F-FDG PET/CT) imaging reveals heightened EAT tracer uptake in AF patients, reflecting enhanced local inflammatory activity [128]. HIF-1α-mediated upregulation of pro-inflammatory cytokines (IL-6, TNF-α) drives atrial electrical remodeling, increasing arrhythmia susceptibility [129]. TNF-α disrupts pulmonary vein cardiomyocyte calcium handling via sarco/ER calcium ATPase 2 (SERCA2) downregulation, promoting delayed afterdepolarizations [130, 131].

Cardiac-specific TNF-α overexpression reduces connexin 40 expression and induces connexin 43 mislocalization, impairing atrial conduction velocity [132]. IL-6 exacerbates electrophysiological dysfunction by increasing calcium current and reducing SERCA2 expression [129]. An in vitro study demonstrates that IL-6 downregulates connexin 40/43 expression in HL-1 cardiomyocytes, suggesting its dynamic gap junction regulation [133]. Adipocyte-derived leptin activates sympathetic neurons to enhance neuropeptide Y (NPY) secretion, potentiating electrophysiological instability by increasing Na^+/Ca^{2+} exchanger activity and calcium/calmodulin-dependent protein kinase II (CaMKII) overactivity [134].

EAT demonstrates a stronger association with AF incidence than waist circumference or waist/hip ratio [135]. Patients with AF exhibit increased EAT volume, and higher EAT burden correlates with elevated post-ablation recurrence rates [136]. Atrial fibrosis acts as a critical driver of AF pathogenesis through dual mechanisms: slowing atrial conduction velocity and promoting structural remodeling [129]. Increased EAT volume, combined with cytokine secretion, drives cardiac fibrosis, impairs myocardial conduction velocity, and disrupts intermyocyte electromechanical coupling, establishing a substrate for arrhythmogenesis [137, 138]. Surgical left atrial appendage specimens reveal that EAT fibrotic burden and local inflammatory markers (IL-6, TNF-α) positively correlate with atrial fibrosis severity, constituting the structural substrate for AF pathogenesis [139]. Furthermore, EAT from individuals with obesity secretes pro-inflammatory cytokines and fibrosis factors that shorten action potential duration and induce conduction disturbances in cardiomyocytes [140, 141].

EAT-derived FFAs infiltrate the myocardium, inducing atrial electromechanical remodeling characterized by conduction slowing, intercellular junction disruption, and myocyte disarray, which collectively precipitate conduction delays [142]. Activation of glucagon-like peptide-1 (GLP-1) receptors in EAT enhances fatty acid oxidation, suggesting a potential antiarrhythmic mechanism through ectopic fat reduction [143].

4. Conclusion

Obesity has been established as an independent risk factor for CVD. Hypertrophic adipose tissue serves as a primary source of metabolic inflammation, driven by adipocyte-immune cell crosstalk that perpetuates chronic inflammatory cascades, ultimately leading to cardiomyocyte injury, endothelial dysfunction, and CVD progression [144]. As such, comprehensive weight management strategies remain critical therapeutic interventions to mitigate CVD advancement, with targeted attenuation of obesity-associated metabolic inflammation offering potential to delay or prevent CVD onset.

Appendices and nomenclature

18 F-FDG PET/CT	18-fluorodeoxyglucose-positron emission tomography/computed tomography
ACS	Acute coronary syndrome
AF	Atrial fibrillation
AMPKα1	Adenosine monophosphate-activated protein kinase α1
Ang II	Angiotensin II

ANXA1	Annexin A1
ApoE	Apolipoprotein E
ASCVD	atherosclerotic cardiovascular disease
ET-1	Endothelin-1
AT1R	Angiotensin type 1 receptor
ATM	Adipose tissue macrophage
BLT1	Leukotriene B4 receptor 1
BMI	Body mass index
BMP4	Bone morphogenetic protein 4
cGMP	Cyclic guanosine monophosphate
CLS	Crown-like structures
COX-1	Cycloxygenase-1
CVD	Cardiovascular disease
CXCL2	C-X-C motif chemokine ligand 2
DAMPs	Damage associated molecular patterns
EAT	Epicardial adipose tissue
eNOS	Endothelial NO synthase
ER	Endoplasmic reticulum
EVs	Extracellular vesicles
FABP4	Fatty acid-binding protein 4
FFA	Free fatty acid
GLP-1	Glucagon-like peptide 1
HFD	High-fat diet
HFpEF	Heart failure with preserved ejection fraction
HIF-1α	Hypoxia inducible factor-1α
HUVECs	Human umbilical vein endothelial cells
ICAM-1	Intercellular adhesion molecule-1
IL	Interleukin
IRE1α	Inositol-requiring enzyme 1α
JNK	c-Jun N-terminal kinase
LCFAs	long-chain saturated fatty acids
LCN2	Lipocalin 2
LDL	Low-density lipoprotein
LDLR	Low-density lipoprotein receptor
LPS	Lipopolysaccharide
LTB4	Leukotriene B4
MCP-1	Monocyte chemoattractant protein-1
MCT1	monocarboxylate transporter 1
MEK1	Mitogen-activated protein kinase kinase 1
MLKL	Mixed lineage kinase domain-like protein
MYCBP2	MYC binding protein 2
NF-κB	Nuclear factor-κB
NLRP3	NOD-like receptor thermal protein domain associated protein 3
NO	Nitric oxide
NOX	NADPH oxidase
PDLIM7	PDZ and LIM domain 7
PGC-1β	Proliferator-activated receptor gamma coactivator-1β
PHD2	Prolyl hydroxylase domain-containing 2

PKA	Protein kinase A
PKG	Protein kinase G
PPARγ	Peroxisome proliferator-activated receptor γ
PVAT	Perivascular adipose tissue
RBP4	Retinol-binding protein 4
RIPK1	Receptor-interacting protein kinase 1
ROS	Reactive oxygen species
SAT	Subcutaneous adipose tissue
SERCA2	Sarco/endoplasmic reticulum calcium ATPase 2
SIRPα	Signaling regulatory protein α
SREBP1c	Sterol regulatory element-binding protein-1
TAB1	TAK1 binding protein 1
TAK1	Transforming growth factor-β-activated kinase 1
TLR4	Toll-like receptor 4
TNF-α	Tumor necrosis factor-α
Treg	Regulatory T cells
VAT	Visceral adipose tissue
VCAM-1	Vascular cell adhesion molecule
ZO-1	Zonula occludens-1

Acknowledgments

This project was supported by Grant 32171174 from the National Natural Science Foundation of China; by Grants 2023A03J0531 and 2024A03J0658 from the Joint Funds of the Guangzhou Science and Technology Project.

Conflict of interest

The author declares no conflicts of interest.

Author details

Jiafu Ouyang[1#], Wen Lu[2#], Yubing Fan[3], Zhishan Jiang[4], Qian Du[5*] and Donghui Liu[1,2*]

1 Department of Geriatrics, Guangzhou First People's Hospital, School of Medicine, South China University of Technology, Guangzhou, China

2 Department of Cardiology, Ziyun County People's Hospital, Anshun, China

3 Department of General Practice, Guangzhou First People's Hospital, School of Medicine, South China University of Technology, Guangzhou, China

4 Department of Clinical Nutrition, Guangzhou First People's Hospital, School of Medicine, South China University of Technology, Guangzhou, China

5 Department of Cardiology, Guangzhou Red Cross Hospital, Medical College of Jinan University, Guangzhou, China

[#] J.O. and W.L. contributed equally to this work.

*Address all correspondence to: eyliudh@scut.edu.cn and duqian1213@126.com.

References

[1] Ahmed B, Konje JC. The epidemiology of obesity in reproduction. Best Practice and Research: Clinical Obstetrics and Gynaecology. 2023;**89**:102342

[2] Collaborators GBDAB. Global, regional, and national prevalence of adult overweight and obesity, 1990-2021, with forecasts to 2050: A forecasting study for the global burden of disease study 2021. Lancet. 2025;**405** (10481):813–838

[3] Bakinowska E, Krompiewski M, Boboryko D, Kielbowski K, Pawlik A. The role of inflammatory mediators in the pathogenesis of obesity. Nutrients. 2024;**16**(17):2822

[4] Kajimura S, Spiegelman BM, Seale P.Brown and Beige fat: Physiological roles beyond heat generation. Cell Metabolism. 2015;**22**(4):546–559

[5] Wang W, Seale P.Control of brown and beige fat development. Nature Reviews Molecular Cell Biology. 2016;**17** (11):691–702

[6] McLaughlin T, Craig C, Liu LF, Perelman D, Allister C, Spielman D, et al. Adipose cell size and regional fat deposition as predictors of metabolic response to overfeeding in insulin-resistant and insulin-sensitive humans. Diabetes 2016;**65**:1245–1254

[7] Zhang YX, Ou MY, Yang ZH, Sun Y, Li QF, Zhou SB. Adipose tissue aging is regulated by an altered immune system. Frontiers in Immunology. 2023;**14**:1125395

[8] Liu L, Peng J, Zang D, Zhang Y, Wu Z, Song C, et al. The Chinese visceral adiposity index: A novel indicator more closely related to cardiovascular disease than other abdominal obesity indices among postmenopausal women. Journal of Translational Medicine 2024;**22**:855

[9] Souza A, Troschel AS, Marquardt JP, Hadzic I, Foldyna B, Moura FA, et al. Skeletal muscle adiposity, coronary microvascular dysfunction, and adverse cardiovascular outcomes. European Heart Journal. 2025;**46**:1112–1123

[10] Rafeh R, Viveiros A, Oudit GY, El-Yazbi AF.Targeting perivascular and epicardial adipose tissue inflammation: Therapeutic opportunities for cardiovascular disease. Clinical Science. 2020;**134**(7):827–851

[11] Valenzuela PL, Carrera-Bastos P, Castillo-Garcia A, Lieberman DE, Santos-Lozano A, Lucia A.Obesity and the risk of cardiometabolic diseases. Nature Reviews Cardiology. 2023;**20** (7):475–494

[12] Yang C, Deng C, Xia J, Wang S, Zhang L, Liu Z, et al. Peri-coronary adipose tissue attenuation and its association with plaque vulnerability and clinical outcomes in coronary artery disease using combined CCTA and OCT. Scientific Reports. 2025;**15**(1):16520

[13] Unamuno X, Gomez-Ambrosi J, Ramirez B, Rodriguez A, Becerril S, Valenti V, et al. NLRP3 inflammasome blockade reduces adipose tissue inflammation and extracellular matrix remodeling. Cellular and Molecular Immunology 2021;**18**:1045–1057

[14] Ye RZ, Richard G, Gevry N, Tchernof A, Carpentier AC.Fat cell size: Measurement methods,

pathophysiological origins, and relationships with metabolic dysregulations. Endocrine Reviews. 2022;**43**(1):35–60

[15] AlZaim I, de Rooij L, Sheikh BN, Borgeson E, Kalucka J.The evolving functions of the vasculature in regulating adipose tissue biology in health and obesity. Nature Reviews Endocrinology. 2023;**19**(12):691–707

[16] Todorcevic M, Manuel AR, Austen L, Michailidou Z, Hazlehurst JM, Neville M, et al. Markers of adipose tissue hypoxia are elevated in subcutaneous adipose tissue of severely obese patients with obesity hypoventilation syndrome but not in the moderately obese. International Journal of Obesity. 2021;**45**:1618–1622

[17] Agabiti-Rosei C, Saxton SN, De Ciuceis C, Lorenza Muiesan M, Rizzoni D, Agabiti Rosei E, et al. Influence of perivascular adipose tissue on microcirculation: A link between hypertension and obesity. Hypertension 2024;**81**:24–33

[18] Wueest S, Rapold RA, Rytka JM, Schoenle EJ, Konrad D.Basal lipolysis, not the degree of insulin resistance, differentiates large from small isolated adipocytes in high-fat fed mice. Diabetologia. 2009;**52**(3):541–546

[19] Lee YS, Kim JW, Osborne O, Oh DY, Sasik R, Schenk S, et al. Increased adipocyte O2 consumption triggers HIF-1alpha, causing inflammation and insulin resistance in obesity. Cell 2014;**157**:1339–1352

[20] Bays HE, Kirkpatrick CF, Maki KC, Toth PP, Morgan RT, Tondt J, et al. Obesity, dyslipidemia, and cardiovascular disease: A joint expert review from the obesity medicine association and the national lipid association. Journal of Clinical Lipidology 2024;**18**:e320–e50

[21] Kawasaki N, Asada R, Saito A, Kanemoto S, Imaizumi K. Obesity-induced endoplasmic reticulum stress causes chronic inflammation in adipose tissue. Scientific Reports. 2012;**2**:799

[22] Fang L, Liu C, Jiang ZZ, Wang M, Geng K, Xu Y, et al. Annexin A1 binds PDZ and LIM domain 7 to inhibit adipogenesis and prevent obesity. Signal Transduction and Targeted Therapy. 2024;**9**:218

[23] Hildebrandt X, Ibrahim M, Peltzer N.Cell death and inflammation during obesity: "Know my methods, WAT (son)". Cell Death and Differentiation. 2023;**30**(2):279–292

[24] Luk CT, Chan CK, Chiu F, Shi SY, Misra PS, Li YZ, et al. Dual role of caspase 8 in adipocyte apoptosis and metabolic inflammation. Diabetes 2023;**72**:1751–1765

[25] Karunakaran D, Turner AW, Duchez AC, Soubeyrand S, Rasheed A, Smyth D, et al. RIPK1 gene variants associate with obesity in humans and can be therapeutically silenced to reduce obesity in mice. Nature Metabolism 2020;**2**:1113–1125

[26] Saeed WK, Jun DW, Jang K, Oh JH, Chae YJ, Lee JS, et al. Decrease in fat de novo synthesis and chemokine ligand expression in non-alcoholic fatty liver disease caused by inhibition of mixed lineage kinase domain-like pseudokinase. Journal of Gastroenterology and Hepatology 2019;**34**:2206–2218

[27] Tilg H, Ianiro G, Gasbarrini A, Adolph TE.Adipokines: Masterminds of

metabolic inflammation. Nature Reviews Immunology. 2025;**25**(4):250–265

[28] Weisberg SP, McCann D, Desai M, Rosenbaum M, Leibel RL, Ferrante Jr AW.Obesity is associated with macrophage accumulation in adipose tissue. Journal of Clinical Investigation. 2003;**112**(12):1796–1808

[29] Antuna-Puente B, Fellahi S, McAvoy C, Feve B, Bastard JP. Interleukins in adipose tissue: Keeping the balance. Molecular and Cellular Endocrinology. 2022;**542**:111531

[30] Kawanishi N, Mizokami T, Yano H, Suzuki K.Exercise attenuates M1 macrophages and CD8+ T cells in the adipose tissue of obese mice. Medicine and Science in Sports and Exercise. 2013;**45**(9):1684–1693

[31] Cancello R, Henegar C, Viguerie N, Taleb S, Poitou C, Rouault C, et al. Reduction of macrophage infiltration and chemoattractant gene expression changes in white adipose tissue of morbidly obese subjects after surgery-induced weight loss. Diabetes 2005;**54**:2277–2286

[32] Kanda H, Tateya S, Tamori Y, Kotani K, Hiasa K, Kitazawa R, et al. MCP-1 contributes to macrophage infiltration into adipose tissue, insulin resistance, and hepatic steatosis in obesity. Journal of Clinical Investigation 2006;**116**:1494–1505

[33] Kamei N, Tobe K, Suzuki R, Ohsugi M, Watanabe T, Kubota N, et al. Overexpression of monocyte chemoattractant protein-1 in adipose tissues causes macrophage recruitment and insulin resistance. Journal of Biological Chemistry 2006;**281**:26602–26614

[34] Ying W, Wollam J, Ofrecio JM, Bandyopadhyay G, El Ouarrat D, Lee YS, et al. Adipose tissue B2 cells promote insulin resistance through leukotriene LTB4/LTB4R1 signaling. Journal of Clinical Investigation 2017;**127**:1019–1030

[35] Spite M, Hellmann J, Tang Y, Mathis SP, Kosuri M, Bhatnagar A, et al. Deficiency of the leukotriene B4 receptor, BLT-1, protects against systemic insulin resistance in diet-induced obesity. The Journal of Immunology 2011;**187**:1942–1949

[36] Bahrami P, Aromolaran KA, Aromolaran AS. Proarrhythmic lipid inflammatory mediators: Mechanisms in obesity arrhythmias. Journal of Cellular Physiology. 2025;**240**(2):e70012

[37] Chen H, Liu Y, Li D, Song J, Xia M. PGC-1beta suppresses saturated fatty acid-induced macrophage inflammation by inhibiting TAK1 activation. IUBMB Life. 2016;**68**(2):145–155

[38] Pal D, Dasgupta S, Kundu R, Maitra S, Das G, Mukhopadhyay S, et al. Fetuin-A acts as an endogenous ligand of TLR4 to promote lipid-induced insulin resistance. Nature Medicine 2012;**18**:1279–1285

[39] Erridge C, Samani NJ. Saturated fatty acids do not directly stimulate Toll-like receptor signaling. Arteriosclerosis, Thrombosis, and Vascular Biology. 2009;**29**(11):1944–1949

[40] Yao J, Wu D, Qiu Y. Adipose tissue macrophage in obesity-associated metabolic diseases. Frontiers in Immunology. 2022;**13**:977485

[41] Castoldi A, Naffah de Souza C, Camara NO, Moraes-Vieira PM. The

macrophage switch in obesity development. Frontiers in Immunology. 2015;**6**:637

[42] Calderon-DuPont D, Torre-Villalvazo I, Diaz-Villasenor A. Is insulin resistance tissue-dependent and substrate-specific? The role of white adipose tissue and skeletal muscle. Biochimie. 2023;**204**:48–68

[43] Lumeng CN, Bodzin JL, Saltiel AR. Obesity induces a phenotypic switch in adipose tissue macrophage polarization. Journal of Clinical Investigation. 2007;**117**(1):175–184

[44] Shan B, Wang X, Wu Y, Xu C, Xia Z, Dai J, et al. The metabolic ER stress sensor IRE1alpha suppresses alternative activation of macrophages and impairs energy expenditure in obesity. Nature Immunology 2017;**18**:519–529

[45] Haase J, Weyer U, Immig K, Kloting N, Bluher M, Eilers J, et al. Local proliferation of macrophages in adipose tissue during obesity-induced inflammation. Diabetologia 2014;**57**:562–571

[46] Cinti S, Mitchell G, Barbatelli G, Murano I, Ceresi E, Faloia E, et al. Adipocyte death defines macrophage localization and function in adipose tissue of obese mice and humans. Journal of Lipid Research. 2005;**46**:2347–2355

[47] Lindhorst A, Raulien N, Wieghofer P, Eilers J, Rossi FMV, Bechmann I, et al. Adipocyte death triggers a pro-inflammatory response and induces metabolic activation of resident macrophages. Cell Death and Disease. 2021;**12**:579

[48] Sotak M, Clark M, Suur BE, Borgeson E.Inflammation and resolution in obesity. Nature Reviews Endocrinology. 2025;**21**(1):45–61

[49] Mishra SP, Wang B, Jain S, Ding J, Rejeski J, Furdui CM, et al. A mechanism by which gut microbiota elevates permeability and inflammation in obese/diabetic mice and human gut. Gut 2023;**72**:1848–1865

[50] Violi F, Cammisotto V, Bartimoccia S, Pignatelli P, Carnevale R, Nocella C.Gut-derived low-grade endotoxaemia, atherothrombosis and cardiovascular disease. Nature Reviews Cardiology. 2023;**20**(1):24–37

[51] Caesar R, Reigstad CS, Backhed HK, Reinhardt C, Ketonen M, Lunden GO, et al. Gut-derived lipopolysaccharide augments adipose macrophage accumulation but is not essential for impaired glucose or insulin tolerance in mice. Gut 2012;**61**:1701–1707

[52] Cani PD, Van Hul M.Gut microbiota in overweight and obesity: Crosstalk with adipose tissue. Nature Reviews Gastroenterology and Hepatology. 2024;**21**(3):164–183

[53] Feng T, Zhao X, Gu P, Yang W, Wang C, Guo Q, et al. Adipocyte-derived lactate is a signalling metabolite that potentiates adipose macrophage inflammation via targeting PHD2. Nature Communications 2022;**13**:5208

[54] Lin Y, Bai M, Wang S, Chen L, Li Z, Li C, et al. Lactate is a key mediator that links obesity to insulin resistance via modulating cytokine production from adipose tissue. Diabetes 2022;**71**: 637–652

[55] Cai H, Wang X, Zhang Z, Chen J, Wang F, Wang L, et al. Moderate l-lactate administration suppresses

adipose tissue macrophage M1 polarization to alleviate obesity-associated insulin resistance. Journal of Biological Chemistry. 2022;**298**(4):101768

[56] Matsuura H, Ichiki T, Inoue E, Nomura M, Miyazaki R, Hashimoto T, et al. Prolyl hydroxylase domain protein 2 plays a critical role in diet-induced obesity and glucose intolerance. Circulation 2013;**127**:2078–2087

[57] Thomou T, Mori MA, Dreyfuss JM, Konishi M, Sakaguchi M, Wolfrum C, et al. Adipose-derived circulating miRNAs regulate gene expression in other tissues. Nature 2017;**542**:450–455

[58] Thery C, Witwer KW, Aikawa E, Alcaraz MJ, Anderson JD, Andriantsitohaina R, et al. Minimal information for studies of extracellular vesicles 2018 (MISEV2018): A position statement of the International Society for Extracellular Vesicles and update of the MISEV2014 guidelines. Journal of Extracellular Vesicles. 2018;7(1): 1535750

[59] Shaikh SR, Beck MA, Alwarawrah Y, MacIver NJ.Emerging mechanisms of obesity-associated immune dysfunction. Nature Reviews Endocrinology. 2024;**20**(3):136–148

[60] Lin YK, Pan YF, Jiang TY, Chen YB, Shang TY, Xu MY, et al. Blocking the SIRPalpha-CD47 axis promotes macrophage phagocytosis of exosomes derived from visceral adipose tissue and improves inflammation and metabolism in mice. Journal of Biomedical Science 2025;**32**:31

[61] Zhang Y, Mei H, Chang X, Chen F, Zhu Y, Han X.Adipocyte-derived microvesicles from obese mice induce M1 macrophage phenotype through secreted miR-155. Journal of Molecular Cell Biology. 2016;**8**(6):505–517

[62] Pan Y, Hui X, Hoo RLC, Ye D, Chan CYC, Feng T, et al. Adipocyte-secreted exosomal microRNA-34a inhibits M2 macrophage polarization to promote obesity-induced adipose inflammation. Journal of Clinical Investigation 2019;**129**:834–849

[63] Liu Y, Lu X, Li X, Du P, Qin G. High-fat diet triggers obesity-related early infiltration of macrophages into adipose tissue and transient reduction of blood monocyte count. Molecular Immunology. 2020;**117**:139–146

[64] Li X, Ren Y, Chang K, Wu W, Griffiths HR, Lu S, et al. Adipose tissue macrophages as potential targets for obesity and metabolic diseases. Frontiers in Immunology. 2023;**14**:1153915

[65] Javaid HMA, Ko E, Joo EJ, Kwon SH, Park JH, Shin S, et al. TNFalpha-induced NLRP3 inflammasome mediates adipocyte dysfunction and activates macrophages through adipocyte-derived lipocalin 2. Metabolism. 2023;**142**:155527

[66] Suganami T, Nishida J, Ogawa Y.A paracrine loop between adipocytes and macrophages aggravates inflammatory changes: Role of free fatty acids and tumor necrosis factor alpha. Arteriosclerosis, Thrombosis, and Vascular Biology. 2005;**25**(10): 2062–2068

[67] Strissel KJ, DeFuria J, Shaul ME, Bennett G, Greenberg AS, Obin MS.T-cell recruitment and Th1 polarization in adipose tissue during diet-induced obesity in C57BL/6 mice. Obesity (Silver Spring). 2010; **18**(10):1918–1925

[68] Feuerer M, Herrero L, Cipolletta D, Naaz A, Wong J, Nayer A, et al. Lean, but not obese, fat is enriched for a unique population of regulatory T cells that affect metabolic parameters. Nature Medicine 2009;**15**:930–939

[69] Nishimura S, Manabe I, Nagasaki M, Eto K, Yamashita H, Ohsugi M, et al. CD8+ effector T cells contribute to macrophage recruitment and adipose tissue inflammation in obesity. Nature Medicine 2009;**15**:914–920

[70] Zuniga LA, Shen WJ, Joyce-Shaikh B, Pyatnova EA, Richards AG, Thom C, et al. IL-17 regulates adipogenesis, glucose homeostasis, and obesity. The Journal of Immunology 2010;**185**:6947–6959

[71] Bruno MEC, Mukherjee S, Powell WL, Mori SF, Wallace FK, Balasuriya BK, et al. Accumulation of gammadelta T cells in visceral fat with aging promotes chronic inflammation. Geroscience 2022;**44**:1761–1778

[72] DeFuria J, Belkina AC, Jagannathan-Bogdan M, Snyder-Cappione J, Carr JD, Nersesova YR, et al. B cells promote inflammation in obesity and type 2 diabetes through regulation of T-cell function and an inflammatory cytokine profile. P Natl Acad Sci USA 2013;**110**:5133–5138

[73] DA W, Winer S, Shen L, Wadia PP, Yantha J, Paltser G, et al. B cells promote insulin resistance through modulation of T cells and production of pathogenic IgG antibodies. Nature Medicine 2011;**17**:610–617

[74] Zhao S, Kusminski CM, Scherer PE. Adiponectin, Leptin and Cardiovascular Disorders. Circulation Research. 2021;**128**(1):136–149

[75] Zhao S, Lin Q, Xiong W, Li L, Straub L, Zhang D, et al. Hyperleptinemia contributes to antipsychotic drug-associated obesity and metabolic disorders. Science Translational Medicine. 2023;**15**: eade8460

[76] Palhinha L, Liechocki S, Hottz ED, Pereira J, De almeida CJ, Moraes-Vieira PMM, et al. Leptin Induces Proadipogenic and Proinflammatory Signaling in Adipocytes. Frontiers in Endocrinology. 2019;**10**:841

[77] Galley JC, Singh S, Awata WMC, Alves JV, Bruder-Nascimento T. Adipokines: Deciphering the cardiovascular signature of adipose tissue. Biochemical Pharmacology. 2022;**206**:115324

[78] Semerena E, Nencioni A, Masternak K. Extracellular nicotinamide phosphoribosyltransferase: Role in disease pathophysiology and as a biomarker. Frontiers in Immunology. 2023;**14**:1268756

[79] Moschen AR, Molnar C, Wolf AM, Weiss H, Graziadei I, Kaser S, et al. Effects of weight loss induced by bariatric surgery on hepatic adipocytokine expression. Journal of Hepatology 2009;**51**:765–777

[80] Kumari B, Yadav UCS. Adipokine Visfatin's Role in Pathogenesis of Diabesity and Related Metabolic Derangements. Current Molecular Medicine. 2018;**18**(2):116–125

[81] Tripathi D, Kant S, Pandey S, Ehtesham NZ. Resistin in metabolism, inflammation, and disease. Febs Journal. 2020;**287**(15):3141–3149

[82] Hsu W-Y, Chao Y-W, Tsai Y-L, Lien -C-C, Chang C-F, Deng M-C, Ho L-T, Kwok CF, Juan -C-C, et al. Resistin induces monocyte–endothelial cell adhesion by increasing ICAM-1 and VCAM-1 expression in endothelial cells via p38MAPK-dependent pathway. Journal of Cellular Physiology 2011;**226**:2181–2188

[83] Yan Y, Wang L, Zhong N, Wen D, Liu L. Multifaced roles of adipokines in endothelial cell function. Frontiers in Endocrinology. 2024;**15**:1490143

[84] Iacobellis G.Epicardial adipose tissue in contemporary cardiology. Nature Reviews Cardiology. 2022;**19**(9):593–606

[85] Horimatsu T, Patel AS, Prasad R, Reid LE, Benson TW, Zarzour A, et al. Remote Effects of Transplanted Perivascular Adipose Tissue on Endothelial Function and Atherosclerosis. Cardiovascular Drugs & Therapy 2018;**32**:503–510

[86] Manka D, Chatterjee TK, Stoll LL, Basford JE, Konaniah ES, Srinivasan R, et al. Transplanted perivascular adipose tissue accelerates injury-induced neointimal hyperplasia: Role of monocyte chemoattractant protein-1. Arteriosclerosis, Thrombosis, and Vascular Biology. 2014;**34**:1723–1730

[87] Song J, Farris D, Ariza P, Moorjani S, Varghese M, Blin M, et al. Age-associated adipose tissue inflammation promotes monocyte chemotaxis and enhances atherosclerosis. Aging Cell. 2023;**22**(2):e13783

[88] Zhang Y, Yang X, Bian F, Wu P, Xing S, Xu G, et al. TNF-alpha promotes early atherosclerosis by increasing transcytosis of LDL across endothelial cells: Crosstalk between NF-kappaB and PPAR-gamma. Journal of Molecular & Cellular Cardiology. 2014;**72**:85–94

[89] Ahmed B, Farb MG, Gokce N. Cardiometabolic implications of adipose tissue aging. Obesity Reviews. 2024;**25**(11):e13806

[90] Sharma BR, Kanneganti TD. NLRP3 inflammasome in cancer and metabolic diseases. Nature Immunology. 2021;**22**(5):550–559

[91] Di Pino A, DeFronzo RA. Insulin Resistance and Atherosclerosis: Implications for Insulin-Sensitizing Agents. Endocrine Reviews. 2019;**40**(6):1447–1467

[92] Ridker PM, Everett BM, Thuren T, MacFadyen JG, Chang WH, Ballantyne C, et al. Antiinflammatory therapy with canakinumab for atherosclerotic disease. New England Journal of Medicine 2017;**377**:1119–1131

[93] Tall AR, Bornfeldt KE. Inflammasomes and Atherosclerosis: A mixed picture. Circulation Research. 2023;**132**(11):1505–1520

[94] Tyrrell DJ, Goldstein DR. Ageing and atherosclerosis: Vascular intrinsic and extrinsic factors and potential role of IL-6. Nature Reviews Cardiology. 2021;**18**(1):58–68

[95] Ridker PM, Devalaraja M, Baeres FMM, Engelmann MDM, Hovingh GK, Ivkovic M, et al. IL-6 inhibition with ziltivekimab in patients at high atherosclerotic risk (RESCUE): A double-blind, randomised, placebo-controlled, phase 2 trial. The Lancet 2021;**397**:2060–2069

[96] Greenstein AS, Khavandi K, Withers SB, Sonoyama K, Clancy O, Jeziorska M, et al. Local inflammation

and hypoxia abolish the protective anticontractile properties of perivascular fat in obese patients. Circulation 2009;**119**:1661–1670

[97] da Costa RM, Fais RS, Dechandt CRP, Louzada-Junior P, Alberici LC, Lobato NS, et al. Increased mitochondrial ROS generation mediates the loss of the anti-contractile effects of perivascular adipose tissue in high-fat diet obese mice. Br J Phar- Macol 2017;**174**:3527–3541

[98] DeVallance E, Branyan KW, Lemaster K, Olfert IM, Smith DM, Pistilli EE, et al. Aortic dysfunction in metabolic syndrome mediated by perivascular adipose tissue TNFalpha- and NOX2-dependent pathway. Experimental Physiology 2018;**103**: 590–603

[99] Kumar RK, Yang Y, Contreras AG, Garver H, Bhattacharya S, Fink GD, et al. Phenotypic changes in T cell and macrophage subtypes in perivascular adipose tissues precede high-fat Diet-Induced hypertension. Frontiers in Physiology. 2021;**12**:616055

[100] Balakumar P, Orayj KM, Khan NA, Shanmugam K, Jagadeesh G. Impact of the local renin-angiotensin system in perivascular adipose tissue on vascular health and disease. Cell Signal. 2024;**124**:111461

[101] Ahmed A, Bibi A, Valoti M, Fusi F. Perivascular adipose tissue and vascular smooth muscle tone: Friends or foes? Cells. 2023;**12**(8):1196

[102] Pahlavani M, Kalupahana NS, Ramalingam L, Moustaid-Moussa N. Regulation and functions of the renin-angiotensin system in white and brown adipose tissue. Comprehensive Physiology. 2017;7(4):1137–1150

[103] DeMarco VG, Aroor AR, Sowers JR.The pathophysiology of hypertension in patients with obesity. Nature Rev Endocrinol. 2014;**10**(6):364–376

[104] Ding J, Yu M, Jiang J, Luo Y, Zhang Q, Wang S, et al. Angiotensin II decreases endothelial nitric oxide synthase phosphorylation via AT(1)R Nox/ROS/PP2A pathway. Frontiers in Physiology. 2020;**11**:566410

[105] Wilcox CS, Wang C, Wang D. Endothelin-1-induced microvascular ROS and contractility in Angiotensin-II-infused mice depend on COX and TP receptors. Antioxidants (Basel). 2019; **8**(6):193

[106] Jialal I, Devaraj S. Subcutaneous adipose tissue biology in metabolic syndrome. Hormone Molecular Biology & Clinical Investigation. 2018;**33**(1)

[107] Neeland IJ, Poirier P, Despres JP. Cardiovascular and metabolic heterogeneity of obesity: Clinical challenges and implications for management. Circulation. 2018; **137**(13):1391–1406

[108] Sorimachi H, Obokata M, Takahashi N, Reddy YNV, Jain CC, Verbrugge FH, et al. Pathophysiologic importance of visceral adipose tissue in women with heart failure and preserved ejection fraction. European Heart Journal. 2021;**42**:1595–1605

[109] Pugliese NR, Paneni F, Mazzola M, De Biase N, Del Punta L, Gargani L, et al. Impact of epicardial adipose tissue on cardiovascular haemodynamics, metabolic profile, and prognosis in heart failure. European Journal of Heart Failure 2021;**23**:1858–1871

[110] Carena MC, Badi I, Polkinghorne M, Akoumianakis I, Psarros C, Wahome

E, et al. Role of human epicardial adipose tissue-derived miR-92a-3p in Myocardial Redox State. Journal of the American College of Cardiology 2023;**82**:317–332

[111] Ren J, Wu NN, Wang S, Sowers JR, Zhang Y. Obesity cardiomyopathy: Evidence, mechanisms, and therapeutic implications. Physiological Reviews. 2021;**101**(4):1745–1807

[112] van Woerden G, van Veldhuisen DJ, Westenbrink BD, de Boer RA, Rienstra M, Gorter TM.Connecting epicardial adipose tissue and heart failure with preserved ejection fraction: Mechanisms, management and modern perspectives. European Journal of Heart Failure. 2022;**24**(12):2238–2250

[113] Obokata M, Reddy YNV, Pislaru SV, Melenovsky V, Borlaug BA. Evidence supporting the existence of a distinct obese phenotype of heart failure with preserved ejection fraction. Circulation. 2017;**136**(1):6–19

[114] Crum Y, Hoendermis ES, van Veldhuisen DJ, van Woerden G, Lobeek M, Dickinson MG, et al. Epicardial adipose tissue and pericardial constraint in heart failure with preserved ejection fraction. ESC Heart Failure 2024;**11**:1698–1706

[115] Cho DH, Park SM.Epicardial adipose tissue and heart failure, friend or Foe? Diabetes & Metabolism Journal. 2024;**48**(3):373–384

[116] ACT N, Strudwick M, van der Geest RJ, ACC N, Gillinder L, Goo SY, et al. Impact of epicardial adipose tissue, left ventricular myocardial fat content, and interstitial fibrosis on myocardial contractile function. Circulation Cardiovascular Imaging. 2018;**11**(8):e007372

[117] Sanders-van Wijk S, van Empel V, Davarzani N, Maeder MT, Handschin R, Pfisterer ME, et al. Circulating biomarkers of distinct pathophysiological pathways in heart failure with preserved vs. reduced left ventricular ejection fraction. European Journal of Heart Failure 2015;**17**:1006–1014

[118] Paulus WJ, Tschope C. A novel paradigm for heart failure with preserved ejection fraction: Comorbidities drive myocardial dysfunction and remodeling through coronary microvascular endothelial inflammation. Journal of the American College of Cardiology. 2013;**62**(4): 263–271

[119] Wu CK, Lee JK, Chiang FT, Yang CH, Huang SW, Hwang JJ, et al. Plasma levels of tumor necrosis factor-alpha and interleukin-6 are associated with diastolic heart failure through downregulation of sarcoplasmic reticulum Ca2+ ATPase. Critical Care Medicine 2011;**39**:984–992

[120] Dronkers J, van Veldhuisen DJ, van der Meer P, Meems LMG. Heart Failure and Obesity: Unraveling Molecular Mechanisms of Excess Adipose Tissue. Journal of the American College of Cardiology. 2024;**84** (17):1666–1677

[121] Schulz R, Heusch G.Tumor necrosis factor-alpha and its receptors 1 and 2: Yin and Yang in myocardial infarction? Circulation. 2009;**119** (10):1355–1357

[122] Chou CH, Hung CS, Liao CW, Wei LH, Chen CW, Shun CT, et al. IL-6 trans-signalling contributes to aldosterone-induced cardiac fibrosis. Cardiovascular Research 2018;**114**:690–702

[123] Griendling KK, Sorescu D, Ushio-Fukai M.NAD(P)H oxidase: Role in cardiovascular biology and disease. Circulation Research. 2000;**86**(5):494–501

[124] Chirinos JA, Akers SR, Trieu L, Ischiropoulos H, Doulias PT, Tariq A, et al. Heart failure, left ventricular remodeling, and circulating nitric oxide metabolites. Journal of the American Heart Association. 2016;**5**(10):e004133

[125] Al-Kaisey AM, Kalman JM. Obesity and atrial fibrillation: epidemiology, pathogenesis and effect of weight loss. Arrhythmia & Electrophysiology Review. 2021;**10**(3):159–164

[126] Aronis KN, Wang N, Phillips CL, Benjamin EJ, Marcus GM, Newman AB, et al. Associations of obesity and body fat distribution with incident atrial fibrillation in the biracial health aging and body composition cohort of older adults. American Heart Journal 2015;**170**:498–505e2

[127] Cabaro S, Conte M, Moschetta D, Petraglia L, Valerio V, Romano S, et al. Epicardial Adipose Tissue-Derived IL-1beta Triggers Postoperative Atrial Fibrillation. Frontiers in Cell and Developmental Biology. 2022;**10**:893729

[128] Mazurek T, Kiliszek M, Kobylecka M, Skubisz-Gluchowska J, Kochman J, Filipiak K, et al. Relation of proinflammatory activity of epicardial adipose tissue to the occurrence of atrial fibrillation. The American Journal of Cardiology 2014;**113**:1505–1508

[129] Ihara K, and Sasano T. Role of Inflammation in the pathogenesis of atrial fibrillation. Frontiers in Physiology. 2022;**13**:862164

[130] Lee SH, Chen YC, Chen YJ, Chang SL, Tai CT, Wongcharoen W, et al. Tumor necrosis factor-alpha alters calcium handling and increases arrhythmogenesis of pulmonary vein cardiomyocytes. Life Sciences 2007;**80**:1806–1815

[131] Kao YH, Chen YC, Cheng CC, Lee TI, Chen YJ, Chen SA. Tumor necrosis factor-alpha decreases sarcoplasmic reticulum Ca2+-ATPase expressions via the promoter methylation in cardiomyocytes. Critical Care Medicine. 2010;**38**(1):217–222

[132] Sawaya SE, Rajawat YS, Rami TG, Szalai G, Price RL, Sivasubramanian N, et al. Downregulation of connexin40 and increased prevalence of atrial arrhythmias in transgenic mice with cardiac-restricted overexpression of tumor necrosis factor. American Journal of Physiology-Heart and Circulatory Physiology. 2007;**292**(3):H1561-H1567

[133] Lazzerini PE, Laghi-Pasini F, Acampa M, Srivastava U, Bertolozzi I, Giabbani B, et al. Systemic inflammation rapidly induces reversible atrial electrical remodeling: The role of interleukin-6-mediated changes in connexin expression. Journal of the American Heart Association. 2019;**8**:e011006

[134] Fan Y, Huang S, Li S, Wu B, Zhao Q, Huang L, et al. The adipose-neural axis is involved in epicardial adipose tissue-related cardiac arrhythmias. Cell Reports Medicine. 2024;**5**(5):101559

[135] Wong CX, Sun MT, Odutayo A, Emdin CA, Mahajan R, Lau DH, et al. Associations of epicardial, abdominal, and overall adiposity with

atrial fibrillation. Circulation Arrhythmia and Electrophysiology. 2016;**9**(12):e004378

[136] Tsao HM, Hu WC, Wu MH, Tai CT, Lin YJ, Chang SL, et al. Quantitative analysis of quantity and distribution of epicardial adipose tissue surrounding the left atrium in patients with atrial fibrillation and effect of recurrence after ablation. The American Journal of Cardiology 2011;**107**: 1498–1503

[137] Nalliah CJ, Bell JR, Raaijmakers AJA, Waddell HM, Wells SP, Bernasochi GB, et al. Epicardial adipose tissue accumulation confers atrial conduction abnormality. Journal of the American College of Cardiology 2020;**76**: 1197–1211

[138] Packer M.Epicardial adipose tissue may mediate deleterious effects of obesity and inflammation on the myocardium. Journal of the American College of Cardiology. 2018;**71**(20): 2360–2372

[139] Abe I, Teshima Y, Kondo H, Kaku H, Kira S, Ikebe Y, et al. Association of fibrotic remodeling and cytokines/ chemokines content in epicardial adipose tissue with atrial myocardial fibrosis in patients with atrial fibrillation. Heart Rhythm: The Official Journal of the Heart Rhythm Society 2018;**15**:1717–1727

[140] Shaihov-Teper O, Ram E, Ballan N, Brzezinski RY, Naftali-Shani N, Masoud R, et al. Extracellular vesicles from epicardial fat facilitate atrial fibrillation. Circulation 2021;**143**: 2475–2493

[141] Venteclef N, Guglielmi V, Balse E, Gaborit B, Cotillard A, Atassi F, et al. Human epicardial adipose tissue induces fibrosis of the atrial myocardium through the secretion of adipo-fibrokines. European Heart Journal. 2015;**36**:795–805a

[142] McCauley MD, Iacobellis G, Li N, Nattel S, Goldberger JJ.Targeting the substrate for atrial fibrillation: JACC review topic of the week. Journal of the American College of Cardiology. 2024;**83**(20):2015–2027

[143] Dozio E, Vianello E, Malavazos AE, Tacchini L, Schmitz G, Iacobellis G, et al. Epicardial adipose tissue GLP-1 receptor is associated with genes involved in fatty acid oxidation and white-to-brown fat differentiation: A target to modulate cardiovascular risk? International Journal of Cardiology. 2019;**292**:218–224

[144] Sattar N, McMurray JJV, McInnes IB, Aroda VR, Lean MEJ.Treating chronic diseases without tackling excess adiposity promotes multimorbidity. The Lancet Diabetes & Endocrinology. 2023;**11**(1):58–62

Chapter 5

Metabolic Syndrome in Pediatric Patients with Chronic Kidney Disease

Miguel Angel Villasis-Keever and Jessie Zurita-Cruz

Abstract

Chronic kidney disease (CKD) in children is a significant public health concern with long-term consequences, particularly due to cardiovascular complications, which are the leading cause of morbidity and mortality in early adulthood. The elevated cardiovascular risk in this population is driven by both traditional factors – such as hypertension, dyslipidemia, obesity, and metabolic syndrome – and nontraditional factors, including chronic inflammation, oxidative stress, vitamin D deficiency, disturbances in bone mineral metabolism, persistent proteinuria, and dysregulated adipocytokine secretion. The pathophysiology is complex and begins in the early stages of CKD, marked by endothelial dysfunction, vascular calcification, and ventricular remodeling. Visceral adiposity, hyperleptinemia, and adiponectin resistance contribute significantly to systemic inflammation and the progression of cardiovascular risk, from left ventricular hypertrophy and arterial stiffness to major cardiovascular events. Early intervention is essential, with a focus on nonpharmacological strategies. Key measures include proper nutrition, weight management, sodium and phosphorus restriction, and regular physical activity. Pharmacological treatments – such as renin–angiotensin–aldosterone system inhibitors, statins, and vitamin D supplementation – should be considered in selected cases, always within a comprehensive and individualized care plan.

Keywords: chronic kidney disease, Pediatric Nephrology, cardiovascular risk, metabolic syndrome, inflammation, adipocytokines

1. Introduction

It has long been recognized that children and adolescents who develop chronic kidney disease (CKD) are at a significantly increased risk of experiencing cardiovascular events in adulthood – even after undergoing kidney replacement therapy or transplantation [1]. Adults aged 25–34 years who are on dialysis due to childhood-onset CKD have been shown to have a 700-fold higher risk of cardiovascular death compared to the general population, highlighting the lasting cardiovascular "footprint" that pediatric CKD can leave into adult life. In this population, the elevated cardiovascular risk is attributed to a combination of traditional risk factors (hypertension, dyslipidemia, obesity/overweight) and nontraditional factors (chronic inflammation, oxidative stress, uremic toxins, disturbances in bone mineral metabolism, endothelial dysfunction, and elevated adipocytokines) [2].

This chapter aims to: 1) describe the cardiovascular risk factors in pediatric patients with kidney disease; 2) review the pathophysiological mechanisms linking CKD to cardiometabolic disorders; 3) analyze the short-, medium-, and long-term prognosis of affected patients; and 4) summarize current therapeutic strategies that may help prevent cardiovascular outcomes in this vulnerable population [1–3].

2. Causes of CKD in children and adolescents

In pediatric populations, the etiology of CKD differs markedly from that in adults. The leading cause is congenital anomalies of the kidney and urinary tract (CAKUT), followed by glomerular diseases [4]. These include nephrotic syndrome and glomerulonephritis, both characterized by persistent proteinuria and frequent exposure to corticosteroids and immunomodulatory agents [2].

Among glomerular causes, nephrotic syndrome is particularly associated with atherogenic dyslipidemia from disease onset, which may persist even after remission and has been linked to increased vascular risk in the second and third decades of life [2, 3]. Glomerulonephritis, on the other hand, combines hypertension and proteinuria with varying degrees of systemic inflammation, contributing to arterial stiffness, endothelial dysfunction, and cardiac remodeling throughout CKD progression, thereby elevating cardiovascular risk [1, 2].

Other, less common causes include kidney stones and nephrocalcinosis, which may lead to chronic obstruction and recurrent inflammation. These conditions are often accompanied by hypertension, further increasing the risk of atherosclerosis [2]. Among hereditary disorders, Alport syndrome and polycystic kidney disease represent a significant proportion of cases and confer heterogeneous cardiometabolic risk profiles due to the interplay of proteinuria, progressive renal impairment, and extrarenal manifestations [1, 4].

While various therapeutic interventions exist to mitigate these conditions, unresolved cases may progress to end-stage CKD, necessitating renal replacement therapy via hemodialysis, peritoneal dialysis, or kidney transplantation. Studies have shown that even post-transplant patients remain at elevated cardiovascular risk [5].

3. Cardiovascular risk factors in pediatric CKD

Numerous factors contributing to increased cardiovascular risk have been identified in children with CKD. Both traditional risk factors – such as hypertension, dyslipidemia, and obesity – and nontraditional ones – including inflammation, oxidative stress, bone mineral metabolism disturbances, adipokine imbalance, and vitamin D deficiency – are present from the early stages of the disease [1, 6].

In children with CAKUT, hypertension is a frequent complication that accelerates arterial stiffness and heightens cardiovascular risk. In nephrotic syndrome, dyslipidemia is the predominant concern, characterized by elevated total cholesterol, LDL cholesterol, and triglycerides, along with reduced HDL cholesterol [2].

Chronic glomerulonephritis is marked by persistent inflammation and hypertension, which are key drivers of endothelial dysfunction, arterial stiffness, and cardiac remodeling – factors that contribute to an adverse cardiometabolic profile [1, 6]. In cases of recurrent nephrolithiasis and nephrocalcinosis, chronic obstruction and inflammation promote hypertension and secondary proteinuria, indirectly increasing long-term cardiovascular risk [2].

Finally, pediatric patients with end-stage CKD who undergo kidney transplantation are at an increased risk of developing overweight/obesity, metabolic syndrome (MS), and hypertension. These complications are often linked to immunosuppressive therapies (e.g., calcineurin inhibitors, mTOR inhibitors), which may lead to subclinical myocardial dysfunction and left ventricular hypertrophy (LVH) within the first months post-transplant [3, 7].

3.1 High blood pressure

High blood pressure (HBP) is the most prevalent cardiovascular risk factor in children with CKD, affecting up to 46% of patients, with higher prevalence observed in advanced stages of the disease [1]. HBP may also be present in early CKD, particularly in cases of congenital urinary tract malformations and glomerular diseases, contributing to accelerated vascular damage [2].

Among pediatric patients undergoing hemodialysis, the prevalence of HBP ranges from 60% to 80% and is strongly associated with LVH and arterial stiffness [4]. Ambulatory blood pressure monitoring has revealed abnormal circadian patterns, such as the absence of nocturnal dipping, which are linked to an increased risk of target organ damage [8].

Poor blood pressure control has been associated with faster CKD progression and increased cardiovascular events during the transition to adulthood [9]. In pediatric kidney transplant recipients, hypertension persists in 40–50% of cases, partly due to immunosuppressive therapy, thereby prolonging cardiovascular risk [5].

3.2 Dyslipidemia

Dyslipidemia in pediatric CKD is typically characterized by hypertriglyceridemia, elevated LDL-C, and reduced HDL-C levels [2]. In nephrotic syndrome, atherogenic lipid profiles are nearly universal during active disease phases and may persist during partial remission [6].

In advanced CKD, lipid abnormalities are present in 50–90% of children and are associated with increased carotid intima-media thickness and arterial stiffness [1, 5]. Post-transplant dyslipidemia affects up to 50% of recipients and is linked to prolonged exposure to glucocorticoids, cyclosporine, tacrolimus, and sirolimus [9].

Beyond its atherogenic role, dyslipidemia contributes to graft deterioration. Valavi et al. reported that hypercholesterolemia is associated with chronic allograft nephropathy over a 48-month follow-up, underscoring its relevance beyond traditional cardiovascular risk [6].

3.3 Obesity and MS

Overweight and obesity are increasingly prevalent among pediatric CKD patients. Prior to transplantation, obesity (based on BMI) is reported in 14–25% of cases, rising to 30–40% within 18 months post-transplant [6, 10]. Abdominal obesity, assessed via waist-to-height ratio, has shown stronger correlations with cardiovascular risk than BMI [10].

Metabolic syndrome significantly increases the likelihood of LVH and subclinical myocardial dysfunction. In a pediatric CKD cohort, MS was independently associated with LVH over a 5-year follow-up [11].

Visceral adiposity not only disrupts lipid metabolism but also serves as a source of proinflammatory adipocytokines (e.g., leptin) and impairs anti-inflammatory signaling (e.g., adiponectin). The leptin/adiponectin ratio has been proposed as a clinical marker of cardiometabolic risk in children receiving renal replacement therapy, predicting persistent dyslipidemia at 12–24 months [12].

3.4 Proteinuria

Proteinuria is both a marker of renal disease progression and an independent cardiovascular risk factor. Urinary protein loss is associated with hypoalbuminemia, hypercoagulability, and lipid abnormalities, all of which contribute to atherosclerosis [13].

In pediatric studies, sustained proteinuria has been linked to increased carotid intima-media thickness and arterial stiffness, independent of renal function [14]. In nephrotic syndrome, the severity of proteinuria predicts the extent of dyslipidemia and the duration of cardiovascular risk [2].

3.5 Bone mineral metabolism disorders and vascular calcification

CKD-related mineral and bone disorder (CKD-MBD) in children is characterized by hyperphosphatemia, hypocalcemia, secondary hyperparathyroidism, and vitamin D deficiency [15]. These abnormalities promote early vascular calcification, even in young patients. Elevated serum phosphorus induces osteoblastic differentiation in vascular smooth muscle cells, contributing to arterial stiffness and LVH [16].

Fibroblast growth factor 23 (FGF-23), a key regulator of phosphate metabolism, rises progressively in CKD and has been associated with an increased risk of LVH in children [17]. Thus, CKD-MBD plays a central role in the pathophysiology of pediatric cardiovascular risk.

3.6 Vitamin D deficiency

Vitamin D deficiency is highly prevalent in children with CKD, with rates exceeding 70% in some studies [18]. Low serum 25(OH)D levels have been associated with dyslipidemia, hypertension, and increased left ventricular mass over 2–5 years of follow-up [19]. Additionally, vitamin D deficiency exacerbates CKD-MBD, further promoting vascular calcification [15].

4. Pathophysiology of the relationship between CKD and cardiometabolic disorders

As shown in **Figure 1**, the association between pediatric CKD and cardiovascular risk is driven by a complex interplay of traditional and nontraditional mechanisms

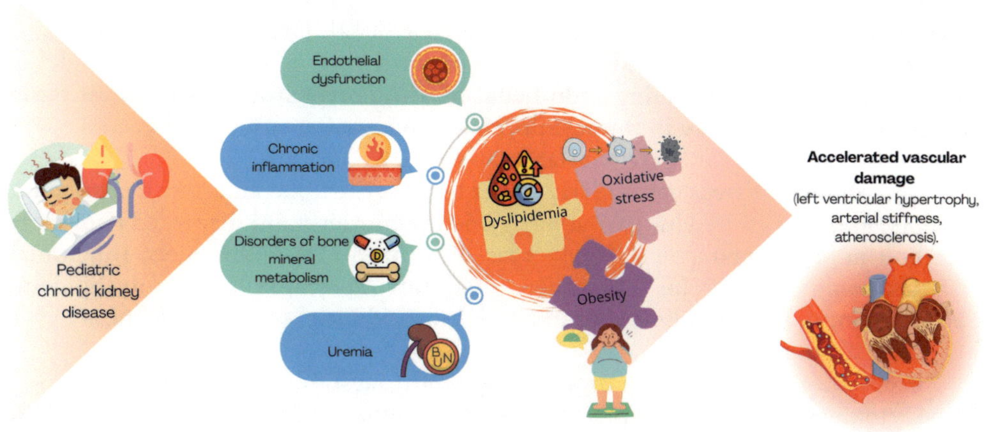

Figure 1.
Pathophysiology of Cardiometabolic Alterations in Pediatric CKD.

that collectively create an environment of accelerated vascular injury [1]. These factors do not act independently: Inflammation exacerbates oxidative stress, uremia promotes endothelial dysfunction, and disturbances in bone mineral metabolism facilitate vascular calcification – forming a vicious cycle of cardiovascular deterioration [2].

Endothelial dysfunction is one of the earliest detectable abnormalities in children with CKD. It results from the combined effects of oxidative stress, chronic inflammation, and the accumulation of uremic toxins [6]. Reduced nitric oxide bioavailability leads to vasoconstriction, platelet aggregation, and vascular smooth muscle proliferation – mechanisms that not only predispose to early atherosclerosis but also increase ventricular afterload, contributing to LVH [3].

Chronic inflammation is characterized by elevated levels of C-reactive protein, interleukin-6, and tumor necrosis factor-alpha, even in early CKD stages [2]. This proinflammatory state is associated with insulin resistance and dyslipidemia, contributing to the development of MS and the progression of cardiovascular disease [11]. In pediatric dialysis patients, recurrent infections and exposure to bioincompatible dialysis membranes further amplify the inflammatory response, accelerating arterial stiffness [20].

Oxidative stress arises from diminished antioxidant enzyme activity and increased production of reactive oxygen species [20]. This imbalance leads to lipoprotein oxidation – particularly of LDL – promoting atherogenesis [1]. Reduced levels of superoxide dismutase and paraoxonase-1 have been documented in CKD, correlating with increased arterial stiffness [21, 22]. Additionally, oxidative stress impairs insulin signaling and promotes peripheral insulin resistance, contributing to metabolic dysfunction [23].

Disturbances in bone mineral metabolism, including hyperphosphatemia, hypocalcemia, and secondary hyperparathyroidism, contribute to early-onset vascular calcification [16]. Elevated serum phosphorus induces osteoblastic transformation of vascular smooth muscle cells, increasing arterial stiffness [1]. Concurrently, elevated FGF-23 and vitamin D deficiency exacerbate vascular and cardiac remodeling [12, 17].

Chronic uremia and prolonged dialysis exposure foster a catabolic and inflammatory state that worsens cardiovascular risk [2]. Uremic toxins, such as indoxyl sulfate and p-cresyl sulfate, induce oxidative stress and mitochondrial dysfunction, directly damaging endothelial cells and myocardial tissue. These toxins also contribute to relative immunosuppression, increasing susceptibility to infections that further intensify inflammation [20].

Lipid abnormalities, particularly in nephrotic syndrome and post-transplant patients, are marked by elevated atherogenic lipoproteins and disrupted cholesterol metabolism [6]. In pediatric CKD, increased oxidized LDL and reduced functional HDL are common, fostering a proatherogenic state. The coexistence of dyslipidemia and proteinuria has been linked to increased carotid intima-media thickness in longitudinal studies [24].

Excess adiposity amplifies these processes through the secretion of adipocytokines [6]. Leptin, typically elevated in advanced CKD, is associated with inflammation, hypertension, and endothelial dysfunction [12]. Adiponectin, although protective in the general population, is paradoxically elevated in CKD, reflecting resistance to its anti-inflammatory effects and correlates with renal progression and cardiovascular risk [25].

Recently, the leptin/adiponectin ratio has emerged as a promising biomarker of persistent dyslipidemia and cardiometabolic risk in children undergoing renal replacement therapy [12]. This ratio reflects the balance between pro- and anti-inflammatory signals in adipose tissue and has shown prognostic value: Higher ratios are associated with an increased likelihood of cardiometabolic complications over 12–24 months of follow-up. This metric appears to offer greater predictive utility than isolated serum levels of leptin or adiponectin [25, 26].

5. Prognosis of CKD patients with cardiometabolic abnormalities

Cardiovascular mortality is the leading cause of death among young adults with childhood-onset CKD, underscoring the significance of subclinical vascular damage that begins in the early stages of the disease. Even after successful kidney transplantation, pediatric patients continue to exhibit markedly elevated cardiovascular risk compared to the general population [4, 7, 27].

5.1 Short-term prognosis (1–3 years)

In pediatric kidney transplant recipients, subclinical myocardial dysfunction can be detected as early as the first month post-transplant, typically assessed via impaired global longitudinal strain. This dysfunction persists at 18 and 30 months, with reported LVH prevalence ranging from 17% to 35%, even in the absence of reduced ejection fraction. The coexistence of obesity, MS, and systolic hypertension significantly increases the likelihood of developing LVH during this period [14, 28].

Among children undergoing dialysis, increased arterial stiffness and carotid intima-media thickness are observed within the first 2–3 years of therapy, indicating that vascular changes begin early after the initiation of renal replacement therapy [24, 29].

5.2 Medium-term prognosis (5–10 years)

Between 5 and 10 years after CKD onset or dialysis initiation, LVH and arterial stiffness become increasingly prevalent. It is estimated that 35–40% of pediatric patients on dialysis or post-transplant develop LVH during this period. On average, LVH develops within 3–7 years of renal replacement therapy and serves as an independent predictor of mortality [27].

Carotid intima-media thickness increases significantly in children with CKD over 5–8 years compared to age-matched healthy controls [24]. In pediatric cohorts, MS has been independently associated with the development of LVH and progressive diastolic dysfunction [11].

In patients with nephrotic syndrome, persistent proteinuria and dyslipidemia lasting more than five years have been linked to increased atherogenic risk and progression to cardiovascular complications, even in the absence of advanced renal impairment [13].

5.3 Long-term prognosis (10–20 years)

Ten to twenty years after the onset of pediatric CKD or kidney transplantation, cardiovascular outcomes worsen considerably. Population-based studies show that cardiovascular mortality in young adults who received renal replacement therapy during childhood is 10 to 30 times higher than that in the general population [27].

Foley et al. reported that adults aged 25–34 years on dialysis have a more than 700-fold increased risk of cardiovascular death compared to their peers without CKD [27]. Clinical manifestations include sudden cardiac death, malignant arrhythmias, acute myocardial infarction, and heart failure – typically emerging in the second and third decades of life [30].

Chronic glomerulonephritis, characterized by sustained inflammation, has been associated with accelerated progression to coronary artery disease and heart failure. Similarly, complicated nephrolithiasis (e.g., nephrocalcinosis, recurrent obstruction) may indirectly contribute to hypertension and vascular damage, amplifying long-term cardiovascular risk [14].

5.4 Very-long-term prognosis (over 20 years)

Pediatric CKD leaves a lasting cardiovascular imprint that extends into mature adulthood. Survivors who began dialysis in childhood may experience major cardiovascular events – such as myocardial infarction and sudden death – 20 to 25 years after disease onset, even following successful kidney transplantation. This excess risk is attributed to cumulative exposure to hypertension, dyslipidemia, chronic inflammation, and other cardiometabolic stressors over time [30, 31] (**Figure 2**).

6. Interventions to prevent/treat MS in CKD patients

According to the KDIGO 2024 Clinical Practice Guideline, individuals with CKD should receive a comprehensive preventive and therapeutic approach that

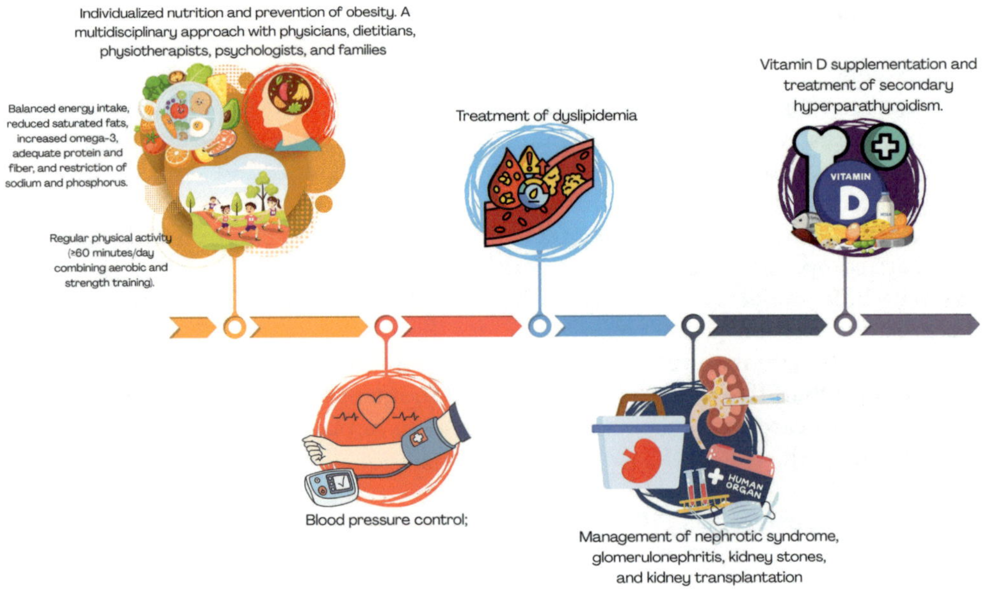

Figure 2.
Comprehensive Treatment of Cardiometabolic Alterations in Pediatric CKD.

integrates both traditional and nontraditional risk factors [32]. This strategy encompasses lifestyle modifications, including regular physical activity – defined as at least 60 minutes of moderate-to-vigorous daily exercise for children and adolescents – reduction of sedentary behavior, and evidence-based nutritional interventions. Additionally, KDIGO advocates for a balanced diet emphasizing a higher intake of plant-based foods, with animal-based products consumed in moderation, and the avoidance of ultra-processed items. Recommended dietary patterns include the Dietary Approaches to Stop Hypertension diet, which is rich in fruits, vegetables, whole grains, and low-fat dairy products, and the Mediterranean diet, characterized by abundant consumption of vegetables, fruits, herbs, nuts, legumes, whole grains, and seafood, complemented by moderate portions of dairy, meat, and eggs.

KDIGO underscores that when these lifestyle interventions are implemented alongside treatments – such as blood pressure management, lipid-lowering therapy, correction of CKD-MBD, and anemia treatment – they yield synergistic effects. This integrated approach offers superior outcomes compared to isolated interventions, contributing to improved cardiovascular health and delayed progression of CKD [32].

6.1 Nonpharmacological measures

Nonpharmacological interventions are the cornerstone of managing cardiometabolic disorders in pediatric CKD, both before and after kidney transplantation. While pharmacological therapies have demonstrated efficacy, lifestyle-based strategies for primary and secondary prevention offer long-term benefits with minimal adverse effects [32–35].

6.1.1 Nutrition

Nutritional management should be tailored to the stage of CKD and the patient's comorbidities, aiming to balance the prevention of malnutrition with the control of excessive weight gain.

- **Energy intake:** Caloric intake must be individualized to support growth and development, avoiding both deficits and excesses. Excess energy intake is associated with increased visceral adiposity and a proinflammatory state, which worsens insulin resistance [32].

- **Fat quality:** Saturated fats should be limited to less than 10% of total caloric intake, and trans fats should be minimized. The consumption of polyunsaturated fatty acids – particularly omega-3s from sources such as fatty fish, flaxseed, and chia – is encouraged due to their triglyceride-lowering and anti-inflammatory properties [33].

- **Carbohydrates:** Emphasis should be placed on complex carbohydrates while limiting simple sugars. A high intake of added sugars is linked to hypertriglyceridemia and increased abdominal fat accumulation [34].

- **Protein:** Protein intake should be adjusted according to the CKD stage. In the early stages, 100–120% of the age-appropriate recommended daily intake is generally advised, with modifications in advanced stages or during dialysis to avoid hyperfiltration [32].

- **Fiber:** Adequate fiber intake (≥14 g per 1,000 kcal) improves insulin sensitivity, supports gut microbiota balance, and may reduce systemic inflammation [33].

- **Sodium:** Moderate sodium restriction (<2 g/day in adolescents) is essential for blood pressure control and volume management, with beneficial effects on LVH [35].

- **Phosphorus and potassium:** Intake should be adjusted based on the CKD stage and laboratory values. Phosphorus restriction is particularly important in managing CKD-MBD and preventing vascular calcification [32].

During corticosteroid therapy and post-transplantation, nutritional strategies should focus on preventing overweight and obesity [25]. Effective approaches include family-centered nutritional education, the use of dietary reminders and food diaries, the replacement of ultra-processed foods with natural, nutrient-dense options, portion control, and regular meal scheduling [32].

6.2 Blood pressure control

Given that hypertension is a major determinant of cardiovascular morbidity and mortality in pediatric CKD, targeted interventions are essential:

- **Lifestyle modifications:** Sodium restriction (<2 g/day in adolescents), weight management, increased physical activity, and improved dietary quality are foundational measures [3].

- **First-line pharmacotherapy:** Angiotensin-converting enzyme inhibitors and angiotensin II receptor blockers are the preferred agents in children with CKD and proteinuria. These medications have been shown to lower blood pressure, reduce proteinuria, and slow the progression of LVH over 2–5 years of follow-up [9].

- **Additional medications:** Beta-blockers, calcium channel blockers, and diuretics may be added based on clinical indications and CKD stage [9, 36].

Studies in pediatric populations have demonstrated that strict blood pressure control (targeting < 50th percentile for age, height, and sex) slows CKD progression and prevents ventricular remodeling over 2–4 years [31]. In transplant recipients, normalization of blood pressure within the first 6–12 months is associated with reduced LVH and improved diastolic function at 3–5 years of follow-up [7].

6.3 Nutritional therapy

Nutritional management is the first-line approach for all patients. Key strategies include the reduction of saturated fats, increased dietary fiber intake, and weight control through balanced energy intake.

Family education is critical, as dietary habits in childhood are largely shaped by caregivers. Empowering families with knowledge and tools for healthy meal planning enhances adherence and long-term outcomes [32].

6.4 Pharmacological therapy

In cases where lifestyle modifications are insufficient, pharmacological treatment may be necessary.

- **Statins:** Statins are the most extensively studied agents for pediatric dyslipidemia. Clinical trials in children and adolescents with familial hypercholesterolemia have shown LDL reductions of 30–50% over 6–12 months, with good safety profiles in follow-ups of up to two years [37]. In pediatric CKD, evidence is limited. Open-label studies have reported similar LDL reductions, though without demonstrated reductions in cardiovascular events [2]. Statins should be reserved for patients with persistent dyslipidemia despite non-pharmacological measures, especially in the presence of additional risk factors such as hypertension, proteinuria, or a family history of premature cardiovascular disease [38].

- **Ezetimibe:** Ezetimibe inhibits intestinal cholesterol absorption and can be added to statin therapy when LDL targets are not achieved. In pediatric populations, it has shown reductions in total and LDL cholesterol within 6–12 weeks [39]. It is considered safe in CKD and does not require dose adjustment for renal function [40].

- **Fibrates:** Primarily indicated for severe hypertriglyceridemia (>500 mg/dL) to reduce the risk of pancreatitis. In small pediatric CKD cohorts, bezafibrate normalized triglyceride levels in approximately one-third of patients over 12 months, although it carries a risk of elevated serum creatinine [41].

- **Bile acid sequestrants:** Agents such as colesevelam and cholestyramine are second-line options for resistant hypercholesterolemia. Pediatric studies have reported 12–13% reductions in total and LDL cholesterol over 6–24 months. However, gastrointestinal side effects often limit their long-term use [42].

6.5 Vitamin D deficiency management

Vitamin D supplementation, either in native or active forms, should be tailored to the stage of CKD and serum 25(OH)D levels. Dietary phosphorus restriction is also recommended, particularly by avoiding phosphate additives and ultra-processed foods. In advanced CKD or dialysis, phosphate binders may be necessary, preferably non-calcium-based agents, to minimize the risk of vascular calcification [43].

Correction of CKD-MBD has implications beyond bone health. It plays a crucial role in preventing cardiac remodeling and vascular calcification over a 5- to 10-year horizon [15, 16, 43].

7. Kidney transplantation and cardiometabolic risk

Kidney transplantation is the preferred treatment for advanced pediatric CKD, offering improved survival and quality of life compared to long-term dialysis [31]. However, cardiometabolic risk remains elevated and may even increase due to immunosuppressive therapy, post-transplant weight gain, and persistent nonmodifiable risk factors [10, 12].

To mitigate these risks, a comprehensive preventive and therapeutic strategy is recommended:

1. **Nutritional support:** Prevents excessive weight gain during the first post-transplant year by reducing the intake of empty calories and controlling sodium consumption [32].

2. **Supervised physical activity:** Aerobic and resistance exercise programs tailored to pediatric transplant recipients have shown improvements in cardiorespiratory fitness and body composition within 6–12 months [44].

3. **Regular monitoring:** Annual evaluations should include blood pressure, lipid profile, endothelial function, and echocardiography to detect early signs of LVH and diastolic dysfunction [6].

4. **Optimization of Immunosuppression:** Minimize glucocorticoid exposure when feasible, monitor calcineurin inhibitor levels, and adjust mTOR inhibitors to reduce adverse metabolic effects [45].

5. **Pharmacological interventions:** Use of statins, ezetimibe, or fibrates should be individualized based on persistent dyslipidemia, with careful monitoring for drug interactions [39].

6. **Cardiovascular rehabilitation:** Multidisciplinary rehabilitation programs – including nutritional counseling, physical therapy, and health education – have demonstrated efficacy in reducing visceral adiposity and improving blood pressure over 12-month follow-ups [46]. These programs should be routinely implemented in pediatric transplant centers.

8. Conclusions

Cardiometabolic disorders are among the most significant complications in children and adolescents with CKD, and they largely account for the elevated cardiovascular mortality observed in early adulthood among individuals with childhood-onset CKD.

Risk factors include both traditional elements – such as hypertension, dyslipidemia, obesity, and MS – and nontraditional contributors, including chronic inflammation, oxidative stress, endothelial dysfunction, disturbances in bone mineral metabolism, uremia, and adipokine imbalance. These factors are often present from the earliest stages of CKD.

The pathophysiology is multifactorial and reflects the interaction of diverse mechanisms, with excess adiposity and adipokine dysregulation playing central roles in mediating cardiovascular risk. These alterations lead to the early development of LVH, arterial stiffness, and subclinical atherosclerosis, which progressively evolve into major clinical outcomes – such as myocardial infarction, heart failure, and sudden cardiac death – typically occurring 10 to 20 years after CKD onset.

Although the long-term prognosis for this population is concerning, it can be significantly improved through timely and sustained intervention. Key strategies include strict blood pressure control, correction of dyslipidemia, comprehensive nutritional management, optimization of immunosuppressive therapy post-transplant, and vitamin D supplementation. However, the evidence supporting the efficacy of lipid-lowering agents in pediatric CKD remains limited and is largely extrapolated from adult studies.

Given these challenges, healthcare professionals must recognize that addressing cardiometabolic alterations in pediatric CKD requires a comprehensive, multidisciplinary, and proactive approach. Early identification and management of these risk factors can substantially improve survival and quality of life, helping to reduce the persistent burden of cardiovascular disease despite advances in renal replacement therapy.

Author details

Miguel Angel Villasis-Keever[1]* and Jessie Zurita-Cruz[2]

1 Mexican Social Security Institute, México City, Mexico

2 UNAM's School of Medicine, National Autonomous University of Mexico, México City, Mexico

*Address all correspondence to: miguel.villasis@gmail.com

References

[1] Tullus K. Dyslipidemia in children with CKD: Should we treat with statins? Pediatric Nephrology. 2012;**27**(3):357–362. DOI: 10.1007/s00467-011-1872-3

[2] Khurana M, Silverstein DM. Etiology and management of dyslipidemia in children with chronic kidney disease and end-stage renal disease. Pediatric Nephrology. 2015;**30**(12):2073–2084. DOI: 10.1007/s00467-015-3075-9

[3] Nelms CL, Shaw V, Greenbaum LA, Anderson C, Desloovere A, Haffner D, et al. Assessment of nutritional status in children with kidney diseases-clinical practice recommendations from the pediatric renal nutrition taskforce. Pediatric Nephrology. 2021;**36**(4):995–1010. DOI: 10.1007/s00467-020-04852-5

[4] Harada R, Hamasaki Y, Okuda Y, Hamada R, Ishikura K. Epidemiology of pediatric chronic kidney disease/kidney failure: Learning from registries and cohort studies. Pediatric Nephrology. 2022;**37**(6):1215–1229. DOI: 10.1007/s00467-021-05145-1

[5] Villasís-Keever MA, Zurita-Cruz JN, Serret-Montoya J, de Leon-herrera AP, Galván-Heredia P, Zepeda-Martínez CDC, et al. Cardiometabolic factors in pediatric patients with chronic diseases. Archives of Medical Research. 2021;**52**(5):535–543. DOI: 10.1016/j.arcmed.2021.01.010

[6] Valavi E, Otukesh H, Fereshtehnejad SM, Sharifian M. Clinical correlation between dyslipidemia and pediatric chronic allograft nephropathy. Pediatric Transplantation. 2008;**12**(7):748–754. DOI: 10.1111/j.1399-3046.2008.00981.x

[7] Sgambat K, Clauss S, Lei KY, Song J, Rahaman SO, Lasota M, Moudgil A. Effects of obesity and metabolic syndrome on cardiovascular outcomes in pediatric kidney transplant recipients: A longitudinal study. Pediatric Nephrology. 2018;**33**(8):1419–1428. DOI: 10.1007/s00467-017-3860-8

[8] Stabouli S, Kotsis V, Zakopoulos N. Ambulatory blood pressure monitoring and target organ damage in pediatrics. Journal of Hypertension. 2007;**25**(10):1979–1986. DOI: 10.1097/HJH.0b013e3282775992

[9] ESCAPE Trial Group; Wühl E, Trivelli A, Picca S, Litwin M, Peco-Antic A, Zurowska A, et al. Strict blood-pressure control and progression of renal failure in children. New England Journal of Medicine. 2009;**361**(17)1639–1650. DOI: 10.1056/NEJMoa0902066

[10] Litwin M, Niemirska A. Metabolic syndrome in children with chronic kidney disease and after renal transplantation. Pediatric Nephrology. 2014;**29**(2):203–216. DOI: 10.1007/s00467-013-2500-1

[11] Drożdż M, Moczulska A, Rudziński A, Drożdż D. Metabolic syndrome as risk factor for left ventricular hypertrophy in children with chronic kidney disease. Frontiers in Endocrinology. 2023;**14**:1215527. DOI: 10.3389/fendo.2023.1215527

[12] Villasís-Keever MÁ, Zurita-Cruz JN, Serret-Montoya J, Barbosa-Cortés L,

Zepeda-Martínez CDC, Alegría-Torres G, et al. The leptin/adiponectin ratio as prognostic marker for dyslipidemia during 1 year of follow-up in pediatric patients receiving kidney replacement therapy. Nutricion Hospitalaria. 2022;**39**(5):977–987. DOI: 10.20960/nh.03890

[13] Chavers BM, Li S, Collins AJ, Herzog CA. Cardiovascular disease in pediatric chronic dialysis patients. Kidney International. 2002;**62**:648–653. DOI: 10.1046/j.1523-1755.2002.00472.x

[14] Mitsnefes MM. Cardiovascular disease in children with chronic kidney disease. Journal of the American Society of Nephrology. 2012;**23**(4):578–585. DOI: 10.1681/ASN.2011111115

[15] Shroff R, Wan M, Nagler EV, Bakkaloglu S, Fischer DC, Bishop N, et al. Clinical practice recommendations for native vitamin D therapy in children with chronic kidney disease stages 2-5 and on dialysis. Nephrology Dialysis Transplantation. 2017;**32**(7):1098–1113. DOI: 10.1093/ndt/gfx065

[16] Goodman WG, Goldin J, Kuizon BD, Yoon C, Gales B, Sider D, et al. Coronary-artery calcification in young adults with end-stage renal disease who are undergoing dialysis. New England Journal of Medicine. 2000;**342**(20):1478–1483. DOI: 10.1056/NEJM200005183422003

[17] Faul C, Amaral AP, Oskouei B, Hu MC, Sloan A, Isakova T, et al. FGF23 induces left ventricular hypertrophy. Journal of Clinical Investigation. 2011;**121**:4393–4408

[18] Shroff R, Egerton M, Bridel M, Shah V, Donald AE, Cole TJ, et al. A bimodal association of vitamin D levels and vascular disease in children on dialysis. Journal of the American Society of Nephrology. 2008;**19**(6):1239–1246. DOI: 10.1681/ASN.2007090993

[19] Parra-Ortega I, Zurita-Cruz JN, Villasis-Keever MA, Klünder-Klünder M, Vilchis-Gil J, Zepeda-Martinez C, et al. Cardiometabolic factors and vitamin D deficiency in pediatric patients with chronic kidney disease. Frontiers in Nutrition. 2024;**11**:1480424. DOI: 10.3389/fnut.2024.1480424

[20] Wang Y, Gao L. Inflammation and cardiovascular disease associated with hemodialysis for end-stage renal disease. Frontiers in Pharmacology. 2022;**13**:800950. DOI: 10.3389/fphar.2022.800950

[21] Samouilidou EC, Liaouri A, Kostopoulos V, Nikas D, Grapsa E. The importance of paraoxonase 1 activity in chronic kidney disease. Renal Failure. 2024;**46**(2):2376930. DOI: 10.1080/0886022X.2024.2376930

[22] Brady TM, Schneider MF, Flynn JT, Cox C, Samuels J, Saland J, et al. Carotid intima-media thickness in children with CKD: Results from the CKiD study. Clinical Journal of the American Society of Nephrology. 2012;7(12):1930–1937. DOI: 10.2215/CJN.03130312

[23] Lindblad YT, Axelsson J, Bárány P, Celsi G, Lindholm B, Qureshi AR, et al. Hyperinsulinemia and insulin resistance, early cardiovascular risk factors in children with chronic kidney disease. Blood Purification. 2008;**26**(6):518–525. DOI: 10.1159/000167799

[24] Doyon A, Hofstetter J, Bayazit AK, Azukaitis K, Niemirska A, Civilibal M, et al. Progression of carotid

intima-media thickness in children of the cardiovascular comorbidity in children with chronic kidney disease study: Risk factors and impact of blood pressure dynamics. Journal of the American Heart Association. 2025;**14**(7):e037563. DOI: 10.1161/JAHA.124.037563

[25] Kuo IC, Wu PH, Lin HY, Niu SW, Huang JC, Hung CC, et al. The association of adiponectin with metabolic syndrome and clinical outcome in patients with non-diabetic chronic kidney disease. PLoS One. 2019;**14**(7):e0220158. DOI: 10.1371/journal.pone.0220158

[26] Zhao S, Kusminski CM, Scherer PE. Adiponectin, leptin and cardiovascular disorders. Circulation Research. 2021;**128**(1):136–149. DOI: 10.1161/CIRCRESAHA.120.314458

[27] Foley RN, Parfrey PS, Sarnak MJ. Clinical epidemiology of cardiovascular disease in chronic renal disease. American Journal of Kidney Diseases. 1998;**32**(Suppl 5):S112–S119. DOI: 10.1053/ajkd.1998.v32.pm9820470

[28] Mitsnefes MM, Kimball TR, Kartal J, Witt SA, Glascock BJ, Khoury PR, et al. Progression of left ventricular hypertrophy in children with early chronic kidney disease: 2-year follow-up study. The Journal of Pediatrics. 2006;**149**(5):671–675. DOI: 10.1016/j.jpeds.2006.08.017

[29] Valdivielso JM, Rodríguez-Puyol D, Pascual J, Barrios C, Bermúdez-López M, Sánchez-Niño MD, et al. Atherosclerosis in chronic kidney disease: More, less, or just different? Arteriosclerosis, Thrombosis, and Vascular Biology. 2019;**39**(10):1938–1966. DOI: 10.1161/ATVBAHA.119.312705

[30] Groothoff JW, Offringa M, Grootenhuis M, Jager KJ. Long-term consequences of renal insufficiency in children: Lessons learned from the Dutch LERIC study. Nephrology Dialysis Transplantation. 2018;**33**(4):552–560. DOI: 10.1093/ndt/gfx190

[31] Francis A, Johnson DW, Melk A, Foster BJ, Blazek K, Craig JC, et al. Survival after kidney transplantation during childhood and adolescence. Clinical Journal of the American Society of Nephrology. 2020;**15**(3):392–400. DOI: 10.2215/CJN.07070619

[32] Kidney Disease: Improving Global Outcomes (KDIGO) CKD Work Group. KDIGO 2024 clinical practice guideline for the evaluation and management of chronic kidney disease. Kidney International. 2024;**105**(4S):S117–S314. DOI: 10.1016/j.kint.2023.10.018

[33] Shaw V, Polderman N, Renken-Terhaerdt J, Paglialonga F, Oosterveld M, et al. Energy and protein requirements for children with CKD stages 2-5 and on dialysis-clinical practice recommendations from the Pediatric Renal Nutrition Taskforce. Pediatric Nephrology. 2020;**35**(3):519–531. DOI: 10.1007/s00467-019-04426-0

[34] Corsello A, Trovato CM, Dipasquale V, Proverbio E, Milani GP, Diamanti A, Agostoni C, Romano C. Malnutrition management in children with chronic kidney disease. Pediatric Nephrology. 2025;**40**(1):15–24. DOI: 10.1007/s00467-024-06436-z

[35] Sethna CB, Merchant K, Reyes A. cardiovascular disease risk in children with kidney disease. Seminars in

Nephrology. 2018;**38**(3):298–313. DOI: 10.1016/j.semnephrol.2018.02.009

[36] Flynn JT, Kaelber DC, Baker-Smith CM, et al. Clinical practice guideline for screening and management of high blood pressure in children and adolescents. Pediatrics. 2017;**140**:e20171904

[37] Wiegman A, Gidding SS, Watts GF, Chapman MJ, Ginsberg HN, Cuchel M, et al. Familial hypercholesterolaemia in children and adolescents: Gaining decades of life by optimizing detection and treatment. European Heart Journal. 2015;**36**(36):2425–2437. DOI: 10.1093/eurheartj/ehv157

[38] Schefelker JM, Peterson AL. Screening and management of dyslipidemia in children and adolescents. Journal of Clinical Medicine. 2022;**11**(21):6479. DOI: 10.3390/jcm11216479

[39] Drastal MS, de Ferranti S, Gooding H. Recent updates on the screening, diagnosis, and management of lipids disorders in children and adolescents. Current Opinion in Pediatrics. 2025;**37**(4):325–332. DOI: 10.1097/MOP.0000000000001460

[40] Mehta A. Managing dyslipidaemia in patients with chronic kidney disease. Indian Heart Journal. 2024;**76**(Suppl 1): S90–S92. DOI: 10.1016/j.ihj.2024.01.012

[41] Lacount S, Tannock LR. Dyslipidemia in Chronic Kidney Disease. In: Feingold KR, Ahmed SF, Anawalt B, editors. Endotext [Internet]. South Dartmouth (MA): MDText.com, Inc. 2000–2005

[42] Arvanitakis K, Chatzikalil E, Antza C, Topalidis C, Kalopitas G, Solomou E, et al. Pediatric familial hypercholesterolemia: Targeting intestinal absorption and other therapeutic strategies. Nutrients. 2025;**17**(14):2357. DOI: 10.3390/nu17142357

[43] KDIGO. Clinical Practice Guideline Update for the Diagnosis, Evaluation, Prevention, and Treatment of CKD-MBD. Kidney International Supplements. 2017;**7**:1–59

[44] Painter P, Krasnoff J, Mathias R. Exercise capacity and physical fitness in pediatric dialysis and kidney transplant patients. Pediatric Nephrology. 2007;**22**(7):1030–1039. DOI: 10.1007/s00467-007-0458-6

[45] Loupy A, Sablik M, Khush K, Reese PP. Advancing patient monitoring, diagnostics, and treatment strategies for transplant precision medicine. The Lancet. 2025;**406**(10501):389–402. DOI: 10.1016/S0140-6736(25)00195-3

[46] Johansen KL, Painter P. Exercise in individuals with CKD. American Journal of Kidney Diseases. 2012;**59**(1):126–134. DOI: 10.1053/j.ajkd.2011.10.008

Chapter 6

Advances in Metabolic Syndrome and Endometriosis: Emerging Insights and Therapeutic Horizons

Shisana M Baloyi

Abstract

Metabolic syndrome and endometriosis are two complex conditions that can significantly impact a woman's quality of life. Research suggests that there may be a link between metabolic syndrome and endometriosis, with some studies indicating that women with endometriosis are more likely to develop metabolic syndrome. The exact mechanisms underlying this association are not yet fully understood. Methods: A selection of articles from Google Scholar, PubMed, and CrossRef, along with a review of recent articles from the literature, was conducted with the aim of providing a comprehensive overview of the current understanding of the interplay between metabolic syndrome and endometriosis. The following topics will be explored: underlying mechanisms, clinical implications, emerging therapeutic strategies for managing metabolic syndrome and endometriosis, and non-invasive methods for diagnosing endometriosis. Results: Women with endometriosis are at a higher risk of developing metabolic syndrome. Screening for metabolic syndrome and its components (e.g., high triglycerides, hypertension, insulin resistance) is recommended to prevent long-term health complications. Lifestyle interventions (diet, exercise) may help reduce metabolic syndrome risk in women with endometriosis. Addressing both conditions can improve fertility outcomes and overall health for infertile women. Conclusions: Healthcare providers should consider a comprehensive approach to managing endometriosis, including screening and treatment for metabolic syndrome. Early intervention and lifestyle modifications can potentially improve health outcomes for women with endometriosis and metabolic syndrome.

Keywords: chronic inflammation, hormonal imbalances, insulin resistance, biomarkers, metabolic syndrome

1. Introduction

Metabolic syndrome (MetS) and endometriosis are two complex, multifactorial conditions that significantly impact women's health across the globe. MetS is defined as a cluster of interrelated metabolic abnormalities –

including central obesity, insulin resistance, hypertension, hyperglycemia, and dyslipidemia – that substantially increase the risk of type 2 diabetes mellitus (T2DM) and cardiovascular disease [1]. Endometriosis, on the other hand, is a chronic gynecological disorder characterized by the presence of endometrial-like tissue outside the uterus, resulting in inflammation, pelvic pain, infertility, and impaired quality of life [2].

Although historically studied in isolation, recent research suggests that these conditions may be interconnected, with metabolic dysregulation influencing endometriosis development and progression, and endometriosis conferring a heightened risk for cardiometabolic disorders [3]. This chapter examines the prevalence, mechanisms, interplay, clinical implications, and therapeutic strategies of MetS and endometriosis, with an emphasis on reproductive health and emerging treatment horizons.

2. Prevalence of metabolic syndrome and endometriosis

2.1 Endometriosis prevalence

Endometriosis affects approximately 10% of women and girls of reproductive age worldwide, equating to around 190 million individuals [4]. Despite this high prevalence, diagnostic delays of 7–10 years are common, often due to the normalization of menstrual pain and the lack of non-invasive diagnostic tools [2].

2.2 Metabolic syndrome prevalence

The prevalence of MetS varies depending on the diagnostic criteria used. The National Cholesterol Education Program's Adult Treatment Panel III (ATP III), the International Diabetes Federation (IDF), and the Joint Interim Statement (JIS) offer slightly differing cut-offs for waist circumference, glucose, and lipid abnormalities [5]. Global estimates suggest that between 12.5% and 31.4% of adults meet the criteria for MetS, with prevalence increasing in parallel with rising obesity and sedentary lifestyles [1].

2.3 Comorbidity between mets and endometriosis

Recent epidemiological studies, including analyses of the U.S. National Health and Nutrition Examination Survey (NHANES), demonstrate that women with endometriosis have 1.5-fold higher odds of developing MetS compared to those without [3]. This association highlights the need for integrated care approaches and early metabolic screening in women diagnosed with endometriosis.

3. Pathophysiological mechanisms

3.1 Mechanisms in metabolic syndrome

MetS is driven by insulin resistance, visceral obesity, and adipose tissue dysfunction, leading to elevated free fatty acids, chronic low-grade inflammation, and dysregulated adipokine secretion [6]. This inflammatory milieu exacerbates vascular dysfunction and accelerates atherosclerosis.

3.2 Mechanisms in endometriosis

Endometriosis is fueled by estrogen dominance, chronic peritoneal inflammation, angiogenesis, and impaired immune surveillance [7]. Reactive oxygen species and iron overload in lesions further perpetuate oxidative stress and tissue injury [8].

3.3 Shared mechanisms

Key shared pathways between MetS and endometriosis include chronic inflammation (TNF-α, IL-6), hormonal imbalance (estrogen dominance, insulin signaling), oxidative stress, and genetic predisposition with polymorphisms linked to immune and metabolic regulation [9]. These shared mechanisms are illustrated in **Figure 1**, which highlights the overlapping inflammatory, hormonal, and oxidative stress pathways linking metabolic syndrome and endometriosis. The diagnotic frameworks and core features of both metabolic syndrome and endometriosis are summarized in **Figure 2**.

4. Interplay between metabolic syndrome and endometriosis

The relationship between MetS and endometriosis is bidirectional. Metabolic disturbances may exacerbate endometriosis lesion growth via hyperinsulinemia, dyslipidemia, and inflammation [10]. Conversely, endometriosis has been prospectively linked to hypertension, hypercholesterolemia, and increased cardiovascular risk, suggesting systemic metabolic consequences [11].

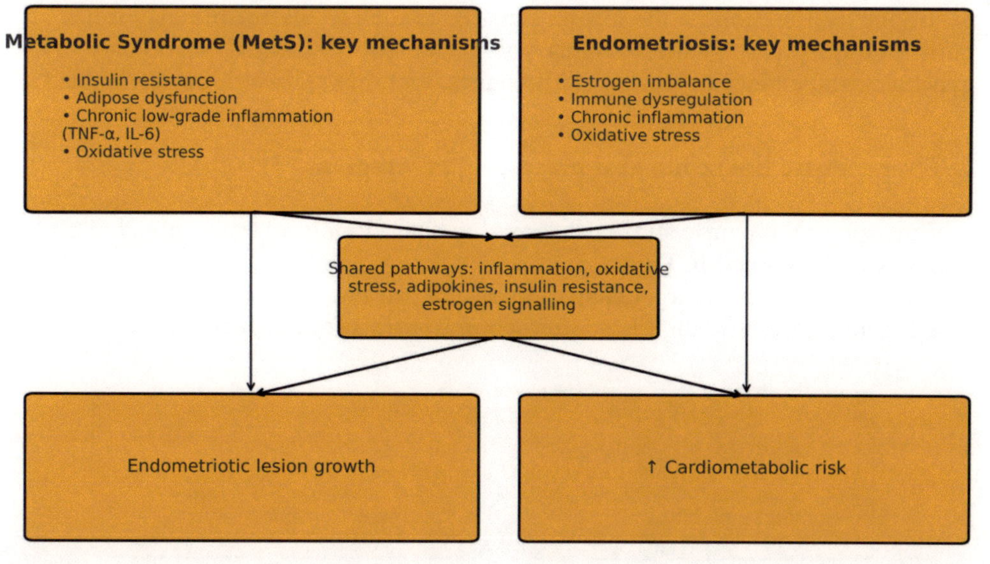

Figure 1.
Shared pathophysiology of metabolic syndrome and endometrios.

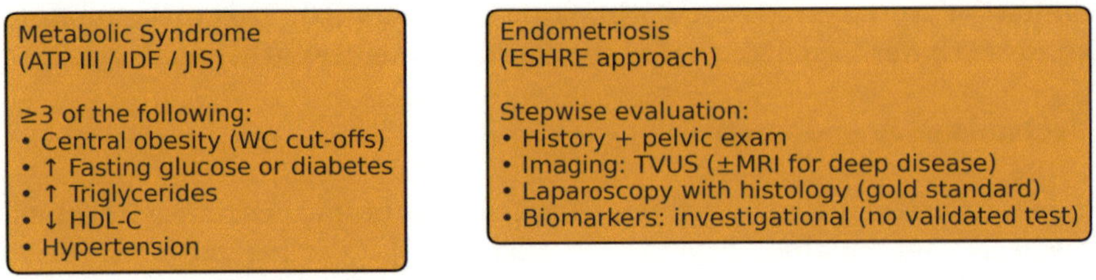

Figure 2.
Diagnostic criteria of metabolic syndrome and endometriosis.

5. Impact on reproductive health

Both MetS and endometriosis profoundly impair reproductive health. Endometriosis accounts for up to 50% of infertility in women with subfertility due to anatomical distortion, poor oocyte quality, and altered endometrial receptivity [12]. MetS impairs ovulation and pregnancy outcomes through insulin resistance and obesity [13].

When combined, these conditions increase the risk of infertility, miscarriage, gestational diabetes, preeclampsia, preterm birth, and placenta previa [14, 15]. Mental health burdens are also heightened, with women experiencing increased depression, anxiety, and a diminished quality of life [16].

6. Clinical implications

From a clinical perspective, women with endometriosis should be screened for MetS and vice versa. Integrated diagnostic models, incorporating both gynecological and metabolic assessments, are needed. Prognostically, co-occurrence worsens reproductive outcomes, elevates cardiovascular risk, and complicates treatment decisions [17].

Therapeutically, hormonal treatments for endometriosis may aggravate metabolic dysfunction, while insulin sensitizers such as metformin may improve both conditions [13]. Multidisciplinary management is essential, involving gynecologists, endocrinologists, cardiologists, and mental health professionals [18].

7. Therapeutic horizons and emerging strategies

Emerging therapeutic strategies targeting shared molecular and metabolic pathways are outlined in **Figure 3**.

Emerging therapies target shared disease pathways: metabolic modulators (metformin, glycolytic inhibitors, mitochondrial-targeted drugs) [19, 20],

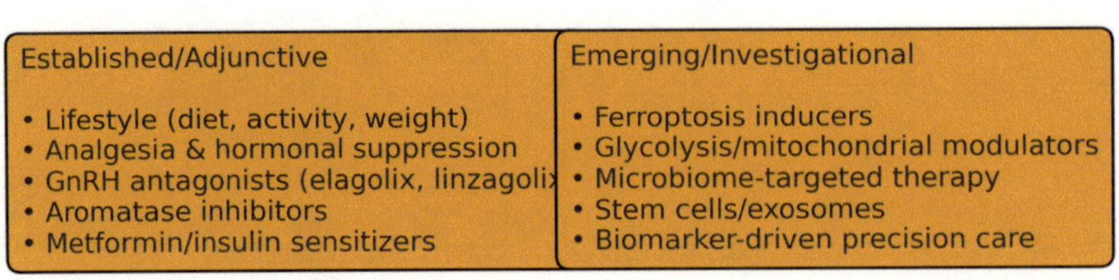

Figure 3.
Therapeutic horizons in metabolic syndrome and endometriosis.

ferroptosis inducers (preclinical) [21], hormonal refinements (oral GnRH antagonists, aromatase inhibitors) [22, 23], regenerative medicine (stem cell/exosome-based) [24, 25], microbiome interventions [26], and precision medicine using biomarkers/genomics [9].

8. Management of reproductive health and infertility

A comprehensive clinical algorithm for fertility management in women with co-existing metabolic syndrome and endometriosis is illustrated in **Figure 4**.

8.1 Evaluation

Women should undergo a complete fertility assessment [27] alongside a metabolic evaluation [5]. EFI (endometriosis fertility Index) scoring assists in prognosis for endometriosis [28]. The EFI is a clinical tool and validated scoring system that predicts non-assisted reproductive technologies pregnancy following surgical evaluation when the patient has functional gametes and uterus used. The following are the parameters considered in the EFI scoring[28]:

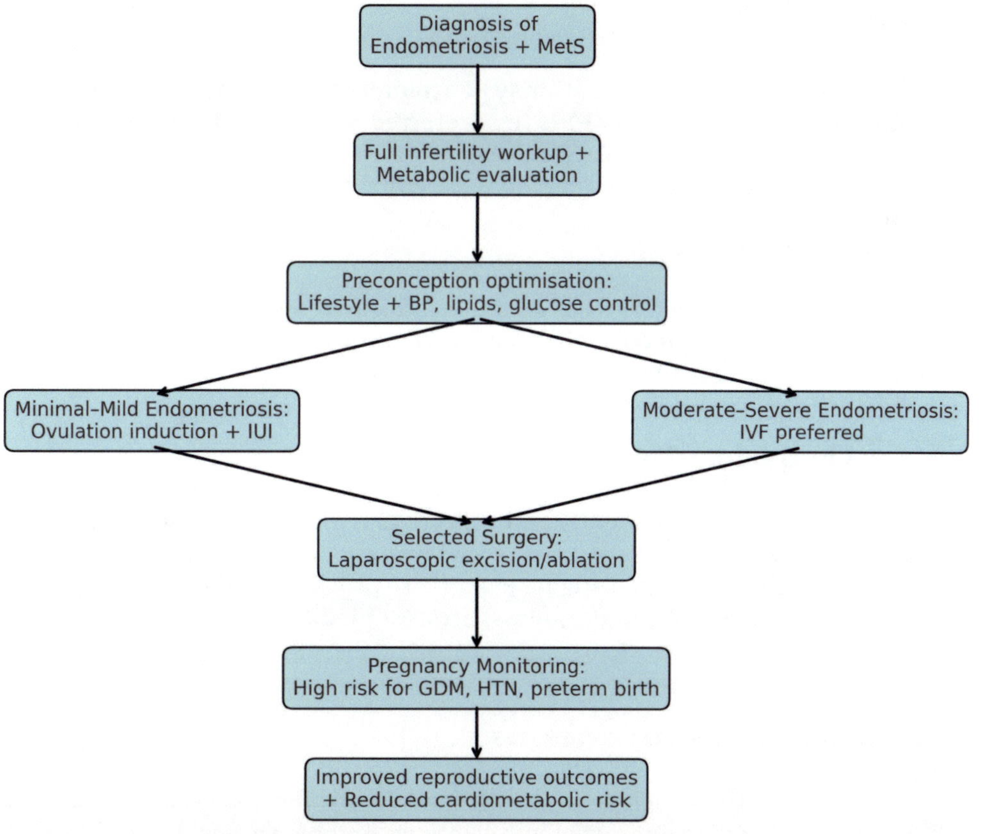

Figure 4.
Clinical management algorithm for fertility in co-occurrence of mets and endometriosis.

1. Historical factors (50%): This includes: Age: 2 points for ≤ 35 years, 1 point for 36–39 years, and 0 points for ≥ 40 years. Years of infertility: 2 points for ≤ 3 years and 0 points for > 3 years. Prior pregnancy: 1 point for yes and 0 points for no.

2. Surgical findings (30%): This assesses the extent of endometriosis and adhesions, with scores ranging from 0 to 5 points based on the severity of the condition and damage to the tubes.

3. rAFS scores (20%): The revised American Fertility Society (rAFS) staging system evaluates the extent of endometriosis.

   The EFI score ranges from 0 to 10 and correlates with estimated pregnancy rates at 1 and 3 years. For instance:

   EFI score 9–10: 67% pregnant at 1 year and 75% at 3 years.

   EFI score 7–8: 39% pregnant at 1 year and 66% at 3 years.

   EFI score 0–3: 10% pregnant at 1 and 3 years.

8.2 Preconception care

Optimization of cardiometabolic health through lifestyle modification and metabolic control is essential before conception [29].

8.3 ART

Intrauterine Insemination (IUI) may be attempted in minimal-to-mild disease, while In Vitro Fertilization (IVF) is the preferred option in advanced endometriosis [30]. In MetS, ART success is improved by prior weight and metabolic optimization [31].

8.4 Pregnancy management

Women face heightened risks of gestational diabetes mellitus (GDM), hypertensive disorders, preterm birth, and adverse neonatal outcomes [15]. Multidisciplinary antenatal monitoring is mandatory.

9. Mental health impacts and quality of life

Both conditions, independently and collectively, impair quality of life, causing high levels of depression, anxiety, and social dysfunction [32, 33]. Chronic pain, infertility, and obesity-related stigma exacerbate psychological burdens [34]. Interventions include CBT, mindfulness, lifestyle modification, and patient-centered care [35].

10. Emerging therapeutic strategies

Therapeutic horizons include metabolic modulators, ferroptosis inducers, stem cell therapies, microbiome-targeted interventions, and biomarker-driven

DOI: http://dx.doi.org/10.5772/intechopen.1013379

personalized medicine. Integration of these approaches into clinical practice requires robust clinical trial validation [20, 36].

11. Management of reproductive health in co-occurrence

Women with both MetS and endometriosis require tailored fertility management. Assisted reproductive technology (ART) strategies should be chosen according to the disease stage and metabolic status, with an emphasis on preconception optimization [18]. Surgery may aid fertility in select cases but carries the risk of ovarian reserve depletion [37].

12. Diagnosis of endometriosis

There are various methods proposed for the diagnosis of endometriosis, including clinical history and physical examination, radiological diagnostic imaging, surgical visualization with histopathological confirmation, and blood-based biomarkers (ongoing research) [38, 39]. **Table 1** summarizes strengths, limitations, and diagnostic accuracy.

12.1 Delay in endometriosis diagnosis

Diagnostic delays of 4–12 years are well-documented [41–43], exacerbated in resource-limited settings [43, 44]. This delay has significant clinical and socioeconomic consequences, including substantial productivity losses and healthcare costs [42]. Laparoscopy with histology remains the gold standard, although it is costly and invasive [45]. While potential biomarkers exist, none have been validated for routine clinical use, particularly in African populations [46].

12.2 Clinical examination

Routine clinical vaginal examination alone is insufficient for definitive diagnosis, though it may assist in localizing lesions and determining disease severity [40]. Symptoms are non-specific and vary with lesion location; common features include chronic pelvic pain, severe dysmenorrhea, dyspareunia, cyclical GI/urinary symptoms, dyschezia, and infertility in 30–50% of cases, with ~ 20–25% asymptomatic [47, 48].

13. Biomarkers for endometriosis

Promising but not yet clinically validated biomarkers include circulating microRNAs (miRNAs), CA-125, CA19-9, MIF, and inflammatory cytokines; performance is inconsistent across studies [49–60]. The inflammatory nature of endometriosis, with elevated peritoneal cytokines, guides biomarker research [61]. Accurate, non-invasive biomarkers could reduce delays and burden [46, 62]. **Table 2** depicts the summaries of the studies conducted to investigate an overview of endometriosis biomarkers and their limitations[46, 51, 53, 55].

Diagnostic method	Advantages/ benefits	Limitations	Sensitivity (Sn)	Specificity (Sp)	Notes
Clinical history and physical exam	Non-invasive; inexpensive; useful for initial suspicion and directing work-up	Non-specific symptoms; low reliability for staging or mapping disease	76–98% (history); 18–88% (exam)	20–58% (history); 76–100% (exam)	Suggests presence; advanced disease may be detected on exam
Ultrasound (transvaginal/ abdominal)	Widely available; anatomic mapping; high accuracy for ovarian endometrioma; dynamic assessment (sliding sign)	Operator-dependent; limited for superficial peritoneal disease; exam may be uncomfortable	OE: ~ 93%; DE: ~ 79%; SE: 65–79%	OE: ~ 96%; DE: ~ 94%; SE: 91–95%	Principal pelvic imaging modality; excellent for cystic disease and DIE mapping with expertise
MRI	High-resolution, reproducible images; excellent for deep endometriosis and extrapelvic sites; preoperative mapping	Static assessment; protocol variability; bowel depth assessment imperfect; higher cost and limited access	76–95% (overall; subtype-dependent)	87–98% (overall; subtype-dependent)	Useful for severe disease and extrapelvic involvement; complements ultrasound
CT/plain radiography	CT helpful for alternative diagnoses in acute abdomen; plain films rarely contributory	Not preferred for endometriosis; nonspecific findings for endometriomas; radiation exposure (CT)	–	–	Use selectively to rule out other conditions; not a primary diagnostic tool for endometriosis
Laparoscopy with histology (gold standard)	Definitive diagnosis; allows simultaneous treatment and lesion mapping	Invasive; surgical risk; diagnostic accuracy varies with surgeon experience and lesion heterogeneity	High (visual 90–94%; definitive with histology)	High (definitive with histology)	Decision based on symptoms, exam, and imaging; histology confirms
Biomarkers (blood/saliva/ menstrual)	Potential non-invasive triage tools; objective measures	No validated single marker; variability with cycle and lab methods; limited phenotype discrimination	Varies by marker/ panel	Varies by marker/ panel	Promising panels (e.g., miRNAs) under investigation; not yet for routine diagnosis

Sources: Pascoal et al. [38]; Woodward et al. [39]; Hudelist et al. [40].

Table 1.
Summary of current diagnostic modalities for endometriosis.

13.1 MicroRNAs (miRNA)

miRNAs regulate gene expression and may serve as diagnostic indicators [63]. Dysregulated miRNAs (e.g., miR-200b family, let-7b, miR-135a, miR-125b-5p) have been linked to endometriosis pathogenesis and show diagnostic potential in serum/

Biomarker type	Biomarker(s)	Sample/fluid	Key findings	Limitations
Glycoprotein	CA-125, CA19-9	Serum	Elevated particularly in moderate–severe disease; widely studied legacy markers	Non-specific; elevated in many gynecologic/ inflammatory conditions
Immune/ inflammatory	CA-125 + neutrophil-to-lymphocyte ratio (NLR)	Serum	Combination improved diagnostic value vs. CA-125 alone	Needs reproducibility; thresholds vary across studies
Multi-marker panels	CA-125 + MIF ± MCP-1 + leptin	Serum	Panels can improve accuracy in subsets of patients	Small cohorts; require external validation
Transcriptomics/ proteomics	Gene/protein panels	Endometrium	Altered expression profiles distinguish cases from controls	Primarily research setting; standardization lacking
miRNAs	Multiple circulating miRNAs	Serum/ plasma	Consistent dysregulation patterns; potential for non-invasive testing	Heterogeneity among panels; no clinical validation yet
Menstrual effluent	Transcriptomic markers	Menstrual blood	Promising, patient-friendly source for molecular testing	Experimental; protocols not standardised

Sources: Baloyi [46], Xavier et al. [53]; Cho et al. [54]; Seeber et al. [55]; Fassbender et al. [56]; Wang et al. [57]; Warren et al. [58]; Vanhie et al. [59].

Table 2.
Studies investigating biomarkers for endometriosis – overview and limitations.

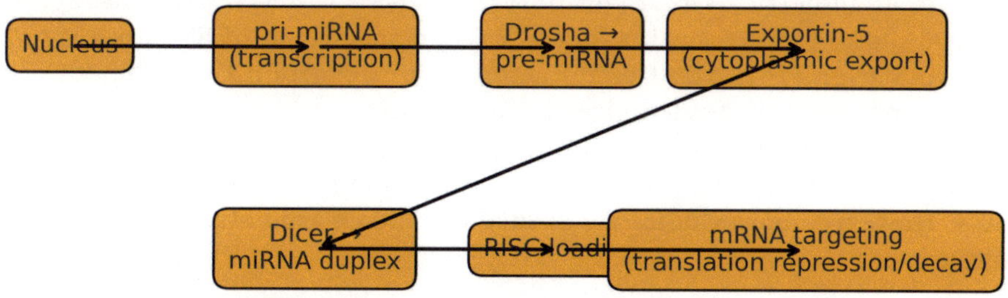

Figure 5.
MicroRNA biogenesis and mechanism of action [65].

plasma profiling [49–52, 64–67]. **Figure 5** depicts microRNA biogenesis and the mechanism of action [65]. Summaries of reported sensitivity/specificity appear in **Tables 3** and **4** [66].

13.2 Hormonal markers

Hormone-related markers (estradiol, progesterone, leptin, LH, activin) have shown variable results; none are consistent for diagnosis [61, 66, 68]. Aromatase

Source (year)	Dysregulated miRNA(s)	Sensitivity (%)	Specificity (%)	Notes
Maria et al. (2010)	miR-200a, miR-200b, miR-141	84.4	66.7	
Maria et al. (2010)	miR-22	90.0	90.0	
Jia et al. [50]	miR-17-5p	60.0	80.0	Downregulated
Jia et al. [50]	miR-20a	60.0	90.0	Downregulated
Jia et al. [50]	miR-145	70.0	96.0	
Wang et al. (2013)	miR-122	80.0	76.0	
Wang et al. (2013)	miR-199a	78.3	76.0	
Wang et al. (2013)	miR-141-5p	71.7	96.0	
Suryawanshi et al. (2013)	miR-195, miR-16	88.0	60.0	
Suryawanshi et al. (2013)	miR-191, miR-200a-3p	71.9	70.8	
Rekker et al. (2015)	miR-200b-3p	70.8	90.6	
Rekker et al. (2015)	miR-141-3p	71.9	70.8	
Cosar et al. [52]	miR-125b	100.0	96.0	Array-based analysis

Sources: Jia et al. [50]; Cho et al. [51]; Cosar et al. [52]; Vanhie et al. [59]; Anastasiu et al. [66].

Table 3.
Diagnostic performance of dysregulated circulating miRNAs in endometriosis (selected studies).

expression has been proposed but remains debated [69–71]. Prolactin may be elevated in endometriosis-related infertility [72, 73]. Meta-analysis suggests aromatase shows pooled sensitivity of 79% and specificity of 89%, but it requires further validation [74]. Additional mechanistic background on aromatase and estrogen synthesis is provided elsewhere [75–78].

The combined diagnostic precision [74] of the studies investigating hormonal use as biomarkers for the non-invasive diagnosis of endometriosis is summarised in **Table 4**. However, more studies are needed to validate aromatase as a biomarker for endometriosis.

14. Conclusion

Women with endometriosis should be screened for metabolic syndrome and its components to prevent long-term health complications. Women with endometriosis are at a higher risk of developing metabolic syndrome, characterised by high triglycerides, hypertension, and insulin resistance. Lifestyle interventions, such as diet and exercise, may help reduce the risk of metabolic syndrome in women with endometriosis. By addressing both endometriosis and metabolic syndrome, healthcare providers can improve fertility outcomes and overall health for infertile women with these conditions.

Index test	No. of studies	Sample size	Sensitivity (95% CI)	Specificity (95% CI)	PLR (95% CI)	NLR (95% CI)	DOR (95% CI)
Aromatase	13	858	0.79 (0.71–0.86)	0.89 (0.82–0.94)	7.22 (4.26–12.24)	0.23 (0.16–0.33)	31.27 (15.70–62.29)
HCG/LH receptor	1	45	0.30 (0.18–0.46)	0.80 (0.65–0.90)	1.49 (0.64–3.47)	0.82 (0.33–2.09)	1.56 (0.24–10.19)
ER-α	1	90	0.75 (0.66–0.83)	0.47 (0.34–0.60)	1.41 (1.09–1.82)	0.54 (0.36–0.81)	2.62 (1.42–4.84)
ER-β	1	90	0.65 (0.56–0.74)	0.68 (0.55–0.80)	2.05 (1.39–3.04)	0.51 (0.38–0.69)	4.03 (2.14–7.58)
Serum prolactin	2	187	0.45 (0.38–0.52)	0.92 (0.85–0.97)	4.86 (2.40–9.82)	0.59 (0.39–0.91)	10.22 (4.35–24.05)
EST	1	68	0.69 (0.51–0.83)	0.30 (0.16–0.49)	0.98 (0.72–1.35)	1.04 (0.51–2.11)	0.95 (0.34–2.66)
17β-HSD2	1	53	0.73 (0.60–0.84)	0.48 (0.33–0.63)	2.38 (0.04–138.12)	0.53 (0.36–0.79)	3.22 (0.18–56.39)

Abbreviations: OE, ovarian endometriosis; DE, deep endometriosis; SE, superficial endometriosis; DIE, deep infiltrating endometriosis; PLR, positive likelihood ratio; NLR, negative likelihood ratio; DOR, diagnostic odds ratio.

Table 4.
Grouped diagnostic accuracy of hormonal biomarkers for endometriosis [74].

Author details

Shisana M Baloyi
School of Medicine, Faculty of Health Sciences, University of Limpopo, Polokwane, South Africa

*Address all correspondence to: shisana.baloyi@ul.ac.za

References

[1] Grundy SM. Metabolic syndrome update. Trends in Cardiovascular Medicine. 2016;**26**(4):364–373

[2] Zondervan KT, Becker CM, Missmer SA. Endometriosis. Lancet. 2020;**395**(10227):730–743

[3] Hu Z, Li S, Liu L, Xu X, Song Y, Wei Y, et al. Endometriosis and risk of metabolic syndrome: Cross-sectional and Mendelian randomization study. Human Reproduction 2020;**35**: 2105–2111

[4] World Health Organization. Endometriosis: Fact Sheet. 2021. [Accessed: 2025-September-02]

[5] Alberti KGMM, Eckel RH, Grundy SM, Zimmet PZ, Cleeman JI, Donato KA, et al. Harmonizing the metabolic syndrome: A joint interim statement. Circulation 2009;**120**:1640–1645

[6] Esser N, Legrand-Poels S, Piette J. Inflammation as a link between obesity, metabolic syndrome and type 2 diabetes. Diabetes Research and Clinical Practice. 2014;**105**(2):141–150

[7] Bulun SE. Endometriosis. The New England Journal of Medicine. 2019;**380** (13):1244–1256

[8] Guo SW, Wang Y. Sources of heterogeneities in estimating the prevalence of endometriosis in infertile and previously fertile women. Fertility and Sterility. 2006;**86**(6):1584–1595

[9] Rahmioglu N, Nyholt DR, Morris AP, Missmer SA, Montgomery GW, Zondervan KT. Genetic variants underlying risk of endometriosis. Human Reproduction Update. 2019;**25**(2):228–248

[10] Vercellini P, Vigano P, Somigliana E, Fedele L. Endometriosis: Pathogenesis and treatment. Nature Reviews Endocrinology. 2014;**10** (5):261–275

[11] Kvaskoff M, Mu F, Terry KL, Harris HR, Poole EM, Farland LV, et al. Endometriosis: A high-risk population for major chronic diseases? Human Reproduction Update 2021;**27**:821–845

[12] de Ziegler D, Borghese B, Chapron C. Endometriosis and infertility: Pathophysiology and management. The Lancet. 2010;**376** (9742):730–738

[13] Palomba S, Santagni S, Falbo A, La Sala GB. Complications and challenges associated with PCOS: Current perspectives. International Journal of Women's Health. 2015;7:745–763

[14] Zullo F, Spagnolo E, Saccone G, Acunzo M, Xodo S, Ceccaroni M, et al. Endometriosis and obstetric complications. Fertility and Sterility 2017;**108**:667–672

[15] Liu L, Zhang W, Liu Y, Huang Q, Liang Y. Endometriosis and adverse pregnancy outcomes: A systematic review and meta-analysis. Reproductive Biology and Endocrinology. 2018;**16** (1):82

[16] Facchin F, Barbara G, Dridi D, Alberico D, Buggio L, Somigliana E, et al. Mental health in women with endometriosis. Human Reproduction 2015;**30**:1119–1125

[17] Farland LV, Prescott J, Sasamoto N, Tobias DK, Gaskins AJ, Stuart JJ, Carusi DA, Chavarro JE, Horne AW, Rich-Edwards JW, Missmer SA. Endometriosis and risk of adverse pregnancy outcomes. Obstetrics and Gynecology. 2019;**134**(3):527–536

[18] ESHRE Guideline Group on Endometriosis. ESHRE guideline: Endometriosis. Human Reproduction Open. 2022;**2022**(2): hoac009

[19] Cheng J, Li C, Ying Y, Lv J, Qu X, McGowan E, Lin Y, Zhu X. Metformin alleviates endometriosis and potentiates endometrial receptivity via decreasing VEGF and MMP9 and increasing leukemia inhibitor factor and HOXA10. Frontiers in Pharmacology. 2022;**13**:750208

[20] Zhao Y, Sun H, Feng M, Zhao J, Zhao X, Wan Q, Cai D. Metformin is associated with reduced cell proliferation in human endometrial cancer by inbibiting PI3K/AKT/mTOR signaling. Gynecological Endocrinology. 2018;**34**(5):428–432

[21] Li Y, Zeng X, Lu D, Yin M, Shan M, Gao Y. Erastin induces ferroptosis via ferroportin-mediated iron accumulation in endometriosis. Human Reproduction. 2021;**36**(4):951–964

[22] Taylor HS, Giudice LC, Lessey BA, Abrao MS, Kotarski J, Archer DF, Diamond MP, Surrey E, Johnson NP, Watts NB, Gallagher JC. Treatment of endometriosis-associated pain with elagolix, an oral GnRH antagonist. New England Journal of Medicine. 2017;**377** (1):28–40

[23] Donnez J, Taylor HS, Taylor RN, Akin MD, Tatarchuk TF, Wilk K, Gotteland JP, Lecomte V, Bestel E. Treatment of endometriosis-associated pain with linzagolix, an oral gonadotropin-releasing hormone–antagonist: A randomized clinical trial. Fertility and Sterility. 2020;**114**(1):44–55

[24] Maruyama T, Yoshimura Y. Stem cell theory for the pathogenesis of endometriosis. Frontiers in Bioscience. 2012;**4**:2754–2763

[25] Yao Y, Chen R, Wang G, Zhang Y, Liu F. Exosomes derived from mesenchymal stem cells reverse EMT via TGF-β1/Smad pathway and promote repair of damaged endometrium. Stem Cell Research and Therapy. 2019;**10** (1):225

[26] Ata B, Yildiz S, Turkgeldi E, Brocal VP, Dinleyici EC, Moya A. The Endobiota Study. Scientific Reports. 2019;**9**:2204

[27] Practice Committee of the American Society for Reproductive Medicine. Endometriosis and infertility: A committee opinion. Fertility and Sterility. 2012;**98**(3):591–598

[28] Adamson GD, Pasta DJ. Endometriosis fertility index. Fertility and Sterility. 2010;**94** (5):1609–1615

[29] Legro RS, Dodson WC, Kunselman AR, Stetter CM, Kris-Etherton PM, Williams NI. Delayed fertility therapy after preconception weight loss in obese women with PCOS. The Journal of Clinical Endocrinology and Metabolism. 2015;**100** (4):1619–1628

[30] Barnhart K, Dunsmoor-Su R, Coutifaris C. Effect of endometriosis on IVF. Fertility and Sterility. 2002;**77** (6):1148–1155

[31] Bellver J, Pellicer A, García-Velasco JA. Obesity and ART outcomes. Reproductive BioMedicine Online. 2010;**21**(4):433–446

[32] Culley L, Law C, Hudson N, Denny E, Mitchell H, Baumgarten M, et al. The social and psychological impact of endometriosis. Human Reproduction Update 2013;**19**:625–639

[33] Nnoaham KE, Hummelshoj L, Webster P, d'Hooghe T, de Cicco Nardone F, de Cicco Nardone C, Jenkinson C, Kennedy SH, Zondervan KT, Study WERFG. Impact of endometriosis on quality of life and work productivity: A multicenter study across ten countries. Fertility and Sterility. 2011;**96**(2):366–373

[34] Moradi M, Parker M, Sneddon A, Lopez V, Ellwood D. Impact of endometriosis on women's lives: A qualitative study. BMC Women's Health. 2014;**14**(1):1–12

[35] Stefanaki C, Bacopoulou F, Livadas S, Kandaraki A, Karachalios A, Chrousos GP, Diamanti-Kandarakis E. Impact of a mindfulness stress management program on stress, anxiety, depression and quality of life in women with polycystic ovary syndrome: A randomized controlled trial. Stress. 2015;**18**(1):57–66

[36] Johnson NP, Hummelshoj L. World Endometriosis Society Montpellier Consortium. Consensus on current management. Human Reproduction. 2022;**37**(3):400–410

[37] Raffi F, Metwally M, Amer S. The impact of excision of ovarian endometrioma on ovarian reserve: A systematic review and meta-analysis. The Journal of Clinical Endocrinology and Metabolism. 2012;**97**(9):3146–3154

[38] Pascoal E, Wessels JM, Aas-Eng MK, Abrao MS, Condous G, Jurkovic D, et al. Strengths and limitations of diagnostic tools for endometriosis. Ultrasound in Obstetrics & Gynecology 2022;**60**:309–327

[39] Woodward PJ, Sohaey R, Mezzetti Jr TP. Endometriosis: Radiologic-pathologic correlation. RadioGraphics. 2001;**21**(1):193–216

[40] Hudelist G, Fritzer N, Staettner S, Tammaa A, Tinelli A, Sparic R, et al. TVUS vs clinical exam in deep endometriosis. Ultrasound in Obstetrics & Gynecology 2011;**37**:480–487

[41] Ballard K, Lowton K, Wright J. What's the delay? Fertility and Sterility. 2006;**86**(5):1296–1301

[42] Schenken RS. Delayed diagnosis of endometriosis. Fertility and Sterility. 2006;**86**(5):1305–1306

[43] Hudelist G, Fritzer N, Thomas A, Niehues C, Oppelt P, Haas D, et al. Diagnostic delay in Austria and Germany. Human Reproduction 2012;**27**:3412–3416

[44] Ghai V, Jan H, Shakir F, Haines P, Kent A. Diagnostic delay in the United Kingdom. Journal of Obstetrics and Gynaecology. 2020;**40**(1):83–89

[45] Vercellini P, Vigano P, Somigliana E, Fedele L. Endometriosis: Pathogenesis and treatment. Nature Reviews Endocrinology. dup. of ref 10; cited once. 2014; **10**(5):261–275.

[46] Baloyi S. Non-invasive diagnosis of endometriosis: The quest for a diagnostic biomarker. Obstetrics and Gynaecology Forum. 2020;**30**(1):1–2

[47] Ballard KD, Seaman HE, de Vries CS, Wright JT. Symptomatology and diagnosis. BJOG. 2008;**115** (11):1382–1391

[48] Bulletti C, Coccia ME, Battistoni S, Borini A. Endometriosis and infertility. Journal of Assisted Reproduction and Genetics. 2010;**27**(8):441–447

[49] Naqvi H, Mamillapalli R, Krikun G, Taylor HS. Endometriosis located proximal to or remote from the uterus differentially affects uterine gene expression. Reproductive Sciences. 2016;**23**(2):186–191

[50] Jia SZ, Yang Y, Lang J, Sun P, Leng J. Plasma miR-17-5p, miR-20a and miR-22 in endometriosis. Human Reproduction. 2013;**28**(2):322–330

[51] Cho S, Mutlu L, Grechukhina O, Taylor HS. Circulating microRNAs as potential biomarkers for endometriosis. Fertility and Sterility. 2015;**103** (5):1252–1260

[52] Cosar E, Mamillapalli R, Ersoy GS, Cho S, Seifer B, Taylor HS. Serum microRNAs as diagnostic markers. Fertility and Sterility. 2016;**106** (2):402–409

[53] Xavier P, Beires J, Belo L. CA-125 and CA19-9 cut-offs. European Journal of Obstetrics and Gynecology and Reproductive Biology. 2005;**123** (2):254–255

[54] Cho S, Cho H, Nam A, Kim HY, Choi YS, Park KH, Cho DJ, Lee BS. Neutrophil-to-lymphocyte ratio as an adjunct to CA-125 for the diagnosis of endometriosis. Fertility and Sterility. 2008;**90**(6):2073–2079

[55] Seeber B, Sammel MD, Fan X. Marker panel to predict endometriosis. Fertility and Sterility 2008;**89**(5), 1073–1080

[56] Fassbender A, Vodolazkaia A, Saunders P, Lebovic D, Waelkens E, De MB, et al. Combined mRNA microarray and proteomics. Human Reproduction 2012;**27**:2020–2029

[57] Wang L, Huang W, Ren C, Zhao M, Jiang X, Fang X. Serum microRNA profile in endometriosis. Reproductive Sciences. 2016;**23**(10):1359–1370

[58] LA W, Shih A, SM R, Seckin T, Blau B, Simons SS, et al. Menstrual effluent analysis. Molecular Medicine. 2018;**24**:1

[59] Vanhie A, O D, Peterse D, Kyama C, Fassbender A, Meuleman C, et al. Plasma miRNAs as biomarkers. Human Reproduction. 2019;**34**:1650–1660

[60] Nisenblat V, et al. Blood Biomarkers for Endometriosis (Cochrane). 2016. [details needed: full citation]

[61] Giudice LC, Kao LC. Endometriosis. The Lancet. 2004;**364** (9447):1789–1799

[62] Agrawal S, Tapmeier TT, Rahmioglu N, Kirtley S, Zondervan KT, Becker CM. The miRNA Mirage. International Journal of Molecular Sciences. 2018;**19**(2):599

[63] Santamaria X, Taylor H. MicroRNA and gynecological reproductive diseases. Fertility and Sterility. 2014;**101**(6):1545–1551

[64] Eggers JC, Martino V, Reinbold R, Sd S, Kiesel L, Schüring AN, et al. miR-200b and endometriotic cells.

Reproductive BioMedicine Online 2016;**32**:434–445

[65] Ryan B, Joilin G, Williams JM. Plasticity-related microRNA. Frontiers in Molecular Neuroscience. 2015;**8**:4

[66] Anastasiu CV, Moga MA, Neculau AE, Bălan A, Scârneciu I, Dragomir RM, et al. Biomarkers for non-invasive diagnosis. International Journal of Molecular Sciences 2020;**21**:1750

[67] Condrat CE, Thompson DC, Barbu MG, Bugnar OL, Boboc A, Cretoiu D, et al. miRNAs as Biomarkers in Disease. Cells. 2020;**9**:276

[68] Liu Y, Shi X, Xu B, Wang Z, Chen Y, Deng M. Differential expression of plasma derived exosomal miRNAs in polycystic ovary syndrome as a circulating biomarker. Biomedical Reports. 2023;**19**(6):92

[69] Kitawaki J, Noguchi T, Amatsu T, Yamamoto T, Okada H, Honjo H. Aromatase P-450 in endometrial biopsy. Fertility and Sterility. 1999;**72** (6):1100–1106

[70] Dheenadayalu K, Mak I, Gordts S, Campo R. Aromatase mRNA in eutopic endometrium not specific. Fertility and Sterility. 2002;**78**(4):825–829

[71] Kitawaki J, Noguchi T, Amatsu T, Maeda K, Tsukamoto K, Yamamoto T, et al. Aromatase in endometriotic/adenomyotic tissues. Biology of Reproduction 1997;**57**:514–519

[72] Cunha-Filho JSLD, Gross JL, Lemos NA, Brandelli A, Castillos M, Passos EP. Hyperprolactinemia and luteal insufficiency in infertile patients with mild and minimal endometriosis. Hormone and Metabolic Research. 2001;**33**(04):216–220

[73] Lima AP, Moura MD, Rosa E Silva AAM. Prolactin and cortisol in endometriosis. Brazilian Journal of Medical and Biological Research. 2006;**39**(8):1121–1127

[74] Gao Y, Liu X, Gu Y, Song D, Ding M, Liao L, Wang J, Ni J, He G. The effect of bisphosphonates on fracture healing time and changes in bone mass density: A meta-analysis. Frontiers in Endocrinology. 2021;**12**:688269

[75] Simpson ER, Mahendroo MS, Means GD, Kilgore MW, Hinshelwood MM, Graham-Lorence S, Amarneh B, Ito Y, Fisher CR, Michael MD, Mendelson CR. Aromatase cytochrome P450, the enzyme responsible for estrogen biosynthesis. Endocrine Reviews. 1994;**15**(3):342–355

[76] Coumailleau P, Kah O. Cyp19a1 expression in Xenopus brain. Journal of Neuroendocrinology. 2014;**26** (4):226–236

[77] Bouchoucha N, Samara-Boustani D, Pandey AV, Bony-Trifunovic H, Hofer G, Aigrain Y, et al. Novel CYP19A1 (aromatase) R192H mutation. Molecular and Cellular Endocrinology. 2014;**390**:8–17

[78] Simpson ER. Aromatase: Biologic relevance of tissue-specific expression. In: Seminars in Reproductive Medicine. **22**. New York, NY, USA: Seventh Avenue; 2004. p. 11–23

Chapter 7

The Development of Metabolic Syndrome on Individuals Suffering from Substance Use Disorders: A Systematic Review

Matome Michael Sekhotha, Tlou Russel Senosha and Maanda Ravhutendele

Abstract

The development of substance use disorder (SUD) is a worldwide. People that suffer from SUD has the potential of manifestation of metabolic syndrome (MetS). Obesity/overeating and the development of SUD share numerous similarities. The development of SUD use can lead to a variety of negative health issues, including manifestation of metabolic syndromes. To study will be to investigate the development of metabolic syndrome in individuals suffering from substance use disorders using existing literature. Data from previously published articles were collected and analysed to illustrate the development of metabolic syndrome of people suffer from the development of SUD. Data was collected using different search strategies applying combinations of various keywords related to the MetS and SUD. According to our research, those with SUD had better lipid profiles and reduced body weight and adiposity. Lower blood glucose levels were linked to opiate use in people with diabetes mellitus. Several authors from different countries showed that there were significant differences between people that suffer from SUD that might cause MetS. These were shown by both odds' ratio and hazard ratio in different studies. Given that SUD, diabetes mellitus (DM), and hypertension are among the leading causes of the global burden of disease, the comorbid MetS with drug use is important. There is adequate evidence that show that during administration and/or withdrawal from adulterated drug significance modification of in nourishment choice and intake occur, with negative or positive health consequence.

Keywords: obesity, dyslipidaemia, hypertension cardiovascular disease, heroin, ecstasy, methamphetamine, marijuana, substance use disorder, mental issues

1. Introduction

According to United Nation of Drug and Crime (UNODC) there is a significant public health issues can result from the use of illegal opioids, and these issues have been found in numerous nations worldwide [1]. The risk of death and crude mortality rates for opioid users are significantly higher than those of the global population. In the US, obesity and people suffering from SUD are two major epidemics that pose serious public health concerns [2]. It was discovered that opioid addicts have MetS around the start of the twenty-first century [3]. The metabolic syndrome is a collection of disorders that collectively raise the risk of development of other health outcomes like stroke, Type 2 diabetes (T2DM), and cardiovascular disease (CVDs). An individual's danger of disease and death from cardiovascular diseases (CVDs) and type 2 diabetes is increased when these metabolic abnormalities co-occur [4, 5]. The people that have MetS are likely to acquire one of the MetS symptoms [5, 6]. Whereby T2DM is most predominant for people that suffer from MetS [7–9].

A significant public health burden that affects many individuals globally is the emergence of metabolic syndrome [10]. This health effects due to MetS become much more severe with the persons that suffer from the development of substance use disorder (SUD). Therefore, is crucial to understand the physiological connection between the development of MetS and substance use utilised problem. The same brain circuits that regulate appetite also govern the metabolism of the tainted medications. Thus, the compulsive drug use linked to addiction and the lack of control and excessive food consumption linked to obesity are instances of brain mechanisms [11, 12]

The rising prevalence, declining disability-adjusted life years, and significant socioeconomic impact of substance use and substance use disorders are contributing to their growing status as a global public health issue [13]. As stated by World Drug Report 2021, approximately 13% of 275 million people drug users in the preceding year were diagnosed with substance use disorders. In 2019, substance use disorders claimed about 0.01% were directly attributable to substance use disorders, and illegal drugs [14].

Arnaud and Thomasius [15] and Martini et al. [16] stated that substance use as the regular use of any substance, including alcohol and/or psychoactive drugs, in amounts (or in methods) that are harmful to the user. Substance abuse is frequently linked to varied levels of intoxication, which is linked to changes in perception, judgement, and attention. Alcohol, illegal drug, and prescription medicine usage have all been linked to negative impact on an individual's productivity and health, as well as a significant financial burden on the family and society [17, 18]. Substance abuse and disorders are becoming increasingly frequent over the world, and this is causing an increase in morbidity and mortality. Africa's most commonly used illegal substances such as benzodiazepines, amphetamine-type stimulants, and cannabis with prevalence rates ranging from 5.2% to 13.5% in West and Central Africa [19].

The disruption of brain dopamine (DA) pathways, which drive behavioural responses to external stimuli, resides at the heart of these two ailments [20, 21]. Dopamine neurones are found in the ventral tegmental area (VTA), substantia nigra pars compacta (SN), and other midbrain nuclei that project to the striatal (dorsal striatum and nucleus accumbens, or NAc), limbic (amygdala and hippocampus), and cortical (prefrontal cortex, cingulate gyrus, and temporal pole) regions (Appendix A). They control the motivation and persistence of effort required to carry out survival behaviours [22]. In order to perform their functions, DA neurones use a variety of neurotransmitters and peptides to receive projections from brain regions related to autonomic responses [23] (i.e., the brainstem and hypothalamus), memory (hippocampus) [24], emotional reactivity (amygdala) [25], arousal (thalamus) [26], and cognitive control (prefrontal cortex and cingulate) [26]. As a result, it is not surprising that peptides that effect food intake influence drug reinforcing effects, and that neurotransmitters connected to drug-seeking behaviours are likewise linked to food consumption.

A variety of peripheral and central systems influence the regulation of eating behaviours and, as a result, food reactions, with the hypothalamus playing a particularly important role [27, 28]. This is in stark contrast to medications, which act through direct pharmacological effects in the brain's reward DA pathway (NAc and ventral pallidum). Peripheral signals, including hormones and peptides like insulin, leptin, cholecystokinin (CCK), and tumour necrosis factor- α , as well as nutrients like sugars and lipids, travel to the nucleus solitary tract via vagus nerve afferents and receptors in the hypothalamus and other autonomic and limbic brain regions.

Food is consumed when it is needed thanks to these several signalling channels, even in the event that one of these redundant systems malfunctions. However, after being repeatedly exposed to extremely appetising food, some people may eventually overcome the inhibitory processes [29]. These processes may indicate fullness and start eating excessively despite being overfed, and in the case of humans, they may even become repulsed by this behaviour. Therefore, this loss of control and obsessive eating behaviour, which is similar to the drug consumption patterns observed in addiction, obesity has been referred to as a type of "food addiction" [30].

The system that influences food and drug intake is intricately linked [30]. These intricately relationship may include the following components:

- Food-responsive hormones and peptides
- The hypothalamus' energy homeostatic structures,
- The ventral tegmental area
- Striatum's dopamine reactive system core,
- Different cortical regions responsible for processing affect, motor, and cognitive information

Unlike medications that directly impact the brain's reward dopamine pathway. But food first influences several peripheral and central mechanisms that both directly and indirectly transmit information to the brain's DA reward pathway. In this context, the hypothalamus is especially important, even if it is also closely related to drug reward [31].

When the similar reinforcement is encountered, the brain's DA reward system, which regulates reactions to the environment, makes it more likely that activities that activate it such as eating or using drugs will be repeated [32]. Although there are distinct differences between the biological mechanisms that impair the role of the DA striatal circuits, such as those linked to reward (ventral striatum) and habit formation (dorsal striatum), disruption of the DA reward circuit has been linked to the loss of control observed in both addiction and obesity.

Furthermore, self-control and compulsive consumption (of food or drugs) occur along a dimensional continuum that is highly context-influenced and can range from complete control to no control at all. These are dynamic and adaptable brain processes, as evidenced by the fact that the same person can exercise greater control in some situations than others. A pathological state resembling the idea of addiction can be evoked when these patterns (loss of control and compulsive intake) become inflexible and control the person's behaviour and decisions in spite of their negative effects. However, most people who overeat maintain control over their food intake in some situations but not in others, just as the majority of drug users are not addicted [33–35]. The argument over whether obesity reflects "food addiction," however, ignores the multifaceted character of these two conditions.

2. Objectives

The aim of this research is to investigation the development of metabolic syndrome on individuals suffering from substance use disorders.

The purpose of this systematic review is to assess and synthesise previous studies that focused on the manifestation of metabolic syndrome in people that suffers from the development of SUD.

3. Methodology

Data from previously published articles were collected and analysed to illustrate the development of metabolic syndrome in patients with substance use disorders. This was structured according to Prisma Guidelines (**Table C1**). Different keywords will be used to retrieve articles from different search engines.

4. Registration and protocol

The review was not registered with any organization.

4.1 Study selection

The abstract was initially identified using keywords. If the abstract passes the first condition, the entire article will be downloaded for additional review. The downloaded article will be investigated further to determine its relevance to this project. The piece will be reviewed again to ensure that it addresses the intended issues. The approach, findings, analysis, limitations, and recommendations were examined and documented. The primary goal will be to explore the development of metabolic syndrome in patients who have substance abuse issues. The findings, debate, and conclusion formed the basis for the article's main point.

4.2 Eligibility criteria (inclusion and exclusion criteria)

The total of 37 studies were chosen for full assessment out of the more than 200 abstracts that were screened to ascertain whether all inclusion requirements were satisfied (Appendix B). Due to their failure to satisfy all the inclusion criteria listed below, 56 were finally disqualified (Appendix B). Twenty-one papers were included in this review because they satisfied all inclusion requirements. The review was carried out by five researchers. In order to minimise inter-rater selection bias, a data extraction form was created to gather information from every research.

The study will include nearly all the full-text publications that have been made since the inspection. Additionally, the research needs to fulfil the requirements given in **Table 1**. Articles that satisfied the requirements in **Table 1** were excluded. The publications were published in English and only appeared in peer-reviewed journals. Using comparable keyword sets, studies were taken out of each database. To complete the manuscript compilation, a last search was carried out from 1985 to 2025. Additional articles were discovered by applying a snowball method to those that met one or both requirements listed in **Table 2**.

No	Criterion
1	Disclosure of the inclusion criteria in the publication and review protocol guarantees openness and enables readers to evaluate the review's rigour.
2	**Only studies published in the last 10 year**
3	Other researchers can duplicate the review procedure and guarantee the validity of the results when the criteria are well-defined.
4	Studies like observational studies, qualitative research, or randomised controlled trials (RCTs) are usually included based on their design.
5	The article/s should have the ethical approval
6	The precise results being assessed, such functional abilities, quality of life, or clinical changes in health, are specified.
7	The study participants' attributes, including age, gender, diagnosis, and health status, are specified

Table 1.
An acceptable article was chosen to be featured in the results section using the information.

No	Criterion
1	Do not use the specific intervention being investigated
2	Non peer reviewed literature
3	Outcomes if they are self- reported rather than using objective measures
4	People that use insulin
5	People with have medical history of the metabolic syndrome condition
6	Reviews articles of other reviews that do not provide primary research data.
7	Studies that do not have enough data for analysis or that have unclear or insufficient results

Table 2.
The following exclusion guidelines were used to be removed from the study.

4.3 Information source

The following search engines: Google Scholar, PubMed, Semantic Scholar, Science.gov, and Ref Seek were the first computer-based searches used to find the studies that would form part of this review. Abstracts from EBSCO and Science Direct were also looked up. To fill in the gaps in the information, we tried to contact the authors of any papers with ambiguous or unreported parameters, such as the kind of adulterated drug with an unidentified name. The time frame covered was 2015–2025 Medical meeting abstracts were excluded.

4.4 Search strategies

The following search engines were used to find the published articles: Google, PubMed, Semantic Scholar, Google Scholar, Science.gov, and Ref Seek [36, 37]. The results section of the reviewed articles between 1985 and 2025, 250 were downloaded (Appendix A). The following keyword combination was used to select the relevant article: In order to obtain further information, such as publishing types and dates, any more related or common names were also used [36, 38]. The following keywords and the medical heading (MeSH) were used to build the search strategy: "Adulterated drugs," "Nyaope," "Heroin," "Crystal meth," "Methamphetamine," "Africa," "marijuana," "dagga," and "Cannabis" (Appendix B). in conjunction with the different types of metabolic syndromes conditions in **Figure 1**.

At least two or three keyword combinations were tried to find the pertinent articles. As part of the articles that employed original research data, only twelve (10) were found to be eligible for the study. Thus, to locate any publications that are pertinent to the current manuscripts. For the current manuscripts, we also used

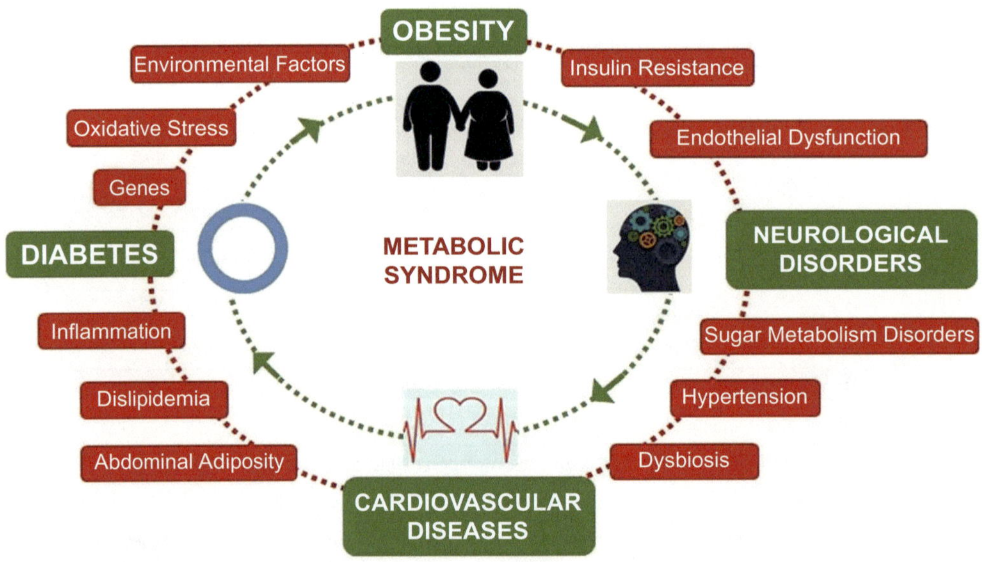

Figure 1.
The type of metabolic syndromes [39].

forward and backward citation searches. As mentioned earlier, we also use authors to search many databases for forward and backward citations. We also used the University of Limpopo library's facilities to seek additional articles.

Therefore, in order to filter the found articles, we modified the results section by utilising the records' title, abstract, and subject indexing. I then use those search phrases along with additional search terms I discovered during my inquiry to plan to find more articles. Furthermore, many search engines were used to locate and validate the search terms. The study was restricted to English-language publications and designed to reflect the metabolic syndrome and the development of the SUD (**Table C1**); all 10 articles were found using various Google search engines (Appendix B). The number of articles used, the author or authors and the year of publication, the city, type of adulterated drug used, statistical analysis, p-value (Confidence interval) and the health outcomes are the variables that will determine the focus; these variables are presented in a tabular format.

4.5 Selection process

Various databases were searched for relevant literature using a general appraisal form for systematic review papers. A variety of subheadings were also utilised for the appraisal worksheet, such as the study's limitations, the year it was published, sample size, outcomes, and the goals, aim, and objectives for the type of substance being used. Using Mendeley and Micro Software reference manager, duplicate entries were removed.

5. Data collection

A structural form was made with the following details to make sure that pertinent data for this systematic review was gathered, as indicated in **Table 2**.

5.1 Supplementary search techniques

We reviewed the bibliographies of all relevant studies to find additional citations. Citation searches (forward and backward) of important relevant papers were performed to locate additional relevant references and evaluate how relevant research are indexed. Because of the novelty of this issue, relevant publications were filtered using medical subject headings (MeSH) for "systematic reviews." Literature searches for future iterations of this living review will be modified on a regular basis to incorporate new papers and ensure that developing relevant findings are included.

5.2 Data items

The current project's components were not categorised as originating from different regions. Thus, the findings will, provide adequate evidences that illustrate the relationship between the development of metabolic syndrome/s and the development of substance use disorder.

5.3 Study risk of bias

The Downs and Black instrument (3) was used to assess bias. To find reporting bias, the tool's multiple domains were used.

5.4 Results of individual synthesis

The outcomes of the manuscripts will be to inform the readers that about the negative health effect of the brain due to the administration of adulterated drug. People that suffer from the development of substance use disorder (SUD) that might lead to the manifestation of metabolic syndrome.

5.5 Biases in reporting

The possibility of bias among the studies that could affect the total quantity of evidence was assessed by looking at the recommendations made by the research. All included papers that complied with the same guidelines were included in the preparation of this review.

5.6 Features of the study

This will cover the kinds of studies that are carried out using either human or animal models.

5.7 Bias risk in research

The Downs and Black tool for evaluating bias risk was used for this (3).

5.8 Findings from individual research

Refer to **Table 2** below.

5.9 Synthesis outcomes

Discussion compelled the results to be synthesised

6. Result

Given that substance use disorders (SUD), diabetes mellitus (DM), and hypertension are among the leading causes of the global burden of disease, the comorbid MetS with drug use is extremely important. The relationship between MetS and SUD, a reciprocal link is suggested. It is believed that substance abuse, genetic susceptibility, and nutritional deficits raise the risk of MetS. Mental health conditions including depression are more common among MetS patients. The development of MetS may result from the use of psychiatric medications for therapy. Psychoactive substances are also frequently used by depressed individuals to "self-medicate" in an attempt to feel better. The table below will them illustrate some of the relationship between MetS and people suffering from SUD due to administration of different types of adulterated drugs.

In a study conducted in the Republic of Macedonia showed that the joint influence of predictor factors, including age, length of heroin addiction, waist circumference, Brinkmann index, BMI, HOMA-IR, HOMA-B, TGl, HDL-C, diastolic and systolic blood pressure, glycemia, and gender, was examined in order to identify the predictors for MetS in [40]. Only the once that showed significant difference of p> 0.05 were presented in this project. For the HD group, the in-dependent factors (duration of HD, Brinkman index, BMI, HOMA-%B, age, HDL-C, diastolic and systolic blood pressure, glycemia, and gender) did not have a statistically significant impact as MetS predictors (**Table 3**). A 1cm increase in waist circumference raises the risk of metabolic syndrome by 3.12 (95% CI 1.41–6.89), making it the variable with the highest predictive value (**Table 2**). HOMA-IR is the second important risk factor since the probability of MetS rises by 1.5 (95% CI 1.02–2.45) for every unit increase. When paired with other predictors, a 1 mmol/l rise in TGl concentration raises the probability of developing MetS by 2.38 (95% CI 1.01–5.61). Although the probability of developing MetS rises by 1.2 (95%CI 0.86 - 1.88) for every year of age gain, this effect is not regarded as significant (p> 0.05). A total of 74.8% of MetS variability was impacted by all independent variables, whereas other factors accounted for 25.2% of MetS variability

In **Table 3**, displays the findings of the multivariate logistic regression analysis conducted by Vallecillo et al. (2018) with the intentions of showing the relationship of development of metabolic syndrome (MetS) amongst individuals with heroin use disorders on methadone therapy. Amongst the participants with heroin use disorder (HUD), BMI was a predictor of metabolic syndrome (odds ratio [OR] 1.49 for a 1 kg/m^2 increase in BMI) (**Table 3**). This study found that there was a higher prevalence of overweight and factors linked to weight fluctuations, including the use of cocaine and psychotropic medicines, as well as mental illness. This furthermore revealed that women were more likely to have abdominal obesity and men to have increased blood pressure.

A study by Seghatoleslam et al. [41] showed people who were experiencing the onset of SUD as a result of administration of heroin. The goal of this research was to compare the prevalence of mental disorders in two common chronic diseases caused by distinct pathologies – drug dependence and diabetes mellitus – to the general population. This was carried out in order to investigate the compatibility of the Symptom CheckList-90-R (SCL-90-R) and General Health Questionnaire-28 (GHQ-28) in identifying mental disorders. According to the GHQ-28 data showed the largest prevalence of mental disorders due to administration of heroin (41.60%, CI 95%: 35–48.1), followed by patients with diabetes mellitus (34.4%, CI 95%: 28.1–46.7) and the normal group (20.90%, CI 95%: 15.4–26.3). Both the Welch test (Welch = 21.507, P <0.01) and the Chi-Square analysis (X^2 = 21.61, P <0.001) showed no significant difference between heroin dependence and diabetic subjects for mental disorder rate (**Table 3**) This study by Seghatoleslam et al. [41], furthermore used a mix of questionnaires to measure the prevalence of mental disorders in patients with heroin dependence, patients with diabetes mellitus, and healthy individuals. SCL90-R and GHQ-28 were used to calculate combined indices, which were classified as negative (without mental disease) and positive (with psychiatric disorder). It was classified as a positive if any instrument identified a person as a positive case. The combined approach's rate of mental disorders in the research populations was shown in **Table 2**. Mental illnesses were present in 52.1% of heroin-dependent people, 49.5% of people with diabetes, and 23.2% of people in the healthy group when the combined index was taken into account. Furthermore, there was a considerable increase in the prevalence of mental disorders among individuals with diabetes mellitus and heroin dependency.

Metabolic syndrome (MetS) was found to be independently linked with lower eGFR, hyperuricemia, serum GGT> 50U/L, and age at admission in multivariate analysis (**Table 1**). In particular, eGFR and MetS had a dose-response effect that was statistically significant; patients with eGFR between 60 and 90 mL/min and those with eGFR <60mL/min were 1.93 (95% CI 1.18–3.15) and 5.61 (95% CI 1.66–19.0) times more likely to have MetS, respectively, than patients with eGFR> 90mL/min [42] (**Table 3**). Additionally, individuals with hyperuricemia (OR 2.28, 95% CI 1.36– 3.82) and those with serum GGT >50U/L (OR 3.67, 95% CI 1.80–7.46) had significantly higher risks of MetS than patients with normal blood GGT levels. Furthermore, for every year of age rise, MetS was strongly correlated with age (OR 1.03; 95% CI 1.01–1.05) [42].

There was a substantial difference between the opium user and non-user in relation to metabolic syndromes in an Iranian study. In **Table 3**, displays the dose-response relationships between incidence type 2 diabetic mellitus (T2DM), Body mass Index (BMI), and waist circumference (WC) and cumulative opium usage (Nalini et al., 2023). Higher nokhod-years (a local unit equal to 0.2g) of opium use among current users were linked to lower waist circumference and BMI as well as a lower risk of incidence type 2 diabetes in both crude and adjusted models (P for trend <0.001), with the correlations being larger among current users than among former users Nalini et al., [43] (**Table 2**). Additionally, cumulative opium usage was associated with inverse dose-response relationships with BMI and waist circumference recorded five years later in the repeated-measurement phase (P for trend< 0.001; **Table 3**). As in the entire cohort, incident T2DM was found in this repeated measurement subsample among 6.5% of present opium users, 9.7% of previous users, and 10.5% of never users [43].

The pooled odds ratio for CVD was 2.27 (95% CI: 2.04–2.53) for males with DUD and 2.98 (95% CI: 2.52–3.52) for women. Both men [v2 (1)=36.14, p<0.001] and women [v2 (1)=42.33, p< 0.001] showed meaningful patterns suggesting that the risk of CVD was comparatively higher in younger age groups than in older ones. When compared to the general population, the odds ratio for having a history of cardiovascular disease (CVD) among DUD patients was 3.29 for men (95% CI 2.81– 3.84) and 5.90 for women (95% CI 4.70–7.35). These were the most notable demographic differences for both genders in the 35–44 age range. The discrepancies between people with and without cardiovascular disease. Patients with CVD reported taking prescription methadone more frequently [odds ratio (OR) = 4.055, p <0.001] and cannabis less frequently (OR = 0.487, p <0.001), and they also had a more severe history of drug use and social maladjustment (**Table 3**). Additionally, the patients were more likely to have a criminal record (OR = 1.306, p <0.001), be referred to methadone therapy (OR = 3.453, p <0.001), inject more frequently (OR = 2.207, p <0.001), or not answer the question about injection (OR = 2.453, p <0.001). Additionally, patients with CVD had lower odds of being men (OR = 0.711, p <0.001), being older (OR = 1.082 per year, p <0.001), and being employed or

7	Hernández-Rubio et al. [46]	Spain	Alcohol	Odd ratio = 8.08 (Univariate)	< 6		2.74; 23.8		metabolic syndrome
				Odd ratio = 3.56 (Univariate) Odd ratio = 3.67 (Multivariate)	> 50 (U/L		1.81; 6.99 1.80; 7.46		
				Odd ratio = 3.36 (Univariate) Odd ratio = 3.67 (Multivariate)			2.07; 5.45 1.80; 7.46		
8	Cusihuaman et al. [44]	Peru	Cannabis	N/A	Baseline = 153 to 225 30 min = 161 to 265 120 min = 150 to 225		184.52; 202 188.95; 209 172.48; 189		High-Density Lipoprotein (HDL), Low-Density Lipoprotein (LDL) and Cholesterol Concentration
					Baseline = 48 to 69 30 min = 48 to 75 120 min = 53 to 144		57.26; 62.8 59.89; 66.6 60.98; 77.3		
					Baseline = 106 to 159 30 min = 82 to 175 120 min = 81 to 166		123.30; 136 121.63; 139 115.81; 129		
9	Nalini et al., [43]	Iran	Opium	N/A	IRR = 0,62 βc = -3,326 βc =-6,354		2,49; 0,77 -3,664; -2,9 -7,224; -5,4		
10	Vallée, [49]	France	Cannabis	N/A	Woman	Men	Woman	Men	Arterial stiffness
					0.01	0.12	-0.13; 0.15	0.03;0.25	
					0.03	-0.02	-0.06; 0.12	-0.11;0.06	
					0.15	0.13	0.11; 0.19	0.08; 0.17	
					0.02	0.08	-0.03; 0.06	0.02; 0.13	
					0.02	0.04	0.01; 0.03	0.01; 0.05	
					0.024	0.01	0.020; 0.028	0.001; 0.02	
					0.27	0.26	0.21; 0.34	0.19; 0.33	
					0.01	0.05	-0.03; 0.07	0.01; 0.11)	

Table 3.
Extraction of data from existing scientific literature to illustrate the relationship between the administration of adulterated drugs and the development of different types of metabolic syndrome

enrolled in school (OR = 0.367, p <0.001). A history of CVD was less common in patients who had never experienced any treatment episodes (OR = 0.377, p <0.001).

The concentration of total cholesterol after using cannabis was 180.95±19.3mg/dL (95%CI 172.5 to 189.5) at 120 minutes and 199.15 ± 23.3mg/dL (95%CI 188.9 to 209.3) at 30 minutes. The baseline and 120-minute total cholesterol concentrations following cannabis usage differed (p = 0.007), however a study in Peru, did not show variations between the baseline and 30-minute concentrations (p = 0.254) [44]. There were also changes in HDL-C concentration following cannabis use (p <0.05), with increases at 30 and 120 minutes (63.25 ± 7.68mg/dL, 95%CI 59.8 to 66.6) (69.15 ± 18.67mg/dL, 95% CI 60.9 to 77.3) (**Table 3**) [44]. Only thirty minutes after consumption did the LDL-C analysis reveal alterations in its concentration (p = 0.002).

A study by Vallée [45], illustrated that the higher arterial stiffness (ASI) levels were linked to heavy lifetime cannabis use in males [b = 0.19 (0.02; 0.35)] but not in women [b = –0.02 (–0.23; 0.19)] after controlling for all factors in sex models (**Table 3**). Following control for all other variables, males [b = 0.17 (0.01; 0.32)] but not women [b = -0.01 (-0.20; 0.18)] who were current cannabis users had higher ASI levels. daily frequency was linked to higher ASI levels in men [b¼0.29 (0.07; 0.51)] but not in women [b = 0.10 (–0.17; 0.37)] among cannabis users (**Table 3**). Ultimately, A study by Vallée [45], discovered that ASI levels were positively correlated with heavy lifetime cannabis use, current cannabis use, and frequency of use in men, but not in women. The epidemiological study on this subject is the first of its kind. By using the ASI assessment, we may conclude that extensive lifetime cannabis use may contribute to men's elevated risk of atherosclerosis and, consequently, cardiovascular events.

7. Discussion

Drug misuse is often associated with significant health risk. While the others authors showed that drug abusers are at a higher risk of the development of metabolic syndrome (**Table 2**). The metabolic syndrome, a group of illnesses that includes high blood pressure [46], excessive blood sugar [47], excess belly fat [48], and abnormal cholesterol levels [49], are more likely to develop in people with substance use problems. Nutritional deficits and the harmful effects of some substances increase this risk. Drug misuse combined with nutritional deficiencies would raise the risk of metabolic syndrome by increasing cell damage, increasing excitotoxicity, decreasing energy generation, and diminishing the cells' antioxidant capability [50, 51]

It worth noting that people that suffers from SUD does not exclude the association of opioid use with IR and MetS, independently of BMI [52] (**Table 2**). MetS is linked to a higher risk of cardiovascular events and diseases; it also has a unique significance in heroin dependence, given that cardiovascular diseases seem to be a more important cause of morbidity and mortality in this population group than infectious diseases.

Numerous reports exist on the connection between the development of metabolic syndrome and administration of adulterated drug. In study in by Pereska et al. [40], showed the relationship between 24 hours insulin resistance (IR24) and MetS amongst people suffering from the development of SUD. This study investigation found that Homeostatic Model Assessment for Insulin Resistance (HOMA-IR) in heroin dependents with MetS (HDM+) was considerably greater than in MSD. These finding suggested that IR in people suffering from SUD [53], but glycemia was insignificantly higher non HDM+ compared to significantly higher insulinemia [40] (**Table 2**). An increasing number of reports have described the intricate mechanism of IR, and some of them even mention the effects of opioids, such as their influence on transport molecules, receptor levels, adipocyte hormones, and insulin-degradation enzymes.

Zinc insufficiency in HD is the main reason why disturbed diet, and its composition might impair glucose control, and a 6-year study found that the length of heroin use was correlated with a drop in zinc concentrations [54]. Zinc is a metal loprotease that is present in the insulin degrading enzyme and is necessary for the catalytic activity of the enzyme. In addition to heroin metabolism's de-sensitizing effect on insulin receptors and induction of insulin resistance, zinc deficiency would decrease the activation of the insulin-degrading enzyme during prolonged heroin use, which could result in decreased hormone degradation [55]. The degree and kind of substance usage, the specific toxicity profile of the drug or substance in question, and the individual's overall risk factor profile all influence the likelihood of causing metabolic syndrome. In general, amphetamines have an impact on the neurological and cardiovascular systems that might cause MetS. Acute methamphetamine misuse can cause CNS symptoms such as agitation and sleeplessness, as well as psychomotor symptoms including excessive speech and hyperactivity, depending on the level of intoxication and duration of use [56, 57]

Methamphetamine (meth), MDE (3,4-methylenedioxyethamphetamine), and "ecstasy" are examples of commonly misused amphetamine medications that alter brain metabolism by causing cerebellar hypermetabolism and cortical hypometabolism [57, 58]. Stimulant activity accounts for a portion of their effects on brain cells, but these drugs' inherent toxicity may also play a role. Meth is a highly addictive and neurotoxic stimulant that is often abused. It results in the death of dopaminergic and serotonergic neurons in the brain, potentially through processes such increased oxidative stress [59] and the production of reactive oxygen and nitrogen species, which raise excitotoxicity and mitochondrial malfunction. When combined with environmental pollutants and nutritional deficiencies, drug addiction can impact cellular defenses and accelerate the progression of disease. Reduced energy production, diminished antioxidant capability, and excitotoxicity would be the main causes of this toxicity and elevated risk of cell damage [60, 61].

Abuse-related drugs impact the metabolism of glucose, one of the cellular energy requirements [62]. The metabolism of fatty and amino acids may also be impacted by such medications. According to positron emission tomography scans, glucose metabolism is higher in meth users' brain regions associated with anxiety and drug cravings but lower in those associated with depressive disorders [63], depression [64], and melancholy [65]. Rats' nucleus accumbens is one example of how long-term cocaine misuse increases cytochrome coxidase and, consequently, metabolic activity in reward regions of the brain. Meth has heart toxicity [56] and immunosuppressive [66] effects in addition to its effects on the neurological system [67]. The adult and developing myocardium are both harmed by meth and cocaine, and both substances can increase each other's toxicity *in vitro* Additionally, in animal trials, meth causes severe cardiac physiology and changes the function of cardiovascular reflexes. Meth can interfere with immune system function, which suppresses mitogen-stimulated lymphocytes and lowers the number of lymphocytes in circulation. In addition to affecting the immune system, it may also increase the likelihood of developing the metabolic syndrome by changing T cells and B-cell proinflammatory cytokine release [68].

Many disorders in the metabolic syndrome are influenced by genetic factors [69]. So, in addition to factors like age, sex, ethnicity, and the kind and severity of drug use, a person's genetic heritage will also affect how likely they are to develop metabolic syndrome as a result of drug misuse. Genetic polymorphism can have a good or detrimental impact, depending on the both development of SUD and acquiring metabolic syndromes Genetic polymorphism can have a good or detrimental impact, depending on the both development of SUD and acquiring metabolic syndromes [70] . Individual responses to the consequences of drug addiction are influenced by the presence or absence of specific alleles or by the existence of faulty alleles. Excessive substance use and substance use disorders (SUDs) are prevalent, significant, and recurrent medical illnesses. They frequently co-occur with other diseases that are the primary causes of disability worldwide. While severe substance use may worsen the course of several of these diseases, there is emerging evidence revealing similar genetic patterns.

The rate at which the drug is metabolized, whether by many genes or by increasing gene expression, determines its efficacy and toxicity, for instance. Epigenetic liability in response to the fetoplacental nutrition supply is likely to influence individual vulnerability [70]. The offspring may be more susceptible to the negative consequences of substance addiction and the emergence of metabolic syndrome if the mother has a nutritional imbalance and a resultant developmental disorder. Certain genetic indicators are linked to alcoholism [71, 72]. The degree of brain damage following long-term alcohol drinking, including in the superior frontal cortex, is likely also influenced by a particular genotype. Thus, the genotype of alcohol dehydrogenase affects the effectiveness of N-methyl-D-aspartate receptors, which in turn can affect neuronal damage and modify amino acid transmission locally [73, 74]

Certain risk factors, such the kind of food consumed, can have an impact on inflammation, intermediate metabolism, and cellular expression, which can both directly and indirectly harm vulnerable people [75]. Genes also influence how severe liver damage is following alcohol usage. The 67th Genes impact advanced alcoholic liver disease and nonalcoholic fatty liver disease in addition to environmental risk factors (level of alcohol consumption) [76]. This may be due to factors that impact the degree of oxidative stress and steatosis, the cytokine levels, the immune response, or the degree of fibrosis.

Alcohol and other substance use disorders (AUD and SUD) are complex diseases that are postulated to have a polygenic inheritance and are often comorbid with other disorders [76]. Alcohol usage and metabolic syndrome are common in the community and commonly coexist. Both are implicated in a wide spectrum of health issues. Oriental populations are also susceptible to alcoholic liver disease due to functional polymorphisms in the genes that produce alcohol dehydrogenases and aldehyde dehydrogenase. The impacted genes are believed to encode angiotensinogen, TNF-, transforming growth factor, CD14 endotoxin receptor, microsomal triglyceride transfer protein, and superoxide dismdismutase which have an underlying role in steatohepatitis and/or fibrosis [76].

The majority of studies on the acute effects of cannabis have been undertaken in recreational users. There is less information coming from clinical studies conducted in medicinal Cannabis users [77]. Despite the prevalence of Cannabis use for neurological illnesses [78], potential metabolic effects [79] have just lately been studied, and medical utility in metabolic. The association between the effects of *Cannabis sativa* and MetS occurred with the discovery of the endocannabinoid system, which emerged as a critical pathway in the regulation of energy balance [80]. It is currently one of the major contenders as a therapeutic target for the treatment of obesity and related disorders, where the hyperactivation and upregulation of Cannabinoid receptors type 1 (CB1) in central and peripheral systems play essential roles in metabolic disorders [81] (**Table 2**). In particular, CB1 is located at the level of the hypothalamic circuits that regulate food intake and the hunger/satiety balance and has been implicated in hyperphagia and weight gain. This has led to new compounds able to selectively block CB1, which have shown utility in weight control in obesity [82, 83], improving cardiovascular [84] risk factors at the experimental level.

Therefore, *Cannabis* preparations have significant therapeutic potential for neurologic [85] and metabolic diseases [79]. However, the use of this plant continues to be controversial, and studies that support its medical use in MetS are required, mainly through controlled clinical studies in MetS patients, rather than only in *Cannabis* users, as well as chemical studies to ameliorate the deleterious effects of *Cannabis* and its components. For this, it is essential to evaluate standardized *Cannabis* products in terms of rational and controlled use. Both CB1 antagonists with restrained passage into the brain and non-psychoactive phytocannabinoids represent a source of new therapeutic agents for the treatment of metabolic abnormalities.

8. Conclusion

Substance misuse is linked to serious health risks. Given the high prevalence of substance use, coexisting substance use and metabolic syndrome is a public health problem. Additionally, research is demonstrating a significant relationship between metabolism, addiction, and circadian rhythms. Along with excessive alcohol use, risk factors that put individuals with AUDs at higher risk for CVD include related bad lifestyle choices such insufficient physical exercise. Habitual substance use, i. e., alcohol, tobacco and betel nut, has been found with an increased risk of metabolic syndrome (MetS) in the general population. A number of population studies have implied that measures of central/abdominal obesity, such as the waist-to-hip ratio, can predict liver-related outcomes more accurately than BMI, including in individuals who consume harmful quantities of alcohol. Many studies even point to synergistic interactions between harmful alcohol use and many metabolic components. The intersection of these epidemics, such as the prevalence of obesity in persons with SUD, has been little explored in the most countries.

9. Limitations of the evidence included in the review.

This review only included literature related to systematic reviews, so articles examining meta-analyses that were not conducted within the context of a systematic review were eliminated. Furthermore, if an article's title or abstract did not clearly identify it as identifying difficulties with systematic reviews, it may have passed through the screening procedure without detection. In the studies included the definition of "'problematic'" systematic reviews may be considered subjective. This review emphasises on the issues with systematic reviews as outputs, rather than the efficiency of the systematic review process, which can be addressed by rapid review products. We set a relatively arbitrary criterion of 85% compliance for reporting or methodological guideline adherence to identify less-than-ideal conduct. The literature searches were restricted to research published after 2000, an arbitrary cut off point before which there were fewer centralised guidelines for systematic review conduct and reporting. Due to the abundance of published data, grey literature in the form of books and PhD theses was excluded from this review for feasibility reasons. A potential research recommendation could involve emphasis on unpublished data, which can assess the implications of publication bias on this review and provide access to even more detailed evaluations of systematic review concerns.

10. Limitations of the review processes used

It may include the following:

- Poor quality of included studies
- Lack of standardized criteria: Different reviewers may use varying standards or interpret guidelines differently.

Implications of the results for practice, policy, and future research.

The practice may include

- Early Detection and Screening
- Lifestyle-based interventions
- Policy changes and public health awareness

Future Research Direction may include

- Precision Medicine Approaches
- Longitudinal Studies
- Study shared biological pathways (e.g., inflammation, stress, HPA axis dysregulation)

Appendices

Appendix A

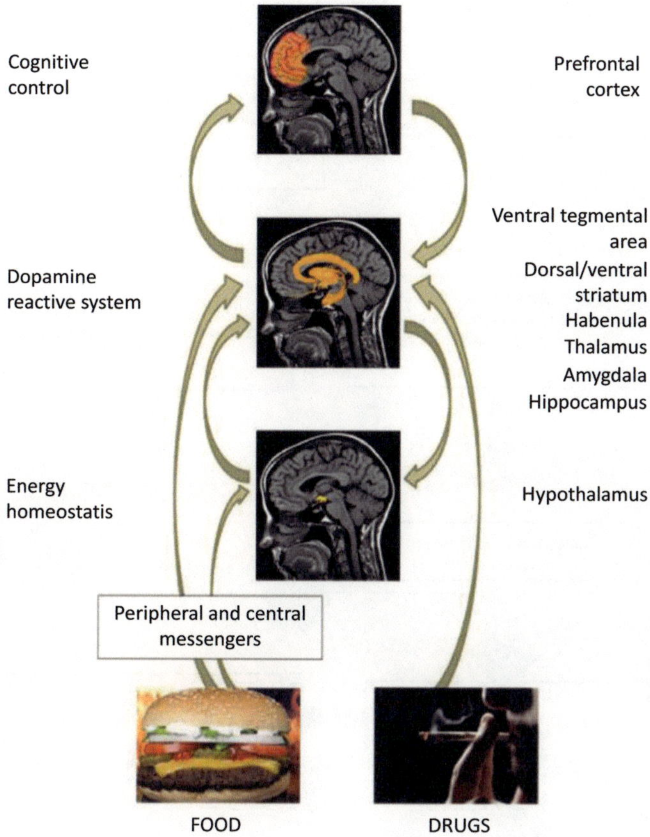

Figure A1.
The interconnection between administration adulterated drug and consumption food [31].

Appendix B

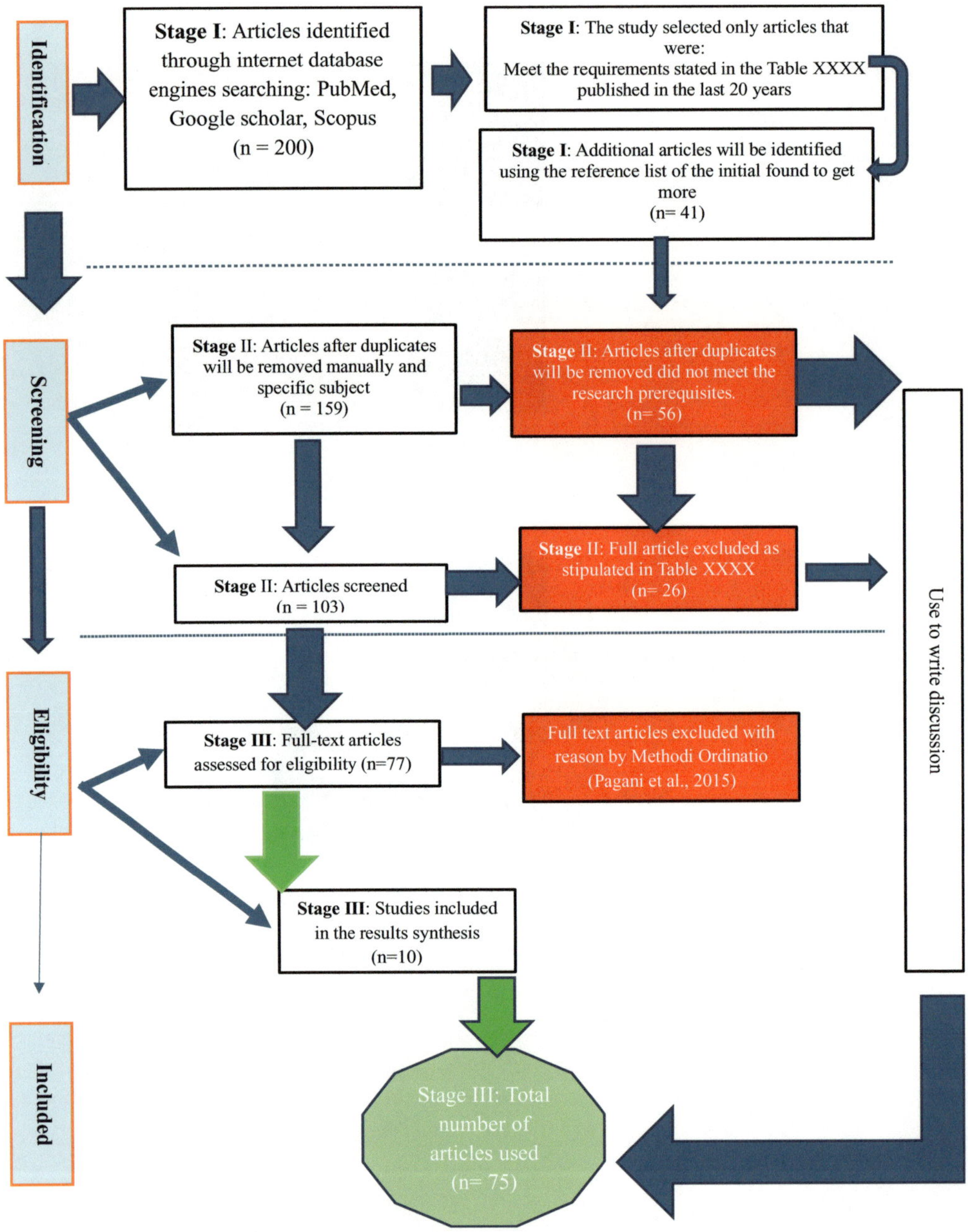

Flow diagram to illustrate the searching strategy.

DOI: http://dx.doi.org/10.5772/intechopen.1011739

Appendix C

Item	Criteria	Answers
	Reporting	
1	Is the aim/objective of the study clearly described?	Yes = 1
2	Are the main outcomes to be measured clearly described in the Introduction or Methods section? If the main outcomes are first mentioned in the Results section, the question should be answered "no".	Yes = 1
3	Are the characteristics of the patients included in the study clearly described? In cohort studies and trials, inclusion and/or exclusion criteria should be given. In case-control studies, a case-definition and the source for controls should be given.	Yes = 1
4	Are the interventions of interest clearly described? Treatmentsand placebo (where relevant) that are to be compared should be clearly described.	No = 0
5	Are the distributions of principal confounders in each group of subjects to be compared clearly described? A list of principal confounders is provided[a].	Partially = 1
6	Are the main findings of the study clearly described? Simple outcome data (including denominators and numerators) should be reported for all major findings so that the reader can check the major analyses and conclusions. (This question does not cover statistical tests which are considered below).	Yes = 1
	Reporting	
7	*Does the study provide estimates of the random variability in the data for the main outcomes?* In non-normally distributed data, the interquartile range of results should be reported. In normally distributed data the standard error, standard deviation or confidence intervals should be reported. If the distribution of the data is not described, it must be assumed that the estimates used were appropriate and the question should be answered yes[b].	No = 0
8	*Have all important adverse events that may be a consequence of the intervention been reported?* This should be answered yes if the study demonstrates that there was a comprehensive attempt to measure adverse events. (A list of possible adverse events is provided).	No = 0
9	*Have the characteristics of patients lost to follow-up been described?* This should be answered "yes" where there were no losses to follow-up or where losses to follow-up were so small that findings would be unaffected by their inclusion. This should be answered "no" where a study does not report the number of patients lost to follow-up.	No = 0
10	*Have actual probability values been reported (e.g. 0.035 rather than < 0.05) for the main outcomes except where the probability value is less than 0.001*[c]	No = 0

Item	Criteria	Answers
	External validity	
11	*Were the subjects asked to participate in the study representative of the entire population from which they were recruited?* The study must identify the source population for patients and describe how the patients were selected. Patients would be representative if they comprised the entire source population, an unselected sample of consecutive patients, or a random sample. Random sampling is only feasible where a list of all members of the relevant population exists. Where a study does not report the proportion of the source population from which the patients are derived, the question should be answered as unable to determine.	Unable to determine = 0
12	*Were those subjects who were prepared to participate representative of the entire population from which they were recruited?* The proportion of those asked who agreed should be stated. Validation that the sample was representative would include demonstrating that the distribution of the main confounding factors was the same in the study sample and the source population.	No = 0
13	*Were the staff, places, and facilities where the patients were treated, representative of the treatment the majority of patients receive?* For the question to be answered yes the study should demonstrate that the intervention was representative of that in use in the source population. The question should be answered no if, for example, the intervention was undertaken in a specialist centre unrepresentative of the hospitals most of the source population would attend.	No = 0
	Internal validity – bias	
14	*Was an attempt made to blind study subjects to the intervention they have received?* For studies where the patients would have no way of knowing which intervention they received, this should be answered "yes" [d].	Unable to determine = 0
15	*Was an attempt made to blind those measuring the main outcomes of the intervention[d]?*	Unable to determine = 0
16	*If any of the results of the study were based on "data dredging", was this made clear?* Any analyses that had not been planned at the outset of the study should be clearly indicated. If no retrospective unplanned subgroup analyses were reported, then answer "yes".	Unable to determine = 0
17	*In trials and cohort studies, do the analyses adjust for different lengths of follow-up of patients, or in case-control studies, is the time period between the intervention and outcome the same for cases and controls?* Where follow-up was the same for all study patients the answer should be "yes". If different lengths of follow-up were adjusted for by, for example, survival analysis the answer should be yes. Studies where differences in follow-up are ignored should be answered "no".	Unable to determine = 0
18	*Were the statistical tests used to assess the main outcomes appropriate?* The statistical techniques used must be appropriate to the data. For example nonparametric methods should be used for small sample sizes. Where little statistical analysis has been undertaken but where there is no evidence of bias, the question should be answered yes. If the distribution of the data (normal or not) is not described it must be assumed that the estimates used were appropriate and the question should be answered "yes".	Unable to determine = 0
19	*Was compliance with the intervention/s reliable?* Where there was noncompliance with the allocated treatment or where there was contamination of one group, the question should be answered no. For studies where the effect of any misclassification was likely to bias any association to the null, the question should be answered "yes".	Unable to determine = 0

Item	Criteria	Answers
	Internal validity – bias	
20	*Were the main outcome measures used accurate (valid and reliable)?* For studies where the outcome measures are clearly described, the question should be answered yes. For studies which refer to other work or that demonstrates the outcome measures are accurate, the question should be answered as "yes".	Unable to determine = 0
	Internal validity – confounding (selection bias)	
21	*Were the patients in different intervention groups (trials and cohort studies) or were the cases and controls (case-control studies) recruited from the same population?* For example, patients for all comparison groups should be selected from the same hospital. The question should be answered unable to determine for cohort and case-control studies where there is no information concerning the source of patients included in the study[d].	Unable to determine = 0
22	*Were study subjects in different intervention groups (trials and cohort studies) or were the cases and controls (case-control studies) recruited over the same period of time?* For a study which does not specify the time period over which patients were recruited, the question should be answered as unable to determine[d].	Unable to determine = 0
23	*Were study subjects randomized to intervention groups?* Studies which state that subjects were randomized should be answered yes except where method of randomization would not ensure random allocation. For example, alternate allocation would score no because it is predictable[d].	Unable to determine = 0
24	*Was the randomized intervention assignment concealed from both patients and health care staff until recruitment was complete and irrevocable?[d]* All nonrandomized studies should be answered no. If assignment was concealed from patients but not from staff, it should be answered "no".	Unable to determine= 0
25	*Was there adequate adjustment for confounding in the analyses from which the main findings were drawn?* This question should be answered no for trials if: the main conclusions of the study were based on analyses of treatment rather than intention to treat; the distribution of known confounders in the different treatment groups was not described; or the distribution of known confounders differed between the treatment groups but was not taken into account in the analyses. In non-randomized studies if the effect of the main confounders was not investigated or confounding was demonstrated but no adjustment was made in the final analyses the question should be answered as no.[d]	Unable to determine = 0
26	*Were losses of patients to follow-up taken into account?* If the numbers of patients lost to follow-up are not reported, the question should be answered as unable to determine. If the proportion lost to follow-up was too small to affect the main findings, the question should be answered yes.	No = 0
	Power	
27*	*Was a power analysis performed?[d]*	No = 0

**Modified from the original form published by Downs and Black.*
[a]Sex, age, hypertrophic lesions, Fitzpatrick skin phototype, and previous treatments were considered principal confounders that should be reported in both controlled and uncontrolled studies.
[b]Studies wherein all individual outcome scores have been reported but not variability parameters the item was answered yes (because variability parameters can be derived retrospectively).
[c]Item was answered 'yes' when no statistical tests were performed.
[d]Item number 14, 15, 21–25, and 27.

Section and Topic	Item #	Checklist item	Location where item is reported
		TITLE	
Title	1	Identify the report as a systematic review.	Pg 1
		ABSTRACT	
Abstract	2	See the PRISMA 2020 for Abstracts checklist.	Pg 1
		INTRODUCTION	
Rationale	3	Describe the rationale for the review in the context of existing knowledge.	Pg 2- 4
Objectives	4	Provide an explicit statement of the objective(s) or question(s) the review addresses.	Pg 4
		METHODS	
Eligibility criteria	5	Specify the inclusion and exclusion criteria for the review and how studies were grouped for the syntheses.	Pg5
Information sources	6	Specify all databases, registers, websites, organisations, reference lists and other sources searched or consulted to identify studies. Specify the date when each source was last searched or consulted.	Pg 6
Search strategy	7	Present the full search strategies for all databases, registers and websites, including any filters and limits used.	Pg 6 - 7
Selection process	8	Specify the methods used to decide whether a study met the inclusion criteria of the review, including how many reviewers screened each record and each report retrieved, whether they worked independently, and if applicable, details of automation tools used in the process.	Pg 7
Data collection process	9	Specify the methods used to collect data from reports, including how many reviewers collected data from each report, whether they worked independently, any processes for obtaining or confirming data from study investigators, and if applicable, details of automation tools used in the process.	Pg 7
Data items	10a	List and define all outcomes for which data were sought. Specify whether all results that were compatible with each outcome domain in each study were sought (e.g. for all measures, time points, analyses), and if not, the methods used to decide which results to collect.	Pg 7
	10b	List and define all other variables for which data were sought (e.g. participant and intervention characteristics, funding sources). Describe any assumptions made about any missing or unclear information.	Pg 7
Study risk of bias assessment	11	Specify the methods used to assess risk of bias in the included studies, including details of the tool(s) used, how many reviewers assessed each study and whether they worked independently, and if applicable, details of automation tools used in the process.	Pg 7
Effect measures	12	Specify for each outcome the effect measure(s) (e.g. risk ratio, mean difference) used in the synthesis or presentation of results.	N/A

Section and Topic	Item #	Checklist item	Location where item is reported
Synthesis methods	13a	Describe the processes used to decide which studies were eligible for each synthesis (e.g. tabulating the study intervention characteristics and comparing against the planned groups for each synthesis (item #5)).	N/A
	13b	Describe any methods required to prepare the data for presentation or synthesis, such as handling of missing summary statistics, or data conversions.	N/A
	13c	Describe any methods used to tabulate or visually display results of individual studies and syntheses.	Pg 8
	13d	Describe any methods used to synthesize results and provide a rationale for the choice(s). If meta-analysis was performed, describe the model(s), method(s) to identify the presence and extent of statistical heterogeneity, and software package(s) used.	N/A
	13e	Describe any methods used to explore possible causes of heterogeneity among study results (e.g. subgroup analysis, meta- regression).	N/A
	13f	Describe any sensitivity analyses conducted to assess robustness of the synthesized results.	N/A
Reporting bias assessment	14	Describe any methods used to assess risk of bias due to missing results in a synthesis (arising from reporting biases).	Pg 8
Certainty assessment	15	Describe any methods used to assess certainty (or confidence) in the body of evidence for an outcome.	N/A
		RESULTS	
Study selection	16a	Describe the results of the search and selection process, from the number of records identified in the search to the number of studies included in the review, ideally using a flow diagram.	Pg 4- 5
	16b	Cite studies that might appear to meet the inclusion criteria, but which were excluded, and explain why they were excluded.	Pg 4- 5
Study characteristics	17	Cite each included study and present its characteristics.	N/A
Risk of bias in studies	18	Present assessments of risk of bias for each included study.	N/A
Results of individual studies	19	For all outcomes, present, for each study: (a) summary statistics for each group (where appropriate) and (b) an effect estimate and its precision (e.g. confidence/credible interval), ideally using structured tables or plots.	Pg 10- 11

Section and Topic	Item #	Checklist item	Location where item is reported
Results of syntheses	20a	For each synthesis, briefly summarise the characteristics and risk of bias among contributing studies.	N/A
	20b	Present results of all statistical syntheses conducted. If meta- analysis was done, present for each the summary estimate and its precision (e.g. confidence/credible interval) and measures of statistical heterogeneity. If comparing groups, describe the direction of the effect.	Pg 10- 14
	20c	Present results of all investigations of possible causes of heterogeneity among study results.	N/A
	20d	Present results of all sensitivity analyses conducted to assess the robustness of the synthesized results.	N/A
Reporting biases	21	Present assessments of risk of bias due to missing results (arising from reporting biases) for each synthesis assessed.	N/A
Certainty of evidence	22	Present assessments of certainty (or confidence) in the body of evidence for each outcome assessed.	N/A
		DISCUSSION	
Discussion	23a	Provide a general interpretation of the results in the context of other evidence.	Pg 14-17
	23b	Discuss any limitations of the evidence included in the review.	
	23c	Discuss any limitations of the review processes used.	
	23d	Discuss implications of the results for practice, policy, and future research.	
		OTHER INFORMATION	
Registration and protocol	24a	Provide registration information for the review, including register name and registration number, or state that the review was not registered.	N/A
	24b	Indicate where the review protocol can be accessed, or state that a protocol was not prepared.	N/A
	24c	Describe and explain any amendments to information provided at registration or in the protocol.	N/A
NSupport	25	Describe sources of financial or non-financial support for the review, and the role of the funders or sponsors in the review.	None
Competing interests	26	Declare any competing interests of review authors.	None
Availability of data, code and other materials	27	Report which of the following are publicly available and where they can be found: template data collection forms; data extracted from included studies; data used for all analyses; analytic code; any other materials used in the review.	N/A

Table C1.
PRISMA guideline.

Author details

Matome Michael Sekhotha*, Tlou Russel Senosha and Maanda Ravhutendele
Department of Physiology and Environmental Health, University of Limpopo, Faculty of Science and Agriculture, School of Molecular and Life Science, Private Bag X 1106, Sovenga, Limpopo, South Africa

*Address all correspondence to: Michael.sekhotha@ul.ac.za

References

[1] UNODC. World Drug Report 2008. Vienna: United Nations: 2008

[2] Manchikanti L, Singh A. Therapeutic opioids: A ten-year perspective on the complexities and complications of the escalating use, abuse, and nonmedical use of opioids. Pain Physician. 2008;**11**: S63–S88

[3] Mattoo S, Chakraborty K, Basu D, Ghosh A, Vijaya Kumar K, Kul-hara P. Prevalence & correlates of metabolic syndrome in alcohol & opioid dependent inpatients. The Indian Journal of Medical Research. 2011;**134**:341–349

[4] Fahed G, Aoun L, Bou Zerdan M, Allam S, Bou Zerdan M, Bouferraa Y, Assi HI, et al. Metabolic syndrome: Updates on pathophysiology and management in 2021. International Journal of Molecular Sciences. 2022;**23**:786

[5] Hayden MR. Overview and New Insights into the metabolic syndrome: Risk factors and emerging variables in the development of Type 2 diabetes and Cerebrocardiovascular disease. Medicina (B Aires). 2023;**59**:561. DOI: 10.3390/medicina59030561

[6] Jaspers Faijer-Westerink H, Kengne AP, Meeks KAC, Agyemang C. Prevalence of metabolic syndrome in sub-Saharan Africa: A systematic review and meta-analysis. Nutrition, Metabolism and Cardiovascular Diseases. 2020;**30**:547–565. DOI: 10.1016/j.numecd.2019.12.012

[7] Roca-Sánchez-Moreno JD, Soto A, Núñez-Muñoz AL, De La Cruz-Vargas JA, Quiñones-Laveriano DM. Comparación de diferentes definiciones de síndrome metabólico y su relación con la estimación del riesgo cardiovascular. Revista de la Facultad de Medicina. 2021;70:e92602. DOI: 10.15446/revfacmed.v70n2.92602

[8] Nwankwo M, Okamkpa CJ, Danborno B. Comparison of diagnostic criteria and prevalence of metabolic syndrome using WHO, NCEP-ATP III, IDF and harmonized criteria: A case study from urban southeast Nigeria. Diabetes & Metabolic Syndrome: Clinical Research & Reviews. 2022; **16**: 102665. DOI: 10.1016/j.dsx.2022.102665

[9] Zong X, Kelishadi R, Kim HS, Schwandt P, Matsha TE, Mill JG, Caserta CA, Medeiros CCM, Kollias A, Whincup PH, Pacifico L, López-Bermejo A, Zhao M, Zheng M, Xi B, et al. A proposed simplified definition of metabolic syndrome in children and adolescents: A global perspective. BMC Medicine. 2024;**22**:190

[10] Noubiap JJ, Nansseu JR, Lontchi-Yimagou E, Nkeck JR, Nyaga UF, Ngouo AT, Tounouga DN, Tianyi F-L, Foka AJ, Ndoadoumgue AL, Bigna JJ, et al. Geographic distribution of metabolic syndrome and its components in the general adult population: A meta-analysis of global data from 28 million individuals. Diabetes Research and Clinical Practice. 2022;**188**:109924. DOI: 10.1016/j.diabres.2022.109924

[11] Gómez-Apo E, Mondragón-Maya A, Ferrari-Díaz M, Silva-Pereyra J, Weller A. Structural brain changes associated with overweight and obesity. Journal of Obesity. 2021;**2021**:1–18. DOI: 10.1155/2021/6613385

[12] Theilade S, Christensen MB, Vilsbøll T, Knop FK. An overview of obesity mechanisms in humans: Endocrine regulation of food intake, eating behaviour and common determinants of body weight. Diabetes Obesity and Metabolism. 2021;**23**:17–35. DOI: 10.1111/dom.14270

[13] Prom-Wormley EC, Ebejer J, Dick DM, Bowers MS. The genetic epidemiology of substance use disorder: A review. Drug and Alcohol Dependence. 2017;**180**:241–259. DOI: 10.1016/j.drugalcdep.2017.06.040

[14] Shao H, Du H, Gan Q, Ye D, Chen Z, Zhu Y, Zhu S, Qu L, Lu J, Li Y, Duan J, Gu Y, Chen M, et al. Trends of the Global burden of disease attributable to cannabis use disorder in 204 Countries and Territories, 1990–2019: Results from the Disease Burden Study 2019. International Journal of Mental Health and Addiction. 2024;**22**:2485–2507

[15] Arnaud N, Thomasius R. Substanzbezogene Störungen und Transitionspsychiatrie. Der Nervenarzt. 2022;**93**:341–350. DOI: 10.1007/s00115-022-01266-6

[16] Martini F, Fregna L, Bosia M, Perrozzi G, Cavallaro R. Fundamental Psychiatry Heal Care Professor. Cham: Springer International Publishing; 2022. 263–295 p. DOI: 10.1007/978-3-031-077 15-9_9

[17] Degenhardt L, Charlson F, Ferrari A, Santomauro D, Erskine H, Mantilla-Herrara A, Whiteford H, Leung J, Naghavi M, Griswold M, Rehm J, Hall W, Sartorius B, Scott J, Vollset SE, Knudsen AK, Haro JM, Patton G, Kopec J, et al. The global burden of disease attributable to alcohol and drug use in 195 countries and territories, 1990–2016: A systematic analysis for the global burden of disease study 2016. The Lancet Psychiatry. 2018;**5**:987–1012

[18] Densley J, McLean R, Deuchar R, Harding S. An altered state? Emergent changes to illicit drug markets and distribution networks in scotland. International Journal of Drug Policy. 2018;**58**:113–120. DOI: 10.1016/J.DRUGPO.2018.05.011

[19] Onaolapo OJ, Olofinnade AT, Ojo FO, Adeleye O, Falade J, Onaolapo AY. Substance use and substance use disorders in Africa: An epidemiological approach to the review of existing literature. World Journal of Psychiatry. 2022;**12**:1268–1286. DOI: 10.5498/wjp.v 12.i10.1268

[20] Kawahata I, Finkelstein DI, Fukunaga K. Dopamine D1–D5 receptors in brain nuclei: Implications for health and disease. Receptors. 2024;**3**:155–181. DOI: 10.3390/receptors3020009

[21] Azizi SA. Monoamines: Dopamine, Norepinephrine, and Serotonin, beyond modulation, "switches" that alter the state of Target Networks. Neurosci. 2022;**28**:121–143. DOI: 10.1177/1073858420974336

[22] Sartika S, Nirbita B. Academic resilience and students engagement in higher education: Study on post-pandemic behaviour. Educational Science Journal. 2023;**27**:29–34

[23] Aksu T, Gopinathannair R, Gupta D, Pauza DH. Intrinsic cardiac autonomic nervous system: What do clinical electrophysiologists need to know about the "heart brain"? Journal of Cardiovascular Electrophysiology. 2021;**32**:1737–1747. DOI: 10.1111/jce.15058

[24] Schwabe L, Hermans EJ, Joëls M, Roozendaal B. Mechanisms of memory under stress. Neuron. 2022;**110**:1450–1467. DOI: 10.1016/j.neuron.2022.02.020

[25] Padgaonkar NT, Phuong Uy J, DePasque S, Galván A, Peris TS. Neural correlates of emotional reactivity and regulation in youth with and without anxiety. Depression and Anxiety. 2021;**38**:804–815. DOI: 10.1002/da.23154

[26] Mashour GA, Pal D, Brown EN. Prefrontal cortex as a key node in arousal circuitry. Trends in Neurosciences. 2022;**45**:722–732. DOI: 10.1016/j.tins.2022.07.002

[27] Watts AG, Kanoski SE, Sanchez-Watts G, Langhans W. The physiological control of eating: Signals, neurons, and networks. Physiological Reviews. 2022;**102**:689–813. DOI: 10.1152/physrev.00028.2020

[28] Yousefvand S, Hamidi F. Role of lateral Hypothalamus area in the central regulation of feeding. International Journal of Peptide Research and Therapeutics. 2022;**28**:83. DOI: 10.1007/s10989-022-10391-4

[29] Bianco V, Veniero D, D'Acunto A, Koch G, Picazio S. Challenging inhibitory control with high- and low-calorie food: A behavioural and TMS study. Frontiers in Nutrition. 2023;**10**. DOI: 10.3389/fnut.2023.1016017

[30] Scholz H From natural behavior to drug screening: Invertebrates as models to study mechanisms associated with alcohol use disorders, 2023; DOI: 10.1007/7854_2022_413

[31] Gutierrez R, Lobo MK, Zhang F, de Lecea L. Neural integration of reward, arousal, and feeding: Recruitment of VTA, lateral hypothalamus, and ventral striatal neurons. IUBMB Life. 2011;**63**:824–830. DOI: 10.1002/iub.539

[32] Lewis RG, Florio E, Punzo D, Borrelli E. The Brain's Reward System in Health and Disease. In: Circadian clock in brain health and disease. Cham: Springer International Publishing; 2021. p. 57–69

[33] Robinson M. Eating ourselves to death: How food is a drug and what food abuse costs. Drug Science Policy Law. 2022;8. DOI: 10.1177/20503245221112577

[34] O'Connor RM, Kenny PJ. Utility of 'substance use disorder' as a heuristic for understanding overeating and obesity. Prog Neuro-Psychopharmacology Biol Psychiatry. 2022; **118**. 110580. DOI: 10.1016/j.pnpbp.2022.110580

[35] Ahmed SH, Avena NM, Berridge KC, Gearhardt AN, Guillem K. food addiction. neuroscience 21st Century. Cham: Springer International Publishing; 2022. pp. 4193–4218 DOI: 10.1007/978-3-030-88832-9_110

[36] Sekhotha M, Daniels W, Muller D, Malatswana S, Mathikhi K, Mokwena T, et al. Nyaope consumption by South African youth-reflections on the neglect of rehabilitation centres for substance use disorder: A systematic review. African Journal for Physical Activity and Health Sciences. 2023;**29**:89–117

[37] Michael Sekhotha MOL, Sekhotha T. The effect of administration of substance abuse among people suffering from substance use disorder on the digestive system: A systematic review. Metabolic Syndrome Lifestyle Biology Risk Factors, IntechOpen. 2024. DOI: 10.5772/intechopen.115034

[38] Daniels W, Sekhotha M, Morgan N, Manilall A. The cytotoxic effects of Nyaope, a heroin-based Street Drug, in SH-SY5Y Neuroblastoma Cells. IBRO Neuroscience Reports. 2024;**16**:280–290. DOI: 10.1016/j.ibneur.2024.01.014

[39] Martemucci G, Fracchiolla G, Muraglia M, Tardugno R, Dibenedetto RS, D'Alessandro AG. Metabolic syndrome: A narrative review from the oxidative stress to the management of related diseases. Antioxidants (Basel, Switzerland). 2023;**12**:2091. DOI: 10.3390/antiox12122091

[40] Pereska Z, Bozinovska C, Dimitrovski C, Cakalarovski K, Chibishev A, Zdravkovska M, Babulovska A, Janicevic D, et al. Heroin dependence duration influences the metabolic parameters: Mechanisms and consequences of impaired insulin sensitivity in hepatitis C virus seronegative heroin dependents. Journal of Addiction Medicine. 2012;**6**:304–310

[41] Seghatoleslam T, Ardakani A, Habil H, Rashid R. Comorbidity of mental disorder in patients with chronic disease: A comparative study of heroin dependence patients and diabetes Mellitus patients. Iranian Journal of Public Health. 2022. doi:10.18502/ijph.v51i1.8305

[42] Hernández-Rubio A, Sanvisens A, Bolao F, Cachón-Suárez I, Garcia-Martín C, Short A, Bataller R, Muga R, et al. Prevalence and associations of metabolic syndrome in patients with alcohol use disorder. Scientific Reports. 2022;**12**:2625

[43] Nalini M, Poustchi H, Roshandel G, Kamangar F, Khoshnia M, Gharavi A, Brennan P, Boffetta P, Dawsey SM, Abnet CC, Malekzadeh R, Etemadi A, et al. Association between incident type 2 diabetes and opium use: Mediation by body mass and adiposity. American Journal of Epidemiology. 2023;**192**:2050–2062

[44] Cusihuaman S, Moya-Salazar J, Wong-Salgado P, Moya-Salazar MM, Cañari B, Chicoma-Flores K, et al. Changes in High-Density Lipoprotein (HDL), Low-Density Lipoprotein (LDL) and cholesterol concentration in Heavy Cannabis users: A single-centre study in Cusco. Peru Processes. 2022;**10**:1597

[45] Vallée A. Association between lifetime cannabis use and arterial stiffness in a middle-aged general population. Journal of Hypertension. 2023;**41**:658–669. DOI: 10.1097/HJH.0000000000003389

[46] Litwin M, Kułaga Z. Obesity, metabolic syndrome, and primary hypertension. Pediatric Nephrology. 2021;**36**:825–837. DOI: 10.1007/s00467-020-04579-3

[47] Kawano Y, Edwards M, Huang Y, Bilate A, Araujo L, Tanoue T, Atarashi K, Ladinsky MS, Reiner SL, Wang HH, Mucida D, Honda K, Ivanov II, et al. Microbiota imbalance induced by dietary sugar disrupts immune-mediated protection from metabolic syndrome. Cell. 2022;**185**:3501–3519

[48] Witczak-Sawczuk K, Ostrowska L, Cwalina U, Leszczyńska J, Jastrzębska-Mierzyńska M, Hładuński M, Witczak-Sawczuk K, Ostrowska L, Cwalina U, Leszczyńska J, Jastrzębska-Mierzyńska M, Hładuński MK. Estimation of the impact of abdominal adipose tissue (Subcutaneous and Visceral) on the occurrence of carbohydrate and Lipid Metabolism Disorders in patients. Nutrients. 2024;**16**:1301

[49] Natesan V, Metabolism KSL. Disorders and Therapeutic Drugs - review. Biomolecules & Therapeutics. 2021;**29**:596–604

[50] Mahboub N, Rizk R, Karavetian M, de Vries N. Nutritional status and eating habits of people who use drugs and/or are undergoing treatment for recovery: A narrative review. Nutrition Reviews. 2021;**79**:627–635. DOI: 10.1093/nutrit/nuaa095

[51] Åberg F, Byrne CD, Pirola CJ, Männistö V, Sookoian S. Alcohol consumption and metabolic syndrome: Clinical and epidemiological impact on liver disease. Journal of Hepatology. 2023;**78**:191–206. DOI: 10.1016/j.jhep.2022.08.030

[52] Saxena J, Chilakapati R, Attia P, Rosenblum D, Weiss S. Body mass index trends among a cohort of subjects enrolled in medication-assisted treatment programmes for opioid use disorder: Racial/ethnic, gender, and age differences. Journal of Food Nutrition and Metabolism. 2023;**5**. DOI: 10.31487/j.JFNM.2022.01.01

[53] Mahboub N, Ayoub E, Mounzer C, Baltagi TK, Papandreou D, de Vries N, Rizk R, et al. Metabolic syndrome as a risk factor among lebanese patients with substance use disorder undergoing treatment for recovery through rehabilitation or Opioid substitution treatment. Clinics and Practice. 2024;**14**:2661–2680

[54] Barman S, Srinivasan K. Diabetes and zinc dyshomeostasis: Can zinc supplementation mitigate diabetic complications? Critical Reviews in Food Science and Nutrition. 2022;**62**:1046–1061. DOI: 10.1080/10408398.2020.1833178

[55] Sousa L, Guarda M, Meneses MJ, Macedo MP, Vicente Miranda H. Insulin-degrading enzyme: An ally against metabolic and neurodegenerative diseases. The Journal of Pathology. 2021;**255**:346–361. DOI: 10.1002/path.5777

[56] Tobolski J, Sawyer DB, Song SJ, Afari ME. Cardiovascular disease associated with methamphetamine use: A review. Heart Failure Reviews. 2022;**27**:2059–2065. DOI: 10.1007/s10741-022-10261-7

[57] Armenta-Resendiz M, Assali A, Tsvetkov E, Cowan CW, Lavin A. Repeated methamphetamine administration produces cognitive deficits through augmentation of GABAergic synaptic transmission in the prefrontal cortex. Neuropsychopharmacology. 2022;**47**:1816–1825. DOI: 10.1038/s41386-022-01371-9

[58] Hwang Z-A, Li C-W, Hsu A-L, Wu CW, Chan WP, Huang M-C. Assessment of resting cerebral perfusion between methamphetamine-associated psychosis and schizophrenia through arterial spin labeling MRI. European Archives of Psychiatry and Clinical Neuroscience. 2025;**275**:873–883. DOI: 10.1007/s00406-024-01857-1

[59] Jîtcă G, Ősz BE, Tero-Vescan A, Vari CE. Psychoactive drugs—from chemical structure to oxidative stress related to dopaminergic neurotransmission. A review. Antioxidants. 2021;**10**:381. DOI: 10.3390/antiox10030381

[60] Lobine D, Sadeer N, Jugreet S, Suroowan S, Keenoo BS, Imran M, Venugopala KN, Ibrahim FM, Zengin G, Mahomoodally MF, et al. Potential of medicinal plants as neuroprotective and

therapeutic properties against Amyloid-β-related toxicity, and glutamate-induced excitotoxicity in human neural cells. Current Neuropharmacology. 2021;**19**:1416–1441

[61] Olufunmilayo EO, Gerke-Duncan MB, Holsinger RMD. Oxidative stress and antioxidants in Neurodegenerative disorders. Antioxidants. 2023;**12**:517. DOI: 10.3390/antiox12020517

[62] Arillotta D, Floresta G, Papanti Pelletier GD, Guirguis A, Corkery JM, Martinotti G, Schifano F, et al. Exploring the potential impact of GLP-1 receptor agonists on substance use, compulsive behavior, and Libido: Insights from social media using a mixed-methods approach. Brain Sciences. 2024;**14**:617

[63] Zhu Q, Jiang G, Lang X, Fu Z, Zhang P, Zheng Y, Zhang X, et al. Prevalence and clinical correlates of abnormal lipid metabolism in first-episode and drug-naïve patients with major depressive disorder with abnormal glucose metabolism. Scientific Reports. 2023;**13**:8078

[64] Wang Q, Li Y, Ren H, Huang Q, Wang X, Zhou Y, Wu Q, Liu Y, Li M, Wang Y, Liu T, Zhang X, et al. Metabolic characteristics, prevalence of anxiety and its influencing factors in first-episode and drug-naïve major depressive disorder patients with impaired fasting glucose. Journal of Affective Disorders. 2023;**324**:341–348

[65] Schulz C, Klaus J, Peglow F, Ellinger S, Kühnel A, Walter M, et al. Blunted anticipation but not consummation of food rewards in depression. medRxiv. 2024; DOI: 10.1101/2024.03.26.24304849

[66] Kalayasiri R, Dadwat K, Thika S, Sirivichayakul S, Maes M. Methamphetamine (MA) use and MA-induced psychosis are associated with increasing aberrations in the compensatory immunoregulatory system, interleukin-1α, and CCL5 levels. Translational Psychiatry. 2023;**13**:361. DOI: 10.1038/s41398-023-02645-6.

[67] Shrestha P, Katila N, Lee S, Seo JH, Jeong J-H, Yook S. Methamphetamine induced neurotoxic diseases, molecular mechanism, and current treatment strategies. Biomedicine & Pharmacotherapy. 2022; **154**: 113591. DOI: 10.1016/j.biopha.2022.113591

[68] Hägglöf T, Vanz C, Kumagai A, Dudley E, Ortega V, Siller M, Parthasarathy R, Keegan J, Koenigs A, Shute T, Leadbetter EA, et al. T-bet+ B cells accumulate in adipose tissue and exacerbate metabolic disorder during obesity. Cell Metabolism. 2022;**34**: 1121–1136.e6

[69] Bovolini A, Garcia J, Andrade MA, Duarte JA. Metabolic syndrome pathophysiology and predisposing factors. International Journal of Sports Medicine. 2021;**42**:199–214. DOI: 10.1055/a-1263-0898

[70] Sanchez-Roige S, Kember RL, Agrawal A. Substance use and common contributors to morbidity: A genetics perspective. EBioMedicine. 2022; **83**: 104212. DOI: 10.1016/j.ebiom.2022.104212

[71] MacKillop J, Agabio R, Feldstein Ewing SW, Heilig M, Kelly JF, Leggio L, Lingford-Hughes A, Palmer AA, Parry CD, Ray L, Rehm J, et al. Hazardous drinking and alcohol use disorders. Nature Reviews Disease Primers. 2022;**8**:80

[72] Hoek AG, van Oort S, Mukamal KJ, Beulens JWJ. Alcohol consumption and cardiovascular disease risk: Placing new data in context. Current Atherosclerosis

Reports. 2022;**24**:51–59. DOI: 10.1007/s11883-022-00992-1

[73] Kashem MA, Šerý O, Pow DV, Rowlands BD, Rae CD, Balcar VJ. Actions of alcohol in brain: Genetics, metabolomics, GABA receptors, Proteomics and Glutamate transporter GLAST/EAAT1. Current Molecular Pharmacology. 2020;**14**:138–149. DOI: 10.2174/18744672136662004 24155244

[74] Kolić D, Kovarik Z. N -methyl- d -aspartate receptors: Structure, function, and role in organophosphorus compound poisoning. BioFactors. 2024;**50**:868–884. DOI: 10.1002/biof.2048

[75] Grados L, Pérot M, Barbezier N, Delayre-Orthez C, Bach V, Fumery M, Anton PM, Gay-Quéheillard J, et al. How advanced are we on the consequences of oral exposure to food contaminants on the occurrence of chronic non communicable diseases? Chemosphere. 2022;**303**:135260. DOI: 10.1016/j.chemosphere.2022. 135260

[76] Juanola O, Martínez-López S, Francés R, Gómez-Hurtado I. Non-alcoholic fatty liver disease: Metabolic, ctors. International Journal of Environmental Research & Public Health. 2021;**18**:5227. DOI: 10.3390/ijerph18105227

[77] Banerjee R, Erridge S, Salazar O, Mangal N, Couch D, Pacchetti B, Sodergren MH, et al. Real World evidence in medical Cannabis research. Therapeutic Innovation & Regulatory Science. 2022;**56**:8–14

[78] Patel AD. Cannabinoids in Neurologic Illnesses. Neurologic Clinics. 2021;**39**:231–241. DOI: 10.1016/j.ncl.2020.09.012

[79] Montoya-Alatriste CA, Alarcon-Aguilar FJ. Cannabis and cannabinoids as an alternative remedy in metabolic syndrome. Brazilian Journal of Pharmaceutical Sciences. 2022;58. doi:10.1590/s2175-97902022e20161

[80] Wiciński M, Fajkiel-Madajczyk A, Kurant Z, Gryczka K, Kurant D, Szambelan M, Malinowski B, Falkowski M, Zabrzyński J, Słupski M, et al. The use of Cannabidiol in metabolic syndrome—an opportunity to improve the patient's health or much ADO about nothing? Journal of Clinical Medicine. 2023;**12**:4620

[81] Han JH, Kim W. Peripheral CB1R as a modulator of metabolic inflammation. The FASEB Journal. 2021;**35**. DOI: 10.1096/fj.202001960R

[82] O'Sullivan SE, Yates AS, Porter RK. The peripheral cannabinoid receptor type 1 (CB1) as a molecular target for modulating Body Weight in Man. Molecules. 2021;**26**:6178. DOI: 10.3390/molecules26206178

[83] Mattelaer N, Van der Schueren B, Van Oudenhove L, Weltens N, Vangoitsenhoven R. The circulating and central endocannabinoid system in obesity and weight loss. International Journal of Obesity. 2024. DOI: 10.1038/s41366-024-01553-z

[84] Dziemitko S, Harasim-Symbor E, Chabowski A. How do phytocannabinoids affect cardiovascular health? An update on the most common cardiovascular diseases. Therapeutic Advances in Chronic Disease. 2023;14. DOI: 10.1177/20406223221143239

[85] Śmiarowska M, Białecka M, Machoy-Mokrzyńska A. Cannabis and cannabinoids: Pharmacology and therapeutic potential. Neurol Neurochir Pol. 2022;**56**:4–13. DOI: 10.5603/PJNNS.a2022.0015

Chapter 8

Reactive Hypoglycemia

Dravecká Ingrid, Galajda Peter and Mokáň Marián

Abstract

Reactive hypoglycemia (RH) is a heterogeneous clinical entity characterized by adrenergic and neuroglycopenic symptoms occurring 1–5 hours after food intake, most commonly following consumption of high-carbohydrate meals. RH can manifest in various forms, including alimentary, idiopathic, prediabetes/diabetes, hormonal, or secondary to congenital enzymatic defects. Pathophysiological mechanisms involve inappropriate insulin secretion, increased incretin response, impaired counter-regulatory hormone activity, or altered glucose metabolism. Diagnostic approaches include a 5-hour oral glucose tolerance test (oGTT) or mixed meal tolerance test (MMTT), although both can produce false-positive or false-negative results. Continuous glucose monitoring (CGM) may aid in detection. Clinical presentation varies from transient adrenergic symptoms to neuroglycopenic signs, and in rare cases, chronic fatigue or mood disturbances. Differential diagnosis must exclude insulinoma, dumping syndromes, and pseudo-hypoglycemia related to adrenergic hyperreactivity or psychiatric factors. Management begins with dietary modification, favoring frequent small meals low in refined carbohydrates, and, when necessary, pharmacologic interventions such as alpha-glucosidase inhibitors, GLP-1 receptor modulators, or somatostatin analogues. In severe or refractory cases, invasive procedures including surgical revision of bariatric procedures may be considered. Awareness of RH and individualized multidisciplinary care are essential, especially in patients with risk factors such as insulin resistance, rapid gastric emptying, or endocrine disorders.

Keywords: reactive hypoglycemia, postprandial hypoglycemia, idiopathic hypoglycemia, alimentary hypoglycemia, insulin resistance, incretin response, oral glucose tolerance test, mixed meal tolerance test, continuous glucose monitoring, dietary management, pharmacologic therapy

1. Introduction

Reactive hypoglycemia (RH) is a condition that is not easily diagnosed. A 5-hour oral glucose tolerance test (oGTT) can be helpful in establishing the diagnosis. The clinical manifestations of hypoglycemia are uncomfortable and often urgent. In the treatment of functional hypoglycemia, dietary interventions are usually effective. Pharmacological treatment is reserved for individuals in whom lifestyle modifications are insufficiently effective [1]. Reactive postprandial hypoglycemia usually occurs

2–5 hours after a high-carbohydrate meal in otherwise healthy individuals. It can present in several forms: alimentary (in 120 minutes), idiopathic (in 180 minutes), and late HR (in 240–300 minutes) [2, 3].

As proposed by Brun et al., reactive (postprandial) hypoglycemia can be divided into several distinct subtypes according to the underlying mechanism, timing, and metabolic context. Four principal forms are typically recognized: early, idiopathic, late (pre-diabetes), and secondary reactive hypoglycemia. Early reactive hypoglycemia usually develops within 1–2 hours after a meal and is attributed to an accelerated gastric emptying or an exaggerated early insulin or incretin response. It is most often observed after gastric surgery or in functional alimentary disorders. Idiopathic reactive hypoglycemia occurs 3–4 hours postprandially in otherwise healthy individuals with normal insulin sensitivity and represents a benign, often self-limited disturbance of postprandial glucose regulation, possibly linked to a mild delay in insulin feedback. The late or pre-diabetic form typically manifests 4–5 hours after a meal and is associated with insulin resistance and delayed, excessive insulin secretion following an exaggerated glucose rise [4]. This variant is regarded as an early indicator of impaired glucose tolerance or incipient type 2 diabetes [4–6]. Secondary or symptomatic reactive hypoglycemia arises due to identifiable underlying causes such as gastrointestinal surgery (dumping syndrome), alimentary hyperinsulinism, metabolic disorders, or gastrointestinal inflammation. Notably, *Helicobacter pylori*-induced gastritis has been linked to postprandial symptomatic hypoglycemia, suggesting that chronic gastric inflammation may contribute to altered glucose-insulin dynamics [7].

2. Etiopathogenesis

It is unclear whether RH is a disorder caused by inappropriate insulin secretion, a consequence of nutritionally unbalanced eating habits, or a psychosomatic condition. The term "reactive hypoglycemia" is recommended for cases of postprandial hypoglycemia that meet Whipple's triad criteria (symptoms related to low blood glucose levels and their resolution after glucose administration). In non-diabetes individuals, blood glucose levels between 2.2 and 3.8 mmol/L are considered hypoglycemic. When diagnosing RH, it is necessary to exclude other potential causes of hypoglycemia, such as gastrointestinal surgery, peptic ulcer disease, hormonal disorders, and alcoholism [8]. Reactive hypoglycemia can be observed in prediabetes stages and in patients living with diabetes as late postprandial hypoglycemia occurring 4–7 hours after a meal (*pre/diabetes RH*), in gastrointestinal dysfunction (*alimentary RH*), and in patients with hormonal deficiencies (*hormonal RH*). However, in a large group of patients, it occurs as *idiopathic RH* [2, 9].

Several etiopathogenetic mechanisms may contribute to postprandial RH:

1. *Inappropriate insulin response to glucose intake, because of insulin resistance or increased secretion of glucagon-like peptide-1 (GLP-1)*. This mechanism is present in all types of RH, including idiopathic RH, where an abnormally rapid increase in glucose leads to prolonged insulin secretion that responds inadequately to the subsequent drop in blood glucose levels.

2. *Renal glycosuria* can contribute to the development of RH in cases of renal tubular damage, for example, due to certain medications or hormonal dysregulation.

3. *Defect in glucagon secretion*, where irregularities in glucagon response to hypoglycemic stimuli have been confirmed in RH.

4. *Increased insulin sensitivity*, which is frequently observed in RH (50–70% of cases). Because it is not compensated by hypoinsulinemia, it cannot be reliably assessed by measuring homeostatic model assessment of insulin resistance (HOMA-IR) [4, 10].

3. Types of postprandial reactive hypoglycemia

3.1 Reactive hypoglycemia in prediabetes and diabetes

Late postprandial RH appears during the 3rd to 5th hour of oGTT. Loss of the first phase of insulin secretion is the first sign of the detrimental effects of hyperglycemia on pancreatic β-cells and insulin-sensitive tissues. This leads to a postprandial increase in blood glucose, which in turn triggers a delayed and excessive second phase of insulin secretion, ultimately resulting in late reactive hypoglycemia. In impaired glucose tolerance (IGT), inhibition of first-phase insulin secretion after oral glucose or a meal causes blood glucose levels to increase at 60–90 minutes (≥8.6 mmol/L), followed by late reactive hypoglycemia due to an exaggerated relative increase in second-phase insulin secretion. Elevated insulin levels persist even after nutrient absorption ceases, at a time when plasma glucose concentration begins to decline [2]. Persistent hyperinsulinemia contributes to the downregulation of post-receptor insulin signaling in skeletal muscle, which reduces insulin sensitivity and promotes the development of type 2 diabetes mellitus (T2DM) [9]. Therefore, late reactive hypoglycemia may serve as a predictor of T2DM. Some individuals with T2DM may experience RH for an extended period before developing overt disease. These individuals often have a positive family history of T2DM or obesity. Patients who experience hypoglycemia during the 4th–5th hour, especially if obese, are at greater risk of developing T2DM than those who experience hypoglycemia during the 3rd hour of the oGTT [2]. Consumption of simple carbohydrates can lead to RH in up to one-third of women with polycystic ovary syndrome, particularly in those who are obese and insulin resistant. Symptoms of hypoglycemia are associated with secretion of cortisol and adrenal androgens [11].

3.2 The role of incretins in insulin resistance and β-cell dysfunction in prediabetes

In non-diabetes individuals, incretins are responsible for 50–70% of total insulin secretion following oral glucose intake [12]. Michaliszyn et al. demonstrated impaired β-cell function in obese adolescents with worsening dysglycemia. Compared with individuals with normal glucose tolerance (NGT), adolescents with impaired glucose tolerance (IGT) had 30% lower β-cell sensitivity to glucose, and those with type 2 diabetes mellitus (T2DM) had 65% lower sensitivity. Youth with IGT or T2DM exhibited 32% and 38% lower incretin effect, respectively, compared to those with NGT, despite similar changes in glucagon-like peptide-1 (GLP-1) and glucose-dependent insulinotropic polypeptide (GIP) levels in response to oral glucose [13]. In prediabetes individuals, a reduced GLP-1 response to oral glucose administration has been observed [12]. The diminished incretin effect in T2DM results in only 20–35% of insulin secretion in response to glucose stimulation [14]. According to Lupoli et al., GLP-1 may contribute to idiopathic RH even in the absence of prediabetes. In individuals with idiopathic RH, the authors confirmed an increase in GLP-1 secretion within the first 30 minutes after oral glucose ingestion, followed by an increase in insulin secretion over the next 90 minutes, suppression of glucagon secretion at 120–180 minutes, and a decline in blood glucose at 240 minutes [15].

3.3 Alimentary reactive hypoglycemia

Reactive hypoglycemia early postprandial (alimentary) occurs 1–2 hours after oGTT. It can be boosted by an accelerated gastric emptying or an excessive incretin effect. It is also possible that rapid gastric evacuation leads to an exaggerated incretin response [2]. Following oral glucose intake, increased secretion of GLP-1 and GIP causes excessive insulin exocytosis with early upregulation of GLUT4 transporters. GLP-1, through subsequent inhibition of glucagon secretion, leads to an inadequate counter-regulatory response to hypoglycemia, resulting in the development of early hypoglycemia [15].

Reactive hypoglycemia can also occur in individuals who fast or follow restrictive diets for various reasons (often self-prescribed weight-loss regimens). These individuals may periodically interrupt their diets by consuming refined sugars ("junk food"), most commonly in the form of soft drinks, sweets, desserts, and similar foods [16]. Reactive hypoglycemia may also occur with simultaneous consumption of alcohol and sugar-containing beverages (e.g., gin and tonic), as this combination disrupts the adrenaline response and markedly suppresses growth hormone secretion in response to induced hypoglycemia [17]. *Helicobacter pylori* (HP)-induced gastritis can also contribute to reactive hypoglycemia; excessive HP colonization promotes insulin secretion stimulated by glucose and mixed meals, likely through increased gastrin secretion. Following HP eradication, a decrease in insulin response at 30 and 60 minutes after oral glucose administration has been observed, along with an increase in blood glucose at 180 minutes after a mixed meal, correlating with reduced gastrin levels [7, 18].

3.4 Postbariatric hypoglycemia

Glucose homeostasis, especially in the postprandial state, is disrupted following gastric surgery, including gastrectomy (e.g., for cancer), Nissen fundoplication, bariatric procedures, and vagotomy. Alimentary hypoglycemia occurs in approximately 15% of patients after gastrectomy and is considered a form of late dumping syndrome. Postprandial hyperinsulinemic hypoglycemia can be observed in patients who have undergone weight-reduction surgeries, gastrectomy, or Roux-en-Y gastric bypass (RYGB), all of which can lead to late dumping syndrome. Dumping syndrome occurs in up to 25% of patients who undergo gastrectomy [19, 20].

Bariatric surgery provides significant metabolic benefits, including weight loss, remission of type 2 diabetes mellitus (T2DM), and a reduction in microvascular and macrovascular events. However, one of the complications of bariatric surgery is postbariatric hypoglycemia, which is characterized as postprandial hyperinsulinemic hypoglycemia occurring 2–4 hours after food intake. Hypoglycemia leads to psychosocial consequences, long-term disruption of work and leisure activities, and an increased risk of motor vehicle accidents. Recurrent hypoglycemia can result in impaired awareness of hypoglycemic symptoms, cognitive dysfunction, cardiac arrhythmias, and increased mortality [21]. Continuous glucose monitoring (CGM) has confirmed the presence of postprandial hypoglycemia in nearly 50% of patients following RYGB or vertical sleeve gastrectomy (SG). Postbariatric hypoglycemia typically manifests more than one year after surgery, with patients usually experiencing hypoglycemic symptoms 1–3 hours after meals. If postprandial hypoglycemia occurs earlier (within less than 6–12 months) after the operation, more than 4 hours after a meal, or during fasting, other potential causes of hypoglycemia should be considered [21, 22]. The risk of developing postbariatric hypoglycemia is higher in non-diabetes individuals with lower HbA1c levels and the presence of hypoglycemia during the preoperative oGTT, indicating compensatory increased β-cell function, greater insulin secretion, and higher insulin sensitivity [23]. Other risk factors for the development of postprandial hypoglycemia after gastrectomy include younger age, lower BMI, and greater weight loss following surgery. Regarding the type of procedure, the risk of postprandial hypoglycemia is higher after Roux-en-Y gastric bypass (RYGB), which shows a similar incidence of hypoglycemia compared with sleeve gastrectomy (SG), although SG is associated with fewer episodes of severe hypoglycemia. The risk of RH is lower following laparoscopic adjustable gastric banding (LAGB), single-anastomosis duodenal-ileal bypass with sleeve gastrectomy (SADI-S), and the duodenal switch (DS). Studies investigating the incidence of hypoglycemia after single-anastomosis gastric bypass (SAGB), also known as one-anastomosis gastric bypass (OAGB) or "mini" gastric bypass, have shown the conflicting results, with findings ranging from low risk to a risk comparable to that observed with RYGB [24–29].

The cause of postbariatric hypoglycemia is the rapid delivery of nutrients into the jejunum, which leads to increased exposure of L-cells in the distal jejunum and proximal ileum to these nutrients and consequently to elevated secretion of incretins that stimulate insulin secretion and glucose utilization. Another mechanism may involve insufficient suppression of basal insulin secretion in response to hypoglycemia, excessive meal-stimulated insulin secretion, and impaired glucagon secretion [18, 21]. Tripyla et al. compared the counter-regulatory hormone response in patients with postbariatric hypoglycemia to that in a control group, confirming significantly lower levels of glucagon and pancreatic polypeptide in the postbariatric hypoglycemia group [30]. In patients after RYGB, alterations in bile acid kinetics have also been described, associated with excessive production of fibroblast growth factor-19 (FGF-19) by ileal enterocytes. In addition to regulating bile acid synthesis in the liver, FGF-19 increases insulin sensitivity by reducing visceral adiposity, enhancing brown adipose tissue activity, and increasing energy expenditure [31]. The clinical presentation ranges from asymptomatic hypoglycemia to impaired quality of life and an increased risk of dementia [22]. It most commonly manifests with neuroglycopenic symptoms several years after surgery [20]. Continuous glucose monitoring (CGM) can be helpful in detecting (but not diagnosing) postbariatric hypoglycemia. Due to varying accuracy and the fact that CGM measures interstitial glucose concentrations, the Society for Endocrinology recommends confirming the findings with capillary blood glucose measurements [32].

Diagnostic criteria for postbariatric hypoglycemia include a drop in blood glucose below 3 mmol/L, fulfillment of Whipple's triad, and exclusion of other causes of hypoglycemia. Dynamic provocative tests are not recommended [21]. In patients with dumping syndrome, the highest insulin concentrations occur 60 minutes after a meal (compared with 90 minutes postprandially in control subjects). Plasma GLP-1 concentrations rise earlier (20 minutes postprandially) and are higher in patients with dumping syndrome compared to controls (30 minutes postprandially). There is a significant negative correlation between early postprandial GLP-1 concentrations and blood glucose levels measured 2 hours after a meal. Thus, reactive hypoglycemia in dumping syndrome following bariatric surgery is caused by increased GLP-1 concentrations that stimulate insulin secretion [33]. In the differential diagnosis, it is important to distinguish early dumping syndrome, which manifests shortly after food intake with dyspeptic symptoms (abdominal pain, bloating, nausea, vomiting, diarrhea, borborygmi) and vasomotor symptoms (fatigue, sweating, palpitations, tachycardia, hypotension, orthostasis, or even syncope) *without* the presence of hypoglycemia. It is caused by the rapid entry of hyperosmolar food into the small intestine, leading to a shift of water from the intravascular compartment, which results in intestinal distension, reduction of intravascular volume, and activation of the autonomic and entero-neuro-endocrine systems. Although early and late dumping syndromes have distinct etiologies, they may coexist in the same patient [24, 34, 35]. According to the recommendations of the Society for Endocrinology, the treatment of postbariatric hypoglycemia begins with comprehensive nutritional management [32]. The treatment cornerstone is dietary modification, which includes consuming smaller, more frequent meals (typically 5–6 meals per day) that are low in carbohydrates and high in protein. It is important to avoid foods with a high glycemic index, prefer slowly absorbed carbohydrates, and limit alcohol consumption. Patients should be educated in self-management, including recognizing hypoglycemia symptoms, responding appropriately (e.g., administering 10–15 g of rapid-acting carbohydrates), and carrying glucose tablets. Regular blood glucose monitoring—especially postprandial glucose—is essential, as well as planning physical activity to minimize the risk of hypoglycemia. If dietary measures alone are insufficient, pharmacological treatment should be initiated. The first-line therapy is the alpha-glucosidase inhibitor:acarbose, which slows carbohydrate absorption and blunts sharp insulin responses. If ineffective, somatostatin analogues such as short-acting octreotide or long-acting pasireotide can be administered to suppress insulin release. In selected patients, diazoxide, which inhibits insulin secretion from pancreatic beta cells, may be considered. In severe cases with recurrent episodes of severe hypoglycemia, a glucagon autoinjector can be prescribed as an emergency treatment [21]. GLP-1 receptor antagonists, such as avexitide (exendin 9-39), represent a promising experimental option for treating postbariatric hypoglycemia in patients unresponsive to dietary and standard pharmacologic interventions. Avexitide blocks the action of endogenous GLP-1, thereby attenuating excessive postprandial insulin secretion. These findings suggest that exaggerated GLP-1 activity plays a key role in the development of postprandial hypoglycemia after gastric bypass surgery and that GLP-1 receptor inhibition may be a potential therapeutic approach [21, 36]. If pharmacological treatment also fails, more invasive options may be considered, such as endoscopic transoral outlet reduction to decrease the gastric outlet size, surgical conversion of the Roux-en-Y gastric bypass to another type of bariatric procedure, or, in exceptional cases, partial pancreatectomy. All treatment decisions should be individualized and supported by a multidisciplinary approach involving endocrinologists, bariatric surgeons, dieticians, and the patient themselves [21].

3.5 Hormonal reactive hypoglycemia

Hypoglycemia typically occurs in endocrine disorders associated with deficiencies in the production of insulin counter-regulatory hormones (glucagon, catecholamines, cortisol, and growth hormone), particularly those affecting the adrenocorticotropic hormone (ACTH)—cortisol axis and catecholamine production. Reactive postprandial hypoglycemia most commonly occurs in patients with hypopituitarism, Addison's disease, or hypothyroidism [37, 38]. Loss of counter-regulatory hormones (ACTH and growth hormone) leads to increased insulin sensitivity, a sudden decrease in insulin requirements, hypoglycemia, or even complete remission of diabetes—a phenomenon known as the Houssay phenomenon. In patients with hypopituitarism, there is progressive failure of hormone secretion in the order: growth hormone (GH) → follicle-stimulating hormone (FSH) and luteinizing hormone (LH) → thyroid-stimulating hormone (TSH) → ACTH. An exception to this sequence is lymphocytic hypophysitis, where ACTH deficiency is observed in 65% of cases as an early and frequent defect [39]. Patients with hypopituitarism may be asymptomatic, but some report fatigue, nausea, vomiting, or neurological symptoms such as headaches or visual disturbances (related to low blood glucose levels). Although it is a rare cause, hypopituitarism can lead to secondary adrenal insufficiency, which, during acute stress, infection, or surgery, can result in the recurrent episodes of hypoglycemia. A specific phenomenon associated with this is the so-called Houssay phenomenon—recurrent hypoglycemia in people living with diabetes due to deficiency of counter-regulatory hormones such as cortisol and growth hormone. This condition increases insulin sensitivity and can cause significant drops in blood glucose even with standard insulin doses [40]. The most common inherited cause of primary adrenal insufficiency is congenital adrenal hyperplasia. Acquired causes include autoimmune (Addison's disease), traumatic (hemorrhage, infarction), infectious (tuberculosis), infiltrative (neuroblastoma), and iatrogenic factors (exogenous steroid use, postoperative states involving the adenohypophysis, adrenalectomy). Typical clinical manifestations include abdominal pain, nausea, and vomiting. Hypoglycemia can have serious consequences if unrecognized and untreated. Symptoms include tremor, palpitations, sweating, hunger, paresthesia, dizziness, weakness, and confusion. In adults, it may present as morning headaches following nocturnal hypoglycemia [41].

Multiple mechanisms contribute to hypoglycemia in hypothyroidism, including reduced basal and stimulated secretion of growth hormone and cortisol, decreased glucagon secretion, slowed insulin clearance, impaired gluconeogenesis, and disrupted glycogenolysis. Additional contributing factors include reduced appetite, delayed gastric emptying, and decreased intestinal glucose absorption. Hypoglycemia usually resolves with thyroid hormone replacement therapy. In treated patients symptoms resolve, insulin secretion decreases by 70%, and the timing of peak insulin secretion coincides with the peak plasma glucose concentration [37]. Growth hormone (GH) deficiency has different effects on glucose homeostasis at various stages of life. In children, it increases insulin sensitivity, leading to spontaneous hypoglycemia due to decreased hepatic glucose output. In adults, GH deficiency is associated with insulin resistance, likely due to increased adiposity, reduced lean body mass, and impaired exercise tolerance [40, 42]. Glucagon is the primary counter-regulatory hormone during hypoglycemia. It raises blood glucose levels by stimulating glycogenolysis and inhibiting glycolysis and glycogen synthesis. Isolated glucagon deficiency with spontaneous hypoglycemia may occur due to autoimmune-mediated failure of pancreatic α-cells or following pancreatectomy [43, 44]. Early postoperative periods after resection of a pheochromocytoma can also lead to reactive hypoglycemia. The cause is secondary increased insulin secretion due to a sudden drop in catecholamines, the administration of beta-blockers, impaired glucagon response to hypoglycemia during catecholamine excess, or preoperative alpha-blockade without concomitant beta-blockade. Additionally, pheochromocytoma can cause hypoglycemia even before surgery due to increased glucose consumption by the rapidly growing tumor or increased insulin secretion mediated by catecholamine stimulation of beta receptors [45–47].

3.6 Idiopathic (functional) reactive hypoglycemia

It typically appears during the 3rd hour of the oGTT, primarily in young and lean individuals [2]. It has also been described in women with mild overweight following significant weight loss. Its occurrence is associated with dietary habits, particularly high-carbohydrate and low-fat diets; alcohol consumption is also a risk factor [4]. The cause and pathophysiology are not fully understood and are likely multifactorial. The hallmark of idiopathic hypoglycemia is increased peripheral insulin sensitivity, observed in 50–70% of cases. Approximately 90% of patients exhibit hyperinsulinism or dysinsulinism (a delay in the insulin peak relative to the timing of the plasma glucose peak). Excessive GLP-1 production also occurs. In about 10% of patients with normal insulin secretion, other abnormalities may cause hypoglycemia, such as impaired timely activation of postprandial glucose production or mild deficiencies of counter-regulatory hormones, which are seen in reactive hypoglycemic patients with hormonal deficits. This type of hypoglycemia is confirmed by the presence of hypoglycemic symptoms related to food intake, documented hypoglycemia during the 3rd hour of the oGTT—usually not dropping below 2.8 mmol/L—and exclusion of other causes of postprandial hypoglycemia. This form of hypoglycemia generally does not progress to diabetes mellitus [2, 4, 48–50]. There is considerable variability in the results of low blood glucose during the oGTT, with reductions below 2.8 mmol/L documented in asymptomatic individuals, and transiently low plasma glucose levels observed during the oGTT in 10–30% of normal subjects. Conversely, in some individuals, even mild postprandial hypoglycemia can trigger a pronounced adrenergic response accompanied by symptoms [48, 49].

3.7 Hypoglycemia versus non-hypoglycemia (pseudo-hypoglycemia)

Many patients report symptoms falsely mimicking hypoglycemia in relation to food intake, but true hypoglycemia and the presence of Whipple's triad are not confirmed. The terms idiopathic postprandial syndrome or adrenergic postprandial syndrome are used to describe this condition, based on the activation of the autonomic adrenergic system as the central mechanism. It occurs more frequently in young, lean women with increased insulin sensitivity, where ingestion of very sweet foods (e.g., chocolate) stimulates insulin release, and even a small drop in blood glucose—still within normal ranges—significantly activates the adrenergic system, leading to typical symptoms (tachycardia, sweating, weakness, or near-syncope). In some cases, such a diagnosis may lead to social advantages or psychological stigmatization [1]. This syndrome is often associated with emotional distress and anxious behavior in the patient. The concurrent presence of a neuropsychiatric disorder in such patients raises suspicion that this condition may underlie the patient's "nonspecific" symptoms. Patients with idiopathic RH and those with psychiatric disorders can exhibit similar adrenergically mediated symptoms and share common personality traits, as assessed by the Minnesota Multiphasic Personality Inventory (MMPI) test. Among patients evaluated for suspected postprandial RH, a 5-hour oGTT failed to confirm hypoglycemia during symptomatic episodes in 45% of cases. Within this group, women outnumbered men by a ratio of 2:1. The predominant symptoms included light-headedness, shakiness, sweating, weakness, and fatigue, which occurred independently of blood glucose levels. MMPI testing in these patients revealed an unusual neurotic triad (a variant of the V-pattern profile), characterized by elevated scores on the hysteria and hypochondriasis scales with a normal depression score. These are predominantly female patients with an increased incidence of hypochondriasis and hysteria, who tend to replace their emotional problems with the somatic complaints and do not respond to psychological treatment nor accept psychological explanations for their symptoms. This V-pattern personality profile is also observed in other psychoneurological disorders, among psychiatric patients, and in less than 2% of the normal population. This personality profile is frequently found even in patients with confirmed reactive hypoglycemia, regardless of whether the condition has an alimentary, hormonal, diabetes, or idiopathic origin. Adrenergic symptoms can also be observed in many cardiovascular, neurological, gastrointestinal, and endocrine diseases. Therefore, patients should initially be evaluated with a focus on these symptoms in relation to possible underlying organ-specific disorders. The diagnosis of reactive hypoglycemia should only be considered if these symptoms occur in connection with eating habits. In highly selected groups of patients suspected of having reactive "functional" hypoglycemia, the actual prevalence of the condition ranges from 2 to 10% [9, 50–52].

The diagnosis of pseudo-hypoglycemia is straightforward: Normal glucose metabolism is confirmed, and no relationship is found between blood glucose levels and the patient's symptoms. Ideally, a 5-hour oGTT should be performed with measurements of glucose, insulin, and C-peptide every 30 minutes [1].

3.8 Congenital enzymatic defects associated with postprandial hypoglycemia

3.8.1 Hereditary fructose intolerance

Hereditary fructose intolerance results from a mutation in the gene encoding fructose-1,6-bisphosphate aldolase, which metabolizes fructose-1-phosphate into glyceraldehyde and dihydroxyacetone phosphate. Increased accumulation of fructose-1-phosphate leads to hepatocellular necrosis in the liver and tubular cell damage in the kidneys. The disease begins to manifest after fructose is introduced into an infant's diet and can present clinically—depending on the amount consumed—with hepatomegaly accompanied by elevated transaminases, or even acute liver failure with ascites and coagulopathy. Gastrointestinal involvement leads to anorexia, vomiting, diarrhea, and gastroesophageal reflux is often present. Laboratory findings may show signs of tubulopathy, hypophosphatemia, and metabolic acidosis. The accumulation of fructose-1-phosphate inhibits glycogenolysis and gluconeogenesis, resulting in late postprandial hypoglycemia, which is present in 30–50% of affected children [53].

3.8.2 Galactosemia

Galactosemia (galactose intolerance) is an autosomal recessive disorder caused by mutations in the genes encoding enzymes of the Leloir pathway:

- galactose-1-phosphate uridyltransferase (GALT)—classic type I,
- galactokinase—type II,
- UDP-galactose 4-epimerase (GALE)—type III.

As a result of these defects, intermediate metabolites (galactitol, galactonate) accumulate, exerting the toxic effects on the brain, liver, kidneys, and the ocular lens. The incidence is approximately 1 in 50,000 live births. Clinical symptoms usually begin between days 3 and 7 of life, and after ingestion of a total of 250–300 mL of breast milk, they manifest as apathy, vomiting, hepatomegaly, and jaundice with rapidly progressive liver and kidney failure and cerebral edema. Bilateral cataracts are frequently present. Postprandial hypoglycemia is also a common symptom. Newborn screening is performed by testing dried blood spots to measure galactose-1-phosphate levels and GALT activity in erythrocytes. Diagnosis is confirmed through genetic testing [54].

4. Clinical presentation of reactive hypoglycemia

Hypoglycemia manifests with adrenergic and/or neuroglycopenic symptoms. Depending on the duration of hypoglycemia, patients may experience fatigue, headache, visual disturbances, slurred speech, psychiatric symptoms, impaired concentration, and altered consciousness. In alimentary RH, symptoms usually appear within 90 minutes to 2 hours after eating, most often after breakfast. Symptoms are transient and typically resolve within 15–30 minutes. Generally, adrenergic symptoms are more common than neuroglycopenic ones and occur depending on individual sensitivity to the degree of blood glucose decline. Seizures and loss of consciousness are uncommon in RH; if present, other causes of hypoglycemia, such as insulinoma, should be considered. Individuals with insulinomas typically experience postabsorptive hypoglycemia in 73% of cases but may also have postprandial hypoglycemia alone in 6% or a combination of both in 21%. Conversely, patients after gastric bypass surgery, who characteristically develop postprandial hypoglycemia, may also experience hypoglycemic symptoms in the fasting state. Postprandial hypoglycemia can also occur in the presence of insulin autoantibodies. Reactive hypoglycemia may also develop 3–5 hours after a meal and is associated with diabetes mellitus, in which the insulin response to glucose is delayed. In such cases, blood glucose rises 2–3 hours after eating, followed by a sharp decline with typical hypoglycemic symptoms. Some patients may present only with chronic complaints such as fatigue, lack of energy, depression, and emotional instability [1].

RH syndromes:

1. *Long QT syndrome*: Characterized by prolonged QT interval on the ECG, hyperinsulinemia, and low potassium levels following oral glucose intake in individuals with RH who carry mutations in the KCN1 gene [55].

2. *Middleton's syndrome*: Patients with normal gastric anatomy may experience symptoms and signs resembling postprandial RH, including early satiety and diarrhea due to the accelerated gastric emptying [34].

5. Diagnosis of reactive hypoglycemia

Despite controversial opinions, the most used diagnostic tool for RH is a 5-hour oral glucose tolerance test (oGTT) [3, 8]. An alternative is the mixed meal tolerance test (MMTT), which more closely mimics a typical meal. However, neither the oGTT nor the MMTT is fully optimal for confirming RH, as both can produce false-positive and false-negative results. A characteristic feature of RH is a drop in blood glucose to ≤3.0 mmol/L. However, symptoms may also occur without glucose falling to 3.0 mmol/L—this is referred to as postprandial syndrome. When confirming a diagnosis of RH, it is essential to exclude other potential causes contributing to hypoglycemia, such as postsurgical states, peptic ulcer disease, hormonal disorders, and alcoholism [2]. Hyperglycemic physiological breakfasts (with >60% carbohydrate content), which resemble normal dietary habits, can serve as a good alternative for outpatient glycemic testing in patients suspected of postprandial hypoglycemia. Using this test, blood glucose levels <3.3 mmol/L were detected in 47.3% of patients studied [42]. The plasma glucose level at which symptoms occur varies individually. It is unclear why some patients experience clinical signs of hypoglycemia during testing even when blood glucose levels are normal, while others have low glucose levels without any accompanying clinical manifestations [2]. In some cases, administration of a mixed meal in the same individual does not induce hypoglycemia, despite the patient exhibiting manifest symptoms after ingesting the same mixed meal without biochemical evidence of hypoglycemia. These observations may be explained by Pavlovian conditioning, the presence of a subconsciously ingrained "idiopathic postprandial syndrome," or the emergence of anxiety about hypoglycemic episodes triggered by the stress of testing or the testing procedure itself [56]. In patients with metabolic disorders, including insulin resistance, testing may reveal effects on lipid profiles—specifically, elevated triacylglycerols and VLDL and reduced HDL cholesterol. Additionally, there is an increased risk of steatohepatitis. These metabolic alterations can also be observed in lean individuals with a normal BMI [2]. Hall et al. investigated the metabolic parameters in 40 hospitalized patients with RH. In 12 individuals, hypoglycemic symptoms and blood glucose levels below 3 mmol/L developed during the 5-hour oGTT. Ten patients experienced hypoglycemic symptoms without a significant drop in blood glucose. Patients diagnosed with RH had statistically significantly lower mean blood glucose levels at the 1st and 2nd hours of the oGTT, as well as lower insulin levels at the 2nd hour, compared with those who did not meet the diagnostic criteria for RH. During the MMTT, clinical symptoms developed in 17 patients, but hypoglycemia was not confirmed [8].

In a cohort of 52 patients with a history of symptomatic postprandial neuroglycopenia, Pant et al. confirmed hypoglycemia during the 5-hour oGTT in 21 individuals. Hypoglycemia occurred in the 3rd hour in nine patients, in the 4th hour in 11 patients, and in the 5th hour in one patient. Fasting insulin levels were significantly higher in individuals with hypoglycemia compared with insulin levels measured during hypoglycemia [3]. The use of continuous glucose monitoring (CGM) can aid in diagnostic accuracy [57].

A clinical diagnosis of reactive hypoglycemia can be made when no other cause is identified and if the patient has nonspecific adrenergic symptoms that are primarily related to the postprandial state and occur after consuming meals high in refined sugars.

6. Treatment

The patient should be educated on the principles of RH occurring after meals and on strategies for its prevention. Regular meals, consumed more frequently in smaller portions with a low glycemic index, are recommended—sometimes even a low-carbohydrate, high-protein diet. Patients with alimentary reactive hypoglycemia respond best to frequent meals with a low glycemic index, distributed in six servings throughout the day. It is advisable to increase intake of fiber, proteins, and fats, which slows carbohydrate absorption [1, 20]. However, dietary measures with reduced carbohydrate intake may sometimes be insufficient for preventing RH, making pharmacological treatment necessary. Pharmacological therapy for RH remains empirical. Alpha-glucosidase inhibitors, sedatives, tranquilizers, anticholinergics, biguanides, diphenylhydantoin, and propranolol have been tried. Calcium channel blockers and somatostatin analogues can reduce the postprandial insulin peak [1].

Alpha-glucosidase inhibitors (voglibose, acarbose, and miglitol), which belong to the group of antidiabetes agents, inhibit carbohydrate absorption, thereby reducing the risk of RH by lowering insulin secretion [58]. They reduce the secretion of the incretin GIP, which is released from K-cells in the duodenum and is stimulated by the absorption of carbohydrates and fats. Acarbose decreases GIP and glucagon levels more markedly after a mixed meal than after an oGTT. Low-dose glitazones (pioglitazone 5 mg) administered to patients with RH associated with impaired glucose tolerance (IGT) have been shown to be effective both for hypoglycemia symptoms and in preventing the progression to diabetes mellitus. DPP-4 inhibitors reduce glucagon levels and attenuate postprandial glucose excursions without the risk of hypoglycemia or weight gain. They may be effective in the treatment of RH, potentially even in prediabetes patients [2]. GLP-1 agonists also have a preventive effect on postprandial RH and prediabetes, particularly in obese individuals. They are associated with improved glucose tolerance and reversal of prediabetes to normal glucose tolerance in more than 50% of patients [59]. Postprandial hypoglycemia in individuals with RYGB can be corrected with the GLP-1 receptor antagonist exendin-(9-39) (Ex9), which reduces abnormally elevated late postprandial insulin secretion [13]. Less selective sodium-glucose cotransporter-2 (SGLT-2) inhibitors, such as canagliflozin, may have beneficial effects on RH by slowing intestinal glucose absorption and consequently lowering the postprandial insulin peak. In postbariatric hypoglycemia, novel approaches such as the use of avexitide (exendin 9-39)—a GLP-1R antagonist—or a glucagon pump are also being explored [44]. Patients with reactive hypoglycemia are uncommon and often not properly understood regarding the symptomatic origins of their condition. Symptoms are frequently triggered by the consumption of refined simple sugars. Dietary history can reveal a relationship between the condition and excessive intake of refined sugars, as well as symptom resolution when the patient consumes a balanced meal. Ingestion of gin and tonic, foods containing sucrose, flour-based meals, or dishes high in refined sugars and/or glucose can provoke reactive hypoglycemia. Refined sugars present in most soft drinks consist of excessive amounts of sucrose and/or glucose, which can mimic the effects of an oGTT. Adding even a small number of refined sugars to a meal significantly increases insulin secretion. Similarly, diets with a high glycemic index cause greater postprandial blood glucose excursions and insulin responses.

The following case reports illustrate the heterogeneous clinical spectrum of reactive and postprandial hypoglycemia, including its association with prediabetes, endocrine disorders, and idiopathic causes. Each case highlights different pathogenetic mechanisms, diagnostic approaches, and therapeutic responses. Special attention is given to the role of oral glucose tolerance testing, fasting tests, and continuous glucose monitoring in evaluating hypoglycemic episodes. These cases underscore the importance of individualized diagnostic assessment and lifestyle-based management in patients presenting with postprandial hypoglycemic symptoms.

DOI: http://dx.doi.org/10.5772/intechopen.1013682

All patients were hospitalized at the 1st Department of Internal Medicine, Faculty of Medicine, Pavol Jozef Šafárik University and University Hospital in Košice, Slovakia.

6.1 Case report 1

6.1.1 Patient with late postprandial hypoglycemia (prediabetes)

A 74-year-old woman with a medical history of metabolic syndrome (obesity, arterial hypertension, hyperlipoproteinemia, and hyperuricemia) complained of a 3-year history of episodes of weakness, tachycardia, nervousness, and sweating, without loss of consciousness. During these episodes, outpatient measurements confirmed low blood glucose levels (2.8–3.5 mmol/L). The patient underwent a 72-hour fasting test, during which the lowest glycemia reached 3.0 mmol/L, with an appropriate suppression of insulin and C-peptide levels. The HOMA-IR index was 4.85 (normal range ≤ 2.0), confirming insulin resistance. A subsequent oral glucose tolerance test (oGTT), extended to 4 hours, revealed hypoglycemia between the 180th and 240th minute, associated with markedly increased insulin secretion following glucose ingestion—see **Table 1**.

The clinical and laboratory findings were interpreted as hypoglycemia in the early stages of diabetes development—prediabetes. A diet with restricted intake of simple carbohydrates was recommended.

6.2 Case report 2

6.2.1 Patient with a history of type 1 diabetes mellitus and Addison's disease—Houssay phenomenon

A 56-year-old man with a history of latent autoimmune diabetes in adults (LADA), Graves-Basedow thyroiditis, and arterial hypertension was admitted to the internal medicine department due to progressive weakness, vomiting, dizziness, and abdominal pain. On physical examination, he was confused, depressed, and tearful, and no pathological findings were noted on physical examination. Blood pressure was 130/80 mmHg (without antihypertensive therapy). The patient reported that he had not administered insulin for approximately 5 years and was not taking or requiring medication for thyroid disease or hypertension.

Laboratory findings revealed the following glycemic profile: 8.7–9.1–6.9–7.4 mmol/L (without insulin administration), HbA1c 9% (75 Mmol/mol) serum sodium 106 mmol/L, potassium 5.4 mmol/L, serum osmolality 226 mOsm/kg, urinary sodium 107 mmol/L, and urinary potassium 57.98 mmol/L. Due to the presence of hyponatremia and hyperkalemia, further testing was performed: serum cortisol 116.8 mmol/L (140–700 nmol/L), ACTH 102.1 pmol/L (2–11 pmol/L), and anti-21-hydroxylase antibodies 77 IU/L (<1.0 IU/L), confirming the diagnosis of Addison's disease.

Time (hour)/parameter	0.	1.	2.	3.	4.
Glycemia (mmol/L)	5.2	7.9	4.8	**3.2**	**2.8**
Insulin (mIU/L)	21.18	**208.8**	**180.5**	**131.4**	36.2

Pathological values are highlighted in bold.

Table 1.
Extended oral glucose tolerance test (oGTT).

The loss of counterregulatory hormones (particularly cortisol) leads to increased insulin sensitivity, a sudden drop in insulin requirements, hypoglycemia, or even a transient remission of diabetes—a phenomenon known as the Houssay phenomenon. The condition was classified as autoimmune polyglandular syndrome type II: Addison's disease, LADA, and Graves-Basedow disease. The patient was treated by replacement therapy with hydrocortisone and fludrocortisone, and due to a subsequent rise in blood glucose levels, insulin therapy was reinitiated using a basal-bolus insulin regimen.

6.3 Case report 3

6.3.1 Patient with idiopathic reactive hypoglycemia

A young 29-year-old woman with a history of thrombophilia underwent a medically induced termination of pregnancy in the 6th month due to a congenital fetal malformation. During the pregnancy (2015), she experienced episodes of weakness and sweating, which resolved after the intake of sweets. These symptoms persisted even after the termination of pregnancy, typically occurring after physical exertion and 30–60 minutes postprandially. Home glucose monitoring during symptomatic episodes revealed values ranging between 3.2–3.6–4.1 mmol/L. She constantly needed to snack, eventually gaining 28 kg over a period of 2.5 years. A prolonged oral glucose tolerance test (oGTT) confirmed hypoglycemia at 180 minutes, with inappropriately elevated insulin secretion at 60 minutes—see **Table 2**.

The condition was assessed as *reactive idiopathic postprandial hypoglycemia* with a flat glycemic curve. The patient was advised on lifestyle modifications including regular meals, adequate physical activity, avoidance of simple carbohydrates, and preference for complex carbohydrates. Following these measures, she lost 10 kg over the course of 3 months; however, occasional episodes of weakness still occurred 1.5–2.5 hours after meals, with measured blood glucose levels between 3.1 and 3.5 mmol/L.

Therefore, the patient was admitted to the internal medicine department for a *72-hour fasting test*, which showed appropriate suppression of insulin and C-peptide levels, along with an increase in counter-regulatory hormones (growth hormone, cortisol). The lowest recorded glycemia was 4.2 mmol/L. Hypoglycemia was not confirmed during CGM monitoring—see **Figure 1**.

Follow-up prolonged oral glucose tolerance test (oGTT) after 8 months of lifestyle modifications (elimination of simple carbohydrates, regular meals, preference for complex carbohydrates) showed no hyperinsulinemia or hypoglycemia—see **Table 3**.

Time (hour)/parameter	**0.**	**1.**	**2.**	**3.**
Glycemia (mmol/L)	4.5	8.1	4.2	**1.75**
Insulin (mIU/L)	18.7	**269.3**	**74.5**	21.66
C-peptide (µg/L)	2.93	15.73	9.4	4.34

C-peptide: reference range: 1.1–4.4 µg/L.
Pathological values are highlighted in bold.

Table 2.
Prolonged oral glucose tolerance test (oGTT).

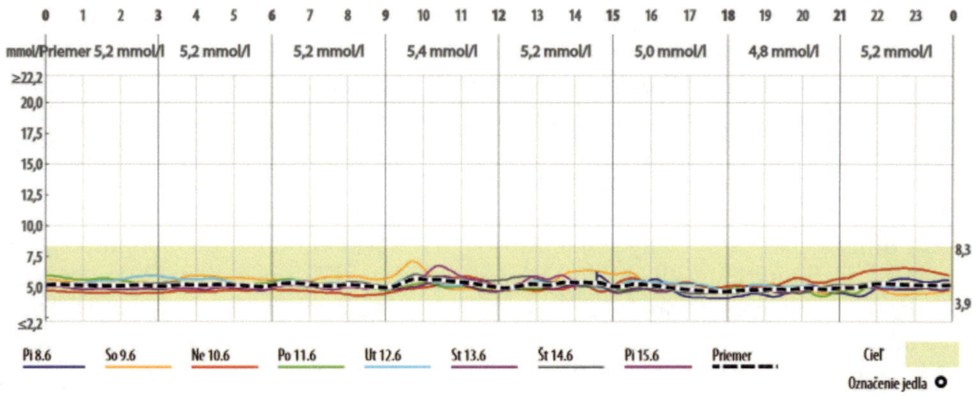

Figure 1.
Continuous glucose monitoring (CGM) without evidence of hypoglycemia.

Time (hour)/parameter	0.	1.	2.	3.
Glycemia (mmol/L)	4.5	6.3	6.5	4.8
Insulin (mIU/L)	18.7	46.74	55.36	11.64
C-peptide (µg/L)	4.48	6.58	6.71	2.46

C-peptide: reference range: 1.1–4.4 µg/L.

Table 3.
Follow-up prolonged oral glucose tolerance test (oGTT) after 8 months.

The clinical condition was assessed as *reactive idiopathic postprandial hypoglycemia*. With lifestyle modifications, the patient's condition has significantly improved, with the lowest recorded glycaemia around 3.2 mmol/L. Overall, she has lost 16 kg after 8 months of dietary and lifestyle adjustments.

7. Conclusion

Reactive hypoglycemia is a complex and multifactorial clinical entity that presents diagnostic and therapeutic challenges. It encompasses a spectrum of conditions ranging from functional (idiopathic) hypoglycemia in healthy individuals to postprandial hypoglycemia associated with prediabetes, gastrointestinal surgery, hormonal deficiencies, or rare congenital enzymatic disorders. Although RH is typically benign and non-life-threatening, it can significantly impact quality of life, lead to misdiagnoses, and, in some cases, serve as an early warning sign of evolving metabolic or endocrine disease.

The pathophysiology of RH involves several interacting mechanisms. These include delayed or excessive insulin secretion, increased insulin sensitivity without compensatory hyperinsulinemia, impaired glucagon or cortisol responses, altered incretin dynamics—especially GLP-1 hypersecretion—and, in some instances, psychological or neuropsychiatric components. Idiopathic RH is commonly observed in young, lean women and is often associated with increased peripheral insulin sensitivity, altered eating patterns, or emotional distress. Conversely, late postprandial hypoglycemia in obese or prediabetes individuals may reflect β-cell dysfunction and an early stage of DMT2, thus serving as a potential predictive marker.

Postbariatric RH has emerged as a clinically significant subtype, particularly RYGB, and is linked to rapid nutrient transit, exaggerated GLP-1 responses, and altered counter-regulatory hormone secretion. These patients may develop recurrent neuroglycopenic symptoms that impair daily functioning and increase the risk of accidents and cognitive decline. CGM can support diagnosis, but confirmatory testing and exclusion of alternative causes remain essential.

Diagnosis of RH relies on clinical correlation with Whipple's triad and the exclusion of other causes of hypoglycemia. Although the 5-hour oGTT is commonly employed, its limitations—including false-positive and false-negative results—necessitate cautious interpretation. MMTT and CGM may provide additional insights in selected cases.

Management of RH prioritizes dietary intervention, which remains the cornerstone of therapy. Patients benefit from education focused on regular meals with a low glycemic index, balanced macronutrient intake, and avoidance of simple sugars and alcohol. In cases refractory to dietary measures, pharmacologic agents such as α-glucosidase inhibitors, DPP-4 inhibitors, or GLP-1 receptor antagonists may be considered. In postbariatric patients, emerging therapies like avexitide (exendin 9-39) show promise in mitigating excessive GLP-1 mediated insulin secretion. More invasive approaches, including endoscopic or surgical interventions, are reserved for severe, treatment-resistant cases.

In conclusion, RH is an under recognized but clinically relevant condition. A thorough understanding of its diverse etiologies, variable presentations, and overlapping pathophysiological pathways is critical for accurate diagnosis and effective management. Given the psychological and metabolic implications, an individualized, multidisciplinary approach—incorporating endocrinology, nutrition, psychology, and, when necessary, surgery—is essential to optimize the patient outcomes and quality of life.

List of abbreviations

ACTH	adrenocorticotropic hormone
BMI	body mass index
CGM	continuous glucose monitoring
T2DM	type 2 diabetes mellitus
DS	duodenal switch
FGF-19	fibroblast growth factor 19
FSH	follicle-stimulating hormone
GIP	glucose-dependent insulinotropic polypeptide
GLP-1	glucagon-like peptide-1
HOMA-IR	homeostatic model assessment of insulin resistance
HP	*Helicobacter pylori*
LADA	latent autoimmune diabetes in adults
LAGB	laparoscopic adjustable gastric banding
LH	luteinizing hormone
MMPI	Minnesota Multiphasic Personality Inventory
MMTT	mixed meal tolerance test
NGT	normal glucose tolerance
oGTT	oral glucose tolerance test
IGT	impaired glucose tolerance

RH	reactive hypoglycemia
RYGB	Roux-en-Y gastric bypass
SADI-S	single anastomosis duodenal-ileal bypass with sleeve gastrectomy
SG	sleeve gastrectomy
TSH	thyroid-stimulating hormone.

Author details

Dravecká Ingrid[1*], Galajda Peter[2] and Mokáň Marián[2]

1 1st Department of Internal Medicine, Faculty of Medicine of Pavol Jozef Šafárik University and University Hospital in Košice, Slovakia

2 1st Department of Internal Medicine, Jessenius Faculty of Medicine of Comenius University in Bratislava, Slovakia

*Address all correspondence to: ingrid.dravecka@upjs.sk

References

[1] Nadeau A. Functional hypoglycemia: Facts and fancies. Canadian Family Physician. 1984;**30**:1333-1335

[2] Altuntaş Y. Postprandial reactive hypoglycemia. Sisli Etfal Hastanesi Tip Bulteni. 2019;**53**(3):215-220. DOI: 10.14744/SEMB.2019.59455

[3] Pant V, Mathema S, Jha S, et al. The detection of postprandial hypoglycemia with 5-hour oral glucose tolerance test. EJIFCC. 2021;**32**(4):451-457

[4] Brun JF, Fedou C, Mercier J. Postprandial reactive hypoglycemia. Diabetes & Metabolism. 2000;**26**(5):337-351

[5] Hamdy O. Hypoglycemia: Practice Essentials, Background, Pathophysiology. eMedicine [Internet]. 28 May 2025. Available from: https://emedicine.medscape.com/article/122122-overview?form=fpf

[6] Cryer PE, Axelrod L, Grossman AB, et al. Evaluation and management of adult hypoglycemic disorders: An Endocrine Society Clinical Practice Guideline. The Journal of Clinical Endocrinology & Metabolism. Mar 2009;**94**(3):709-728. DOI: 10.1210/jc.2008-1410

[7] Açbay O, Celik AF, Kadioğlu P, et al. Helicobacter pylori-induced gastritis may contribute to occurrence of postprandial symptomatic hypoglycemia. Digestive Diseases and Sciences. 1999;**44**(9):1837-1842

[8] Hall M, Walicka M, Panczyk M, et al. Metabolic parameters in patients with suspected reactive hypoglycemia. Journal of Personalized Medicine. 2021;**11**(4):1-13. DOI: 10.3390/jpm11040276

[9] Hofeldt FD. Reactive hypoglycemia. Endocrinology and Metabolism Clinics of North America. 1989;**18**(1):185-201

[10] Leonetti F, Morviducci L, Giaccari A, Sbraccia P, Caiola S, Zorretta D, et al. Idiopathic reactive hypoglycemia: A role for glucagon? Journal of Endocrinological Investigation. 1992;**15**(4):273-278. DOI: 10.1007/BF03348727

[11] Karakas SE. Reactive hypoglycemia: A trigger for nutrient-induced endocrine and metabolic responses in polycystic ovary syndrome. Journal of Clinical Medicine. 2023;**12**(23):7252. DOI: 10.3390/jcm12237252

[12] De León DD, Crutchlow MF, Ham JY, et al. Role of glucagon-like peptide-1 in the pathogenesis and treatment of diabetes mellitus. The International Journal of Biochemistry & Cell Biology. 2006;**38**:845-859. DOI: 10.1016/j.biocel.2005.07.011

[13] Michaliszyn SF, Mari A, Lee S, et al. β-cell function, incretin effect, and incretin hormones in obese youth along the span of glucose tolerance from normal to prediabetes to type 2 diabetes. Diabetes. 2014;**63**:3846-3855. DOI: 10.2337/db13-1951

[14] Holst JJ. The physiology of glucagon-like peptide 1. Physiological Reviews. 2007;**87**:1409-1439. DOI: 10.1152/physrev.00034.2006

[15] Lupoli R, Cotugno M, Griffo E, et al. Role of the entero-insular axis in the pathogenesis of idiopathic reactive hypoglycemia: A pilot study. The Journal of Clinical Endocrinology and Metabolism. 2015;**100**:4441-4446. DOI: 10.1210/jc.2015-3309. Epub 2015 Oct 26

[16] Permutt MA, Kelly J, Berstein R, Alpers DH, Siegel BA, Kipnis DM. Alimentary hypoglycemia in the absence of gastrointestinal surgery. The New England Journal of Medicine. 1973;**288**(23):1206-1210. DOI: 10.1056/NEJM197306072882304

[17] Flanagan D, Wood P, Sherwin R, Debrah K, Kerr D. Gin and tonic and reactive hypoglycemia: What is important-the gin, the tonic, or both? The Journal of Clinical Endocrinology and Metabolism. 1998;**83**(3):796-800. DOI: 10.1210/jcem.83.3.4622

[18] Açbay O, Celik AF, Gündoğdu S. Does helicobacter pylori-induced gastritis enhance food-stimulated insulin release? Digestive Diseases and Sciences. 1996;**41**(7):1327-1331. DOI: 10.1007/BF02088555

[19] Danowitz M, De Leon DD. The role of GLP-1 signaling in hypoglycemia due to hyperinsulinism. Frontiers in Endocrinology (Lausanne). 2022;**13**:863184. DOI: 10.3389/fendo.2022.863184

[20] Coelho T, Freitas A, Carmona Alexandrino H, et al. Roux-en-Y gastric bypass surgery leading to postprandial hypoglycemia: A case report. Cureus. 2022;**14**(12):e32265. DOI: 10.7759/cureus.32265

[21] Hazlehurst J, Khoo B, Lobato CB, Ilesanmi I, Abbott S, Chan T, et al. Society for endocrinology guidelines for the diagnosis and management of post-bariatric hypoglycaemia. Endocrine Connections. 2024;**13**(5):e230285. DOI: 10.1530/EC-23-0285

[22] Carpentieri GB, Gonçalves SEAB, Mourad WM, Pinto LGC, Zanella MT. Hypoglycemia post bariatric surgery: Drugs with different mechanisms of action to treat a unique disorder. Archives of Endocrinology and Metabolism. 2023;**67**(3):442-449. DOI: 10.20945/2359-3997000000598

[23] Lee CJ, Clark JM, Schweitzer M, et al. Prevalence of and risk factors for hypoglycemic symptoms after gastric bypass and sleeve gastrectomy. Obesity (Silver Spring). 2015;**23**(5):1079-1084. DOI: 10.1002/oby.21042. Epub 2015 Apr 10

[24] Sjöström L. Review of the key results from the Swedish obese subjects (SOS) trial - A prospective controlled intervention study of bariatric surgery. Journal of Internal Medicine. 2013;**273**(3):219-234. DOI: 10.1111/joim.12012

[25] Capristo E, Panunzi S, De Gaetano A, Spuntarelli V, Bellantone R, Giustacchini P, et al. Incidence of hypoglycemia after gastric bypass vs sleeve gastrectomy: A randomized trial. The Journal of Clinical Endocrinology and Metabolism. 2018;**103**(6):2136-2146. DOI: 10.1210/jc.2017-01695

[26] Sessa L, Guidone C, Gallucci P, Capristo E, Mingrone G, Raffaelli M. Effect of single anastomosis duodenal-ileal bypass with sleeve gastrectomy on glucose tolerance test: Comparison with other bariatric procedures. Surgery for Obesity and Related Diseases. 2019;**15**(7):1091-1097. DOI: 10.1016/j.soard.2019.04.013

[27] Roslin MS, Dudiy Y, Brownlee A, Weiskopf J, Shah P. Response to glucose tolerance testing and solid high carbohydrate challenge: Comparison between Roux-en-Y gastric bypass, vertical sleeve gastrectomy, and duodenal switch. Surgical Endoscopy. 2014;**28**(1):91-99. DOI: 10.1007/s00464-013-3176-0

[28] Rheinwalt KP, Plamper A, Rückbeil MV, Kroh A, Neumann UP,

Ulmer TF. One anastomosis gastric bypass-mini-gastric bypass (OAGB-MGB) versus Roux-en-Y gastric bypass (RYGB)-a mid-term cohort study with 612 patients. Obesity Surgery. 2020;**30**(4):1230-1240. DOI: 10.1007/s11695-019-04250-3

[29] Ashrafi RA, Ahola AJ, Rosengård-Bärlund M, Saarinen T, Heinonen S, Juuti A, et al. Computational modelling of self-reported dietary carbohydrate intake on glucose concentrations in patients undergoing Roux-en-Y gastric bypass versus one-anastomosis gastric bypass. Annals of Medicine. 2021;**53**(1):1885-1895. DOI: 10.1080/07853890.2021.1964035

[30] Tripyla A, Herzig D, Reverter-Branchat G, et al. Counter-regulatory responses to postprandial hypoglycaemia in patients with post-bariatric hypoglycaemia vs surgical and non-surgical control individuals. Diabetologia. 2023;**66**(4):741-753. DOI: 10.1007/s00125-022-05861-9

[31] Mulla CM, Goldfine AB, Dreyfuss JM, Houten S, Pan H, Pober DM, et al. Plasma FGF-19 levels are increased in patients with post-bariatric hypoglycemia. Obesity Surgery. 2019;**29**(7):2092-2099. DOI: 10.1007/s11695-019-03845-0

[32] McCall AL, Lieb DC, Gianchandani R, et al. Management of individuals with diabetes at high risk for hypoglycemia: An endocrine society clinical practice guideline. The Journal of Clinical Endocrinology and Metabolism. 2023;**108**(3):529-562. Erratum in: J Clin Endocrinol Metab. 2023; 108(3):e44

[33] Gebhard B, Holst JJ, Biegelmayer C, Miholic J. Postprandial GLP-1, norepinephrine, and reactive hypoglycemia in dumping syndrome. Digestive Diseases and Sciences. 2001;**46**(9):1915-1923. DOI: 10.1023/a:1010635131228

[34] Middleton SJ, Balan K. Idiopathic accelerated gastric emptying presenting in adults with post-prandial diarrhea and reactive hypoglycemia: A case series. Journal of Medical Case Reports. 2012;**19**(6):132. DOI: 10.1186/1752-1947-6-132

[35] Laurenius A, Hedberg S, Olbers T. Possible relation between partial small bowel obstruction and severe postprandial reactive hypoglycemia after Roux-en-Y gastric bypass. Surgery for Obesity and Related Diseases. 2019;**15**(6):1024-1028. DOI: 10.1016/j.soard.2019.03.031

[36] Salehi M, Gastaldelli A, D'Alessio DA. Blockade of glucagon-like peptide 1 receptor corrects postprandial hypoglycemia after gastric bypass. Gastroenterology. 2014;**146**(3):669-680. DOI: 10.1053/j.gastro.2013.11.044

[37] Kalra S, Unnikrishnan AG, Sahay R. The hypoglycemic side of hypothyroidism. Indian Journal of Endocrinology and Metabolism. 2014;**18**(1):1-3. DOI: 10.4103/2230-8210.126517

[38] Fernandez CJ, Rajgopal RK, Pappachan JM. Hypoglycaemia associated with critical illness and hormone deficiencies: A narrative review. Journal of Laboratory and Precision Medicine. 2021;**6**:7. DOI: 10.21037/jlpm-2020-ash-01

[39] Rizwan T, Arora G, Alchalabi M, Qureshi F. Hypopituitarism presenting as recurrent episodes of hypoglycemia: Houssay phenomenon. Cureus. 2023;**15**(4):e37530. DOI: 10.7759/cureus.37530

[40] Nishad R, Mukhi D, Menon RK, et al. Growth hormone and metabolic homeostasis. EMJ Diabetes. 2018;**6**:78-87

[41] Lee SC, Baranowski ES, Sakremath R, Saraff V, Mohamed Z. Hypoglycaemia in adrenal insufficiency. Frontiers in Endocrinology (Lausanne). 2023;**14**:1198519. DOI: 10.3389/fendo.2023.1198519

[42] Castillo AR, de Souza AL, Alegre SM, Atala YB, Zantut-Wittmann DE, Garmes HM. Insulin sensitivity is not decreased in adult patients with hypopituitarism without growth hormone replacement. Frontiers in Endocrinology (Lausanne). 2019;**10**:534. DOI: 10.3389/fendo.2019.00534

[43] Quesada I, Tudurí E, Ripoll C, Nadal A. Physiology of the pancreatic alpha-cell and glucagon secretion: Role in glucose homeostasis and diabetes. The Journal of Endocrinology. 2008;**199**(1):5-19. DOI: 10.1677/JOE-08-0290

[44] Craig CM, Lawler HM, Lee CJE, Tan M, Davis DB, Tong J, et al. PREVENT: A randomized, placebo-controlled crossover trial of avexitide for treatment of postbariatric hypoglycemia. The Journal of Clinical Endocrinology and Metabolism. 2021;**106**(8):e3235-e3248. DOI: 10.1210/clinem/dgab103

[45] Butz JJ, Yan Q, McKenzie TJ, Weingarten TN, Cavalcante AN, Bancos I, et al. Perioperative outcomes of syndromic paraganglioma and pheochromocytoma resection in patients with von Hippel-Lindau disease, multiple endocrine neoplasia type 2, or neurofibromatosis type 1. Surgery. 2017;**162**(6):1259-1269. DOI: 10.1016/j.surg.2017.08.002

[46] Habra MA, Núñez R, Chuang H, Ayala-Ramirez M, Rich T, Kyle K, et al. Fatal hypoglycemia in malignant pheochromocytoma: Direct glucose consumption as suggested by (18) F-2-fluoro-2-deoxy-D-glucose positron emission tomography/computed tomography imaging. Endocrine. 2010;**37**(1):209-212. DOI: 10.1007/s12020-009-9300-1

[47] Thonangi RP, Bhardwaj M, Kulshreshtha B. A case report of reactive hypoglycemia in a patient with pheochromocytoma and it's review of literature. Indian Journal of Endocrinology and Metabolism. 2014;**18**(2):234-237. DOI: 10.4103/2230-8210.129120

[48] Palardy J, Havrankova J, Lepage R, Matte R, Bélanger R, D'Amour P, et al. Blood glucose measurements during symptomatic episodes in patients with suspected postprandial hypoglycemia. The New England Journal of Medicine. 1989;**321**(21):1421-1425. DOI: 10.1056/NEJM198911233212101

[49] Barry JA, Bouloux P, Hardiman PJ. The impact of eating behavior on psychological symptoms typical of reactive hypoglycemia. A pilot study comparing women with polycystic ovary syndrome to controls. Appetite. 2011;**57**(1):73-76. DOI: 10.1016/j.appet.2011.03.003

[50] Johnson DD, Dorr KE, Swenson WM, Service FJ. Reactive hypoglycemia. Journal of the American Medical Association. 1980;**243**(11):1151-1155

[51] Anthony D, Dippe S, Hofeldt FD, Davis JW, Forsham PH. Personality disorder and reactive hypoglycemia: A quantitative study. Diabetes. 1973;**22**(9):664-675. DOI: 10.2337/diab.22.9.664

[52] Ford CV, Bray GA, Swerdloff RS. A psychiatric study of patients referred with a diagnosis of hypoglycemia. The American Journal of Psychiatry. 1976;**133**(3):290-294. DOI: 10.1176/ajp.133.3.290

[53] Singh SK, Sarma MS. Hereditary fructose intolerance: A comprehensive review. World Journal of Clinical Pediatrics. 2022;**11**(4):321-329. DOI: 10.5409/wjcp. v11.i4.321

[54] Demirbas D, Coelho AI, Rubio-Gozalbo ME, Berry GT. Hereditary galactosemia. Metabolism. 2018;**83**:188-196. DOI: 10.1016/j.metabol.2018.01.025

[55] Torekov SS, Iepsen E, Christiansen M, et al. KCNQ1 long QT syndrome patients have hyperinsulinemia and symptomatic hypoglycemia. Diabetes. 2014;**63**:1315-1325. DOI: 10.2337/db13-1454

[56] Brun JF, Fédou C, Bouix O, Raynaud E, Orsetti A. Evaluation of a standardized hyperglucidic breakfast test in postprandial reactive hypoglycaemia. Diabetologia. 1995;**38**(4):494-501. DOI: 10.1007/BF00410289

[57] Nguyen Q, Pandya S, Chin K, et al. Use of continuous glucose monitoring in detecting reactive hypoglycemia in individuals without diabetes. Journal of Diabetes Science and Technology. 2018;**12**(6):1244-1245. DOI: 10.1177/1932296818777273

[58] Hücking K, Kostic Z, Pox C, et al. Alpha-glucosidase inhibition (acarbose) fails to enhance secretion of glucagon-like peptide 1 (7-36 amide) and to delay gastric emptying in type 2 diabetic patients. Diabetic Medicine. 2005;**22**:470-476. DOI: 10.1111/j.1464-5491.2005.01451.x

[59] Salamah HM, Marey A, Abugdida M, Abualkhair KA, Elshenawy S, Elhassan WAF, et al. Efficacy and safety of glucagon-like peptide-1 receptor agonists on prediabetes: A systematic review and meta-analysis of randomized controlled trials. Diabetology and Metabolic Syndrome. 2024;**16**(1):129. DOI: 10.1186/s13098-024-01371-3

Chapter 9

Clinical and Etiological Peculiarities of Hypoglycemia in Patients with Diabetes

Simona Georgiana Popa and Andreea Loredana Golli

Abstract

Hypoglycemia is the main limiting factor in the management of diabetes. The current study includes case presentations that highlight the precipitating factors of hypoglycemia in diabetic patients, represented by sepsis, hemodialysis, but also by the failure to anticipate the decrease in insulin requirements during the period of transient remission of diabetes or after the remission of an infectious process, emphasizing the need for permanent adaptation of the therapeutic regimen to the patient's status. The clinical cases also emphasize the usefulness of continuous glycemic monitoring systems in detecting asymptomatic or nocturnal hypoglycemia and in evaluating the Low Blood Glucose Index (LBGI) that indicates the patient's risk of hypoglycemia and the Glycemic Risk Assessment in Diabetes Equation (GRADE) that quantifies the risk and consequences of hypoglycemia.

Keywords: hypoglycemia in sepsis, hypoglycemia in dialysis, continuous glucose monitoring system, remission phase in type 1 diabetes, glucotoxicity remission

1. Introduction

Hypoglycemia is the main limiting factor in the therapeutic management of diabetes, being frequently encountered in patients with diabetes mellitus (DM) treated with insulin or sulfonylureas [1, 2].

Hypoglycemia is defined based on the Whipple triad represented by [1, 2]:

- Autonomic and neuroglycopenic symptoms;
- Low plasma glucose concentration (< 70 mg/dl, 3.9 mmol/l);
- Remission of symptoms after carbohydrate intake.

2. Pathophysiology

Glycemic homeostasis is maintained by multiple physicochemical, metabolic, and hormonal mechanisms that control two opposing processes: glucose production (liver and muscle glycogenolysis, liver and kidney gluconeogenesis) and peripheral glucose consumption (glycolysis) [3].

Thus, hypoglycemia occurs when the amount of glucose used as an energy source (glycolysis) in all tissues is greater than the amount of glucose released into the blood through the absorption of glucose from carbohydrate intake and through endogenous hepatic (glycogenolysis and gluconeogenesis) and renal (gluconeogenesis) production of glucose.

The decrease in plasma glucose concentration below normal triggers adaptive neurohormonal mechanisms that induce a series of metabolic processes that have a role in restoring normoglycemia [4–6].

The acute neurohormonal response induced by hypoglycemia is represented by increased secretion of glucagon from pancreatic alpha cells and catecholamines from the adrenal medulla and from the endings of the sympathetic nervous system. Catecholamines suppress endogenous secretion of insulin from pancreatic beta cells (in conditions where there is an insulin secretory reserve in patients with diabetes).

The late hormonal response, induced by prolonged hypoglycemia, is represented by increased secretion of cortisol from the adrenal cortex and growth hormone from the adenohypophysis.

Restoration of normoglycemia, secondary to the neurohormonal response, is achieved by (**Figure 1**) [7]:

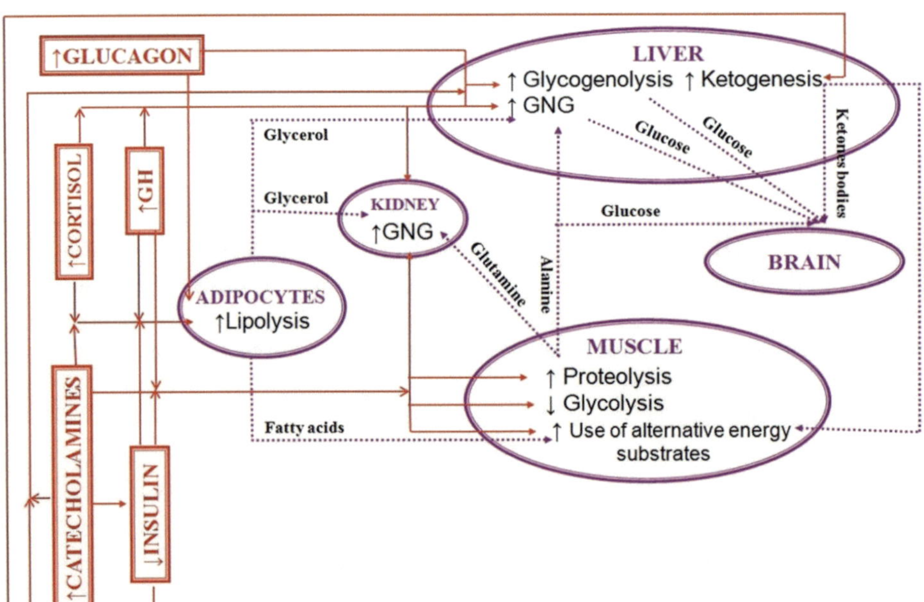

Figure 1.
Metabolic response to hypoglycemia.

- reducing glucose uptake and utilization in peripheral tissues through glycolysis
- promoting the use of alternative sources of glucose (fatty acids, ketone bodies)
- stimulating lipolysis in adipose tissue, by splitting triglycerides, resulting in both a substrate for gluconeogenesis (glycerol) and an alternative source of energy (fatty acids, ketone bodies)
- stimulating proteolysis in muscle, the resulting amino acids (glutamine, alanine) represent a substrate for gluconeogenesis
- promoting ketogenesis, the resulting ketone bodies constitute an energy substrate, especially in the central nervous system
- stimulating endogenous glucose production through hepatic glycogenolysis and hepatic and renal gluconeogenesis.

The neurohormonal response is compromised in patients with type 1 diabetes, in those with long-standing type 2 diabetes, and also in patients with diabetes and a history of severe recurrent hypoglycemia [8–11]. In the context of the functional decline of the pancreatic beta cell and the need for exogenous insulin in type 1 and type 2 diabetes, there is:

- loss of the ability to reduce insulin secretion from the beta cell in response to hypoglycemia
- attenuation of the sympathetic autonomic response (catecholamine secretion) induced by hypoglycemia, secondary to diabetic autonomic neuropathy
- an inhibitory effect of exogenous insulin on glucagon release by pancreatic alpha cells
- unchanged plasma insulin levels in the context of hypoglycemia, secondary to the persistence of exogenous insulin absorption (administered prior to the hypoglycemic episode) or secondary to the stimulation of insulin secretion, independent of the plasma glucose level, determined by sulfonylureas.

The impaired counterregulatory hormone response induced by low blood glucose levels increases the risk of severe hypoglycemia.

Repeated episodes of hypoglycemia induce a reduction in the catecholaminergic response to hypoglycemia (catecholamine secretion is triggered by a much lower blood glucose level), a decrease in sensitivity to hypoglycemia (asymptomatic hypoglycemia), and thus increase vulnerability to hypoglycemia and the recurrence of hypoglycemic episodes [12].

3. Clinical classification of hypoglycemia

Classification of hypoglycemia according to glycemic value [1].

Grade 1: Blood glucose < 70 mg/dl (3.9 mmol/l) and blood glucose ≥ 54 mg/dl (3 mmol/l).

A blood glucose value of 70 mg/dl (3.9 mmol/L) is considered the threshold value for triggering the neuroendocrine response in people without diabetes.

Since patients with DM frequently present with altered counterregulatory response to hypoglycemia or present with unawareness of hypoglycemia, detection of a blood glucose level < 70 mg/dl (3.9 mmol/l) is considered clinically important, regardless of the severity of acute hypoglycemic symptoms.

Grade 2: Blood glucose < 54 mg/dl (3 mmol/l).

A blood glucose value of 54 mg/dl (3.9 mmol/l) is considered the threshold value for the appearance of neuroglycopenic symptoms. Grade 2 hypoglycemia requires immediate action to correct the hypoglycemic event.

Grade 3: Regardless of blood glucose level.

It is characterized by a severe episode characterized by altered mental and/or physical status that requires assistance from another person for recovery.

Classification of hypoglycemia according to severity [2, 13].

Mild hypoglycemia: autonomic symptoms are present that can be corrected by the patient and do not have a negative impact on the patient's comfort;

Moderate hypoglycemia: autonomic and neuroglycopenic symptoms are present that can be corrected by the patient, but have a negative impact on the patient's comfort.

Severe hypoglycemia is defined by the patient's inability to act coherently to correct the hypoglycemia, requiring the intervention of another person to administer glucose, glucagon, or other measures to correct the hypoglycemia. Due to significant neuroglycopenia, convulsions or coma may occur.

Classification of hypoglycemia according to symptoms and blood glucose level [1, 13].

Documented symptomatic hypoglycemia is defined by the presence of symptoms of hypoglycemia accompanied by the detection of a plasma glucose concentration < 70 mg/dl (3.9 mmol/l);

Asymptomatic hypoglycemia is defined by the detection of a plasma glucose concentration < 70 mg/dl (3.9 mmol/l) but not accompanied by symptoms of hypoglycemia. It occurs frequently in patients with long-term DM and predisposes patients to severe hypoglycemia. It can occur in conditions of chronic exposure to low blood glucose levels or the presence of diabetic autonomic neuropathy.

Probable symptomatic hypoglycemia is defined by the presence of symptoms of hypoglycemia that are not accompanied by the determination of the blood glucose level. Many patients opt to treat symptoms by ingesting carbohydrates, but without first determining blood glucose levels.

Relative hypoglycemia is defined as the patient reporting symptoms of hypoglycemia that they interpret as a hypoglycemic episode, but the plasma glucose level at that time is > 70 mg/dl (3.9 mmol/l), disproving hypoglycemia. These episodes may occur in patients with poor metabolic control in whom symptoms of hypoglycemia occurring at blood glucose levels > 70 mg/dl (3.9 mmol/l) may be explained by the rapid decrease in blood glucose from a high value.

It should be noted that, in recent years, the first of the three classifications mentioned above has become established in practice, and it is also used in the annual guidelines of the American Diabetes Association [1].

4. Signs and symptoms of hypoglycemia

Autonomic signs and symptoms: tremors of the extremities, palpitations, cold sweats, anxiety, hunger, nausea, paresthesias, pallor, tachycardia, and increased blood pressure.

Neuroglycopenic signs and symptoms: dizziness, fatigue, headache, confusion, drowsiness, visual disturbances, diplopia, cognitive dysfunction, behavioral disorders (irritability, automatisms, lethargy, aggressiveness), seizures, coma. Neurological signs and symptoms (speech disorders, ataxia, focal neurological deficit, choreoathetosis, transient ischemic attacks) and neuropsychiatric manifestations (automatisms, psychoses) may occur.

Neuroglycopenic clinical manifestations can mimic numerous neurological (epilepsy, brain tumors, meningitis, migraine, stroke, etc.); psychiatric (hysteria, neuroses, schizophrenia, depression, dementia, etc.); endocrine (thyrotoxicosis, pheochromocytoma, etc.); cardiovascular (carotid sinus syncope, orthostatic hypotension, rhythm disorders, etc.); and diseases caused by alcohol intoxication, sedatives, carbon monoxide, etc. The differential diagnosis of neuroglycopenic syndromes is based on the clinical context of onset and blood glucose values.

There is a great variability of symptomatology from one person to another and even in the same person from one episode to another.

In children, behavioral disorders predominate, and in the elderly, neurological symptoms.

5. Precipitating factors of hypoglycemia in patients with diabetes

1.1.*Absolute or relative excess of insulin*:

- Administration errors:
  - o Accidental reversal of the types of insulin administered (administration of basal insulin instead of prandial insulin or vice versa) [1, 14–22].
  - o Exposure, immediately after insulin administration, to high temperatures that increase the rate of insulin absorption.
  - o Accidental injection of insulin into a blood vessel, which can be suspected if drops of blood appear after removing the needle from the skin.
  - o Accidental, deliberate, suicidal, or malicious administration.
- Doses that are too high in relation to insulin requirements
- Reduced clearance of exogenous insulin: chronic kidney disease
- Increased insulin sensitivity (rapid decrease in insulin requirements)
  - o Postpartum

- o Failure to anticipate a decrease in insulin requirements during the recovery period after infections or acute medical or surgical conditions, after weight loss, or during the period of sudden reduction in the dose of corticosteroids.

- o After the decrease in glucotoxicity and lipotoxicity in patients with new-onset diabetes.

- o Transient remission of diabetes ("honeymoon"), which represents the period of variable duration (1–12 months) after the diagnosis of type 1 diabetes, when, in the context of initiating insulin therapy, glucotoxicity improves significantly, and thus the suppression of insulin secretion induced by glucotoxicity is reduced, and the pancreas begins to secrete the remaining insulin reserves.

- Intensive insulin therapy itself (glycemic/HbA1c targets too low). Hypoglycemia in this case is the price paid to maintain optimal metabolic control. Hypoglycemia may be the consequence of aggressive correction of glycemic values above therapeutic targets or of hyperglycemia reactive to hypoglycemia.

2. *Treatment with long-acting insulin secretagogues*: (sulfonylureas) can induce hypoglycemia. Hypoglycemia induced by sulfonylureas can be long-lasting and may recur after initial correction of hypoglycemia due to the persistence of the drug action. Therefore, patients with hypoglycemia secondary to sulfonylureas often require parenteral glucose therapy and must be hospitalized for monitoring. Glucagon is ineffective in the correction of hypoglycemia secondary to sulfonylureas.

3. *Reduced exogenous glucose intake*:

    - Inadequate quantitative carbohydrate intake (intake of insufficient carbohydrates at a meal, vomiting)

    - Lack of synchronization between insulin administration and carbohydrate ingestion (significant delay in carbohydrate intake after administration of prandial insulin or short-acting insulin secretagogues—glinides)

    - Unexpected interruption of oral, enteral, or parenteral nutrition

4. *Reduced endogenous glucose production*:

    - Alcohol ingestion, especially if associated with increased physical exertion (e.g., dancing parties). Alcohol can cause hypoglycemia by inhibiting hepatic gluconeogenesis. Ethanol does not inhibit glycogenolysis, however, and therefore does not cause hypoglycemia in those who have ingested a significant amount of carbohydrates previously, 12–24 hours before alcohol consumption. Alcohol alters the counterregulatory hormonal response (delays the response of glucagon and catecholamines to hypoglycemia and inhibits the response of cortisol and growth hormone to hypoglycemia), thus contributing to the occurrence of fasting hypoglycemia. Acute alcohol ingestion can cause severe asymptomatic hypoglycemia by reducing the appreciation of symptoms and the counterregulatory hormonal response.

- Liver failure—secondary to reduced hepatic glycogenolysis and gluconeogenesis).

5. *Increased glucose utilization*—in case of unforeseen physical exertion associated with the administration of insulin in an area involved in the performance of the effort. The risk of hypoglycemia can be immediate in the case of intense, short-term physical exercise (due to increased glucose consumption at the muscle level) or delayed in the case of prolonged physical exercise (through depletion of muscle and liver glycogen) if carbohydrates are not ingested or the doses of hypoglycemic therapy are not adjusted.

6. *Mixed mechanisms*

    - Renal failure—secondary to reduced renal gluconeogenesis, reduced clearance of insulin or insulin secretagogues, reduced appetite, and food intake. Hypoglycemia may occur during or immediately after hemodialysis, possibly secondary to decreased insulin resistance due to the reduction of uremic toxins by dialysis.

    - Hypoglycemia due to sepsis is secondary to decreased hepatic glucose production in the late stages of sepsis, increased glucose consumption by macrophages, and increased ifnsulin secretion induced by inflammatory cytokines (IL-1, IL-6, TNF-α).

7. *Recurrent hypoglycemia, nocturnal hypoglycemia, or severe hypoglycemia* with a history of frequent episodes. Young children and the elderly on insulin therapy are considered vulnerable to hypoglycemia due to their reduced ability to recognize and report hypoglycemic symptoms and to effectively communicate their needs.

8. *Unawareness hypoglycemia* is defined as the absence of significant hypoglycemic symptoms at blood glucose levels of 50–54 mg/dl and has been reported in 25–40% of patients with type 1 DM and 6–17% of patients with insulin-treated type 2 DM. The frequency of unawareness hypoglycemia may be underestimated, however, because patients who report intact hypoglycemia awareness are often unaware of hypoglycemia that was only identified on CGMS. Recurrent hypoglycemia is the main cause of unawareness hypoglycemia because the adrenomedullary response is impaired, and unawareness hypoglycemia significantly increases the risk of severe hypoglycemia. Factors that can induce asymptomatic hypoglycemia also include psychological stress and sleep, and there is controversy over the impact of exercise and beta-blockers on the risk of asymptomatic hypoglycemia.

    The hyperinsulinemic hypoglycemic clamp is the gold standard in detecting hypoglycemic awareness and reactive hormonal response by assessing hypoglycemic symptoms, identifying glycemic thresholds for the occurrence of hypoglycemic symptoms, and assessing the counterregulatory hormonal profile and hepatic glucose production at different stages of hypoglycemia. In current practice, however, validated hypoglycemia awareness questionnaires are used, such as the Gold, Clarke, Pedersen-Bjergaard, or HypoA-Q119 questionnaires based on patient reporting of experience in detecting hypoglycemic episodes and the glycemic values at which hypoglycemic symptoms occur, as well as the severity, frequency, and impact of hypoglycemic episodes.

9. *Socioeconomic factors*: low economic status, food insecurity, poor medical literacy

6. Usefulness of continuous monitoring systems in the identification of hypoglycemia

Identification of hypoglycemia in patients with diabetes can be achieved by determining the concentration of glucose in plasma or by intermittent self-monitoring of capillary blood, using a glucometer, or continuous self-monitoring of interstitial tissue using a continuous glucose monitoring system. Determination of HbA1c has limited utility in diagnosing hypoglycemia in patients with high glycemic variability (alternating hypoglycemia/hyperglycemia), because HbA1c indicates the average blood glucose levels over a period of approximately three months [1].

The classical methods of assessing glycemic control—determination of blood glucose, HbA1c, mean blood glucose (MBG), and standard deviation (SD) of blood glucose—have proven ineffective in assessing glycemic variability and in identifying the frequency, duration, and severity of hypoglycemia. The introduction of continuous glucose monitoring systems in therapeutic regimens has allowed the quantification of glycemic variability and hypoglycemic episodes and their impact by measuring or calculating specific indices [22–25].

Coefficient of variation (CV) is calculated as a ratio between the standard deviation and the mean blood glucose. CV provides a standardized comparative analysis of patients who have similar mean blood glucose values. According to recent American Diabetes Association (ADA) guidelines, the target value of CV is 0.36, but several studies suggest that a target CV value < 0.33 is more appropriate, providing protection against hypoglycemia.

Mean Amplitude of Glycemic Excursions (MAGE)—calculated based on the mean of the differences between the highest and lowest consecutive glucose values, only for differences greater than the standard deviation. MAGE provides a measure of intraday glycemic variability with high amplitude and low frequency.

Mean daily differences (MODD)—calculated as the mean of the absolute differences between glucose values at corresponding time points on two consecutive days. MODD thus allows for the estimation of glycemic variability between two consecutive days.

Time in range (TIR)—percent of time spent with glycemic values between 70 mg/dl (3.9 mmol/l) and 180 mg/dl (10.0 mmol/l), which represent the target glucose range.

Time below range (TBR)—the percentage of time spent with glycemic values < 70 mg/dl (3.9 mmol/l) and, respectively, < 54 mg/dl (3.0 mmol/l).

Time above the range (TAR)—the percentage of time spent with glycemic values >180 mg/dl (10.0 mmol/l) and, respectively, >250 mg/dl (13.9 mmol/l).

International guidelines recommend that for optimal metabolic control, TIR should be >70%, TBR should be less than 5%, with the mention that the percentage of time with glycemic values in the range of 70–54 mg/dl (3.9–3.0 mmol/l) should be less than 4%, and that with glycemic values <54 mg/dl (3.0 mmol/l) should be less than 1%. Regarding TAR, it must be less than 30%, a percentage that is divided as follows: the percentage of time with glycemic values in the range of 180–250 mg/dl (10.0–13.9 mmol/l) must be less than 25%, and that with glycemic values > 250 mg/dl (13.9 mmol/l) must be less than 5%.

For elderly patients, therapeutic targets are less strict to avoid the risk of hypoglycemia and the consequences of hypoglycemia, taking into account the reduced ability of this category of patients to recognize the symptoms of hypoglycemia, to self-care and self-monitor, but also the greater risks associated with hypoglycemia in the elderly. Thus, in the elderly, the TIR target is > 50%, the target for the percentage of time with glycemic values < 70 mg/dl (3.9 mmol/l) is < 1%, while the target for TAR is > 50%.

J index calculated based on MBG and SD of blood glucose, according to the formula [0.001x(MBG + SD)2], provides information regarding the level of glycemic control. Thus, a J index value between 10 and 20 indicates ideal glycemic control, a J index between 20 and 30 suggests good glycemic control, while a J index value > 30 indicates poor glycemic control.

Low glycemic index (LBGI) and high glycemic index (HBGI). The formulas for LBGI and HBGI are established by converting glucose values into risk scores. If the glucose risk score is less than 0, then the risk is considered LBGI, and if it is above 0, then it is considered HBGI.

The Glycemic Risk Assessment Equation (GRADE) formula transforms glucose values into a risk score, calculates the median, and indicates the risk attributable to hypoglycemia/hyperglycemia. GRADE is calculated according to the formula: [median (425 · {log[log(Gn)] + 0.16}2)], where G is the glycemic value. A GRADE value < 5 indicates good glycemic control.

In order to highlight the utility of CGMS in the assessment of glycemic control, glycemic variability, and, in particular, in the identification of nocturnal or asymptomatic hypoglycemia in patients with type 1 diabetes, we will present several clinical cases.

The patients presented are with type 1 diabetes on basal-bolus insulin therapy or insulin pump therapy and, based on CGMS records, the glycemic mean, SD, CV%, M100, J index, MAGE, MODD, the risk of hypo/hyperglycemia and the risk attributable to hypo/hyperglycemia, as well as the percentage of time spent with glycemic values below target (< 54 mg/dl (3.0 mmol/l) and 54–70 mg/dl (3.0–3.9 mmol/l), respectively), above glycemic target (180–250 mg/dl (10.0–13.9 mmol/l) and > 250 mg/dl (13.9 mmol/l), respectively) and in glycemic target, respectively, were analyzed.

To exemplify the involvement, in the occurrence of hypoglycemia, of specific factors, such as sepsis, socioeconomic factors, chronic kidney disease, hemodialysis, transient remission of type 1 diabetes, and failure to anticipate a decrease in insulin requirements during the recovery period after infections, we will present several suggestive clinical cases below.

6.1 Case 1

A 64-year-old female patient, diagnosed with type 2 diabetes 19 years ago, treated with Glimepiride 1 mg/day (the patient being immobilized, medication and food intake are provided by the caregiver, the last carbohydrate intake and the last dose of Glimepiride being administered the day prior to presentation), who presented to the emergency department unconscious, the venous blood glucose value at the time being 12 mg/dl (0.7 mmol/l).

Personal pathological history includes: peripheral diabetic sensory-motor and vegetative neuropathy, grade 3 hypertension with very high cardiovascular risk, paroxysmal atrial fibrillation, sequelae of ischemic stroke, and mixed dementia.

Clinical examination reveals: a decrease in skin turgor, dry mucous membranes, left hemiplegia post-stroke, presence of a decubitus ulcer with purulent, fetid secretions, at the level of the right buttock, and multiple skin vesicles with hemorrhagic content at the bilateral calcaneal level.

Paraclinical examinations revealed an HbA1c value of 6.56%, absent urinary ketone bodies (during the hypoglycemic episode, suggesting that the hypoglycemia is insulin-mediated), creatinine 0.58 mg/dl, GOT 15 U/l, GPT 11 U/l, presepsin 983 ng/l, microbiological examination of purulent secretions collected from the eschar revealed the presence of *Proteus Mirabilis* and *Escherichia Coli*.

Analyzing the results of the biological examinations, we detect values within normal limits of creatinine, GOT, and GPT, indicating normal renal and hepatic function. Taking into account the presence of the infected eschar, as well as the absence of Glimepiride treatment on the day of presentation, we consider the occurrence of the severe hypoglycemic episode in the context of the septic state, which can induce, through secreted inflammatory cytokines, inhibition of hepatic glucose production, but also increased glucose consumption associated with the bacterial skin infection.

Calcaneal blisters are common complications of diabetes and occur in the context of the existence of peripheral diabetic neuropathy and can have an unfavorable evolution in the sense of extension, infection, rupture, and generation of neuropathic ulcers with a reserved prognosis. The presence of neuropathic ulcers, hemiplegia, eschar, dementia associated with the unfavorable social context—the patient lives alone and depends on the periodic visit of relatives who bring her food and administer her medication, implies an increased risk of severe hypoglycemia caused by the reduction of the patient's mobility and thus the capacity for self-care (poor nutrition, inconsistent meal times, errors in the administration of therapy with increased hypoglycemic risk, etc.), the difficulty of recognizing the symptoms of hypoglycemia, the presence of neuropathy that induces the reduction/absence of autonomic symptoms of hypoglycemia and the difficulty of correcting hypoglycemia in time. Furthermore, symptoms of hypoglycemia, such as confusion, altered mental status, and fatigue, can overlap with manifestations characteristic of dementia, so distinguishing between the two can be difficult.

Also, considering the diagnosis of type 2 diabetes, even in conditions of a long duration of diabetes evolution, the occurrence of severe hypoglycemia indicates that there is still endogenous insulin secretion which, cumulated with the inhibition of hepatic glucose production, increased glucose consumption, therapy with sulfonylureas that have a long duration of action, stimulates insulin secretion independently of glucose concentration and thus maintains suppressed glucagon secretion even in the context of hypoglycemia and associated with the lack of carbohydrate intake, may additionally contribute to the occurrence of severe and prolonged hypoglycemia.

Consequently, the failure to adjust the dose of Glimepiride in relation to the low food intake and the presence of the septic state led to the occurrence of severe hypoglycemia with the abolition of the state of consciousness.

It is necessary to consider the risk of paroxysmal episodes of atrial fibrillation because severe hypoglycemia may increase the risk of arrhythmias. The exact mechanism is not known, but factors that modify the structure of the heart, lead to dysfunction of the autonomic nervous system, and the appearance of inflammation are involved. It is also important to differentiate the symptoms characteristic of hypoglycemia, such as palpitations, vertigo, from the episode of paroxysmal atrial fibrillation.

The patient's management involves stopping the therapy with a high risk of hypoglycemia and opting for a therapy with a minimal risk of hypoglycemia, and it is also important to set less stringent glycemic targets to avoid the risk of severe hypoglycemia.

6.2 Case 2

In the second case, we present a 32-year-old patient with type 1 diabetes, on sensor augmented insulin pump therapy (total daily insulin dose -35 IU insulin/day, basal rate—23.7 IU insulin/day, Insulin-to-Carb Ratio—1 IU insulin/10 g carbohydrates, Insulin Sensitivity Factor—1 IU insulin decreases blood glucose by 30 mg/dL), with multiple micro- and macrovascular diabetic chronic complications and comorbidities, including: diabetic peripheral sensory-motor and vegetative neuropathy with cardiovascular manifestations (orthostatic hypotension), diabetic peripheral arterial disease, sequelae of ischemic stroke, chronic glomerulonephritis, stage 5 chronic kidney disease on renal replacement therapy by hemodialysis (without glucose in the dialysis solution), grade 3 hypertension with very high cardiovascular risk, ankylosing spondylitis and chronic viral hepatitis B.

Clinically, the patient frequently presents during hemodialysis sessions with symptoms such as dizziness, headache, cold sweats, tremors, and visual disturbances, symptoms suggestive of hypoglycemia. Capillary blood glucose monitoring reveals glycemic variability with significant decreases in glycemic values and even symptomatic and documented hypoglycemia (glycemia 58 mg/dl) (3.2 mmol/l) during hemodialysis sessions in the absence of basal rates administration during the hemodialysis session, without administration of a prandial or corrective bolus prior to the start of hemodialysis and in the conditions of uncorrected hydrate intake with prandial bolus during the hemodialysis session.

In addition to the decrease in renal gluconeogenesis and the reduction in insulin clearance specific to chronic kidney disease, hemodialysis is additionally associated with significant improvement in insulin resistance and glucose loss during hemodialysis, which explains the occurrence of frequent hypoglycemia.

From the patient's history, chronic viral hepatitis B led to liver damage through inflammatory processes and fibrotic liver lesions. Thus, glycogen stores and gluconeogenesis are consequently affected, which can contribute to the occurrence of hypoglycemia. Liver dysfunction associated with chronic kidney disease and hemodialysis can complicate diabetes management and glycemic control through significant glycemic variability dominated by hypoglycemia, making it difficult to maintain glycemic values within the target.

Management of these patients involves individualizing glycemic targets and adapting insulin doses on the day of the hemodialysis session to prevent hypoglycemia or a significant decrease in glycemia during hemodialysis sessions.

It was observed that on days without hemodialysis, no hypoglycemia or marked decreases in blood glucose were recorded under the conditions of basal rates administration and ingestion of hydrates appropriately corrected with insulin (**Figure 2**). At 8:00 PM on the day without hemodialysis, a blood glucose value of 158 mg/dl (8.8 mmol/l) is detected following the prandial bolus, and at the same time, on the day with hemodialysis, in the absence of the prandial bolus, a value of 58 mg/dl (3.2 mmol/l) is highlighted, a value that caused the appearance of signs and symptoms specific to hypoglycemia (**Figure 2**).

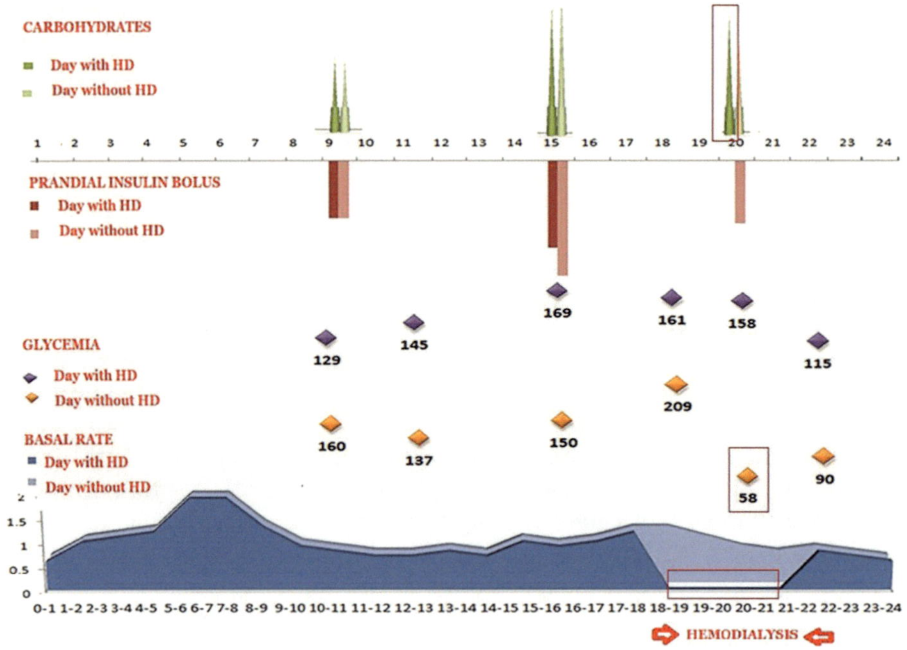

Figure 2.
Carbohydrate intake, prandial insulin bolus, basal rate, and glycemic profile in a day with hemodialysis (HD) and without hemodialysis. Hypoglycemia during a hemodialysis session.

Hypoglycemia was prevented by the intake of carbohydrates, not corrected with insulin, before the hemodialysis session.

Therefore, the following therapeutic plan was chosen for this patient to prevent hypoglycemia during hemodialysis sessions (**Figure 3**).

- intake of 50 g of carbohydrates, uncorrected with a prandial insulin bolus, before starting hemodialysis
- maintaining the snack uncorrected with insulin during the hemodialysis session
- discontinuation of the basal insulin rate for the entire duration of the hemodialysis session.

Thus, it was found that on days when the patient, before but also during the hemodialysis session, had an intake of 50 g of carbohydrates uncorrected with a prandial insulin bolus, the blood glucose value was maintained above the threshold of 70 mg/dl (3.9 mmol/l); thus, hypoglycemia episodes were prevented.

6.3 Case 3

In this case, we present a 59-year-old male patient, diagnosed with type 2 diabetes for 3 years, treated with insulin since diagnosis (0.4 IU insulin/kg/day), insulin therapy being initiated in the context of the presence of glucotoxicity (HbA1c 13.9%) and hepatic cytolysis syndrome (acute viral hepatitis B and toxic-metabolic).

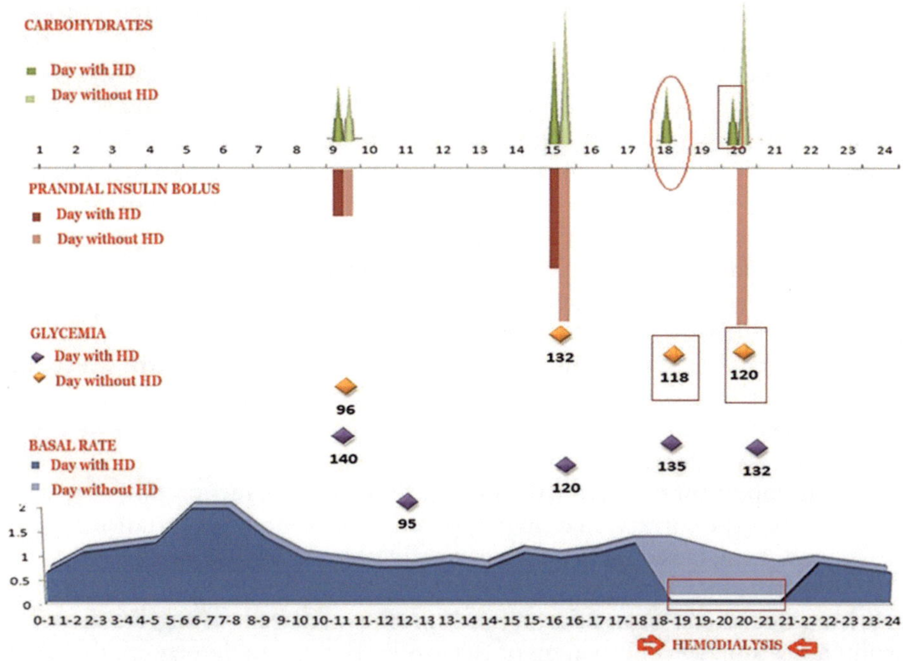

Figure 3.
Carbohydrate intake, prandial insulin bolus, basal rate, and glycemic profile in a day with hemodialysis (HD) and without hemodialysis.

Approximately one year later, the patient presented supra- and subfascial phlegmon on the right thigh associated with extensive cellulitis involving the thigh and upper third of the calf.

For the treatment of the infection, a debridement incision was performed with evacuation of purulent secretions (microbiological examination of the purulent secretion revealed Klebsiella sp., Enterococcus sp., *Escherichia coli*, and methicillin-resistant *Staphylococcus aureus*) and systemic antibiotic therapy.

Considering the HbA1c value (10.34%) dosed during the diagnosis of the phlegmon, the glycemic profile, and the septic context, the insulin doses were titrated progressively up to a requirement of 38 IU insulin/day. The subsequent evolution was favorable with the remission of the infectious phenomena.

The insulin requirement established in the context of the extensive infectious process was no longer titrated regressively after the remission of the infection, the patient presenting at 2-year intervals with weight gain and persistent feeling of hunger occurring both during the day and at night, corrected by the ingestion of carbohydrates without determining the blood glucose at that time.

The paraclinical evaluation in dynamics indicated a progressive decrease in glycated hemoglobin at one year after diagnosis as a result of the initiation of insulin treatment and correction of glucotoxicity, and at 2 years after the remission of the infectious episode, a marked decrease in HbA1c to 6.89%, and a glycemic profile on the first day of hospitalization, under the conditions of administering the same doses of insulin (38 IU insulin/day) from the outpatient setting, characterized by glycemic values < 70 mg/dl (3.9 mmol/l), before lunch and during the night, as a result of the remission of the infection and the lack of adjustment of the insulin requirement.

Regressive titration of insulin doses after the remission of an infectious process is essential to ensure optimal glycemic control and to prevent potential complications. Infectious factors have a significant effect on glycemic control by increasing pro-inflammatory cytokines, oxidative stress, changing the diet, but also altering insulin sensitivity. Although the dose adjustment was performed appropriately during the infectious episode, the period following healing requires a new titration. The low adherence to the periodic clinical evaluation program led to the maintenance of insulin doses higher than the patient's actual insulin requirement (necessarily low in the context of remission of the infectious episode and increased insulin sensitivity), and thus, resulted in recurrent, symptomatic episodes of undocumented hypoglycemia as a result of excessively high insulin doses.

An impediment to obtaining and maintaining good glycemic control is also the patient's history of acute viral hepatitis B, given the role of the liver in gluconeogenesis and storing glucose in the form of glycogen, thus contributing to the additional increase in the risk of hypoglycemia.

Thus, it is important to educate the patient regarding the recognition of hypoglycemia symptoms, the correction of hypoglycemia, but also the importance of glycemic self-monitoring, based on which to correctly titrate insulin doses.

The symptomatology suggestive of frequent episodes of hypoglycemia, the current HbA1c value of 6.89% and the glycemic profiles required the regressive titration of insulin doses and the replacement of the insulin therapy regimen with the administration of basal insulin at a dose of 12 IU/day (0.1 IU/kg/day), with improvement in glycemic profiles and without persistence of hypoglycemia.

6.4 Case 4

We present a 20-year-old female patient, normal weight (BMI: 18.5 kg/m^2), with a personal pathological history of autoimmune thyroiditis, diagnosed with type 1 diabetes mellitus for 11 years, with sensor augmented insulin pump therapy with a basal rate of 22.8 IU/24 hours and prandial boluses of 1.4 IU for 10 g of carbohydrates.

Glycated hemoglobin was 7.75%, a value above the established glycemic targets, HbA1c target in this case, considering the patient's young age, the lack of other comorbidities, and the duration of diabetes, being 6.5% with minimizing hypoglycemic episodes as much as possible.

Based on the CGMS records, over the 90 days, it was observed that the patient used the sensor 80% of the time, with a daily average of 1.9 calibrations. These records revealed a mean blood glucose value of 162 mg/dl (9.0 mmol/l) and an estimated glycated hemoglobin value of 7.2%.

According to the information obtained with the CGMS, the TIR was 62%. The patient also had blood glucose values between 70 and 54 mg/dl (3.9–3.0 mmol/l) in 4% of the time and values lower than 54 mg/dl (3.0 mmol/l) in 1% of the time. Regarding hyperglycemia, 25% of the time, the patient recorded values above 180 mg/dl (10.0 mmol/l), but below 250 mg/dl (13.9 mmol/l), and a percentage of 8% of the time she had significant glycemic excursions above 250 mg/dl (13.9 mmol/l) (**Figure 4**).

It was observed that the patient mainly presents hypoglycemia during the night, but also during the day, which can be explained by both the overcorrection of hyperglycemia that occurred reactively to hypoglycemia and in the context of performing physical exertion without prior supplementation with carbohydrates (**Figures 5–8**).

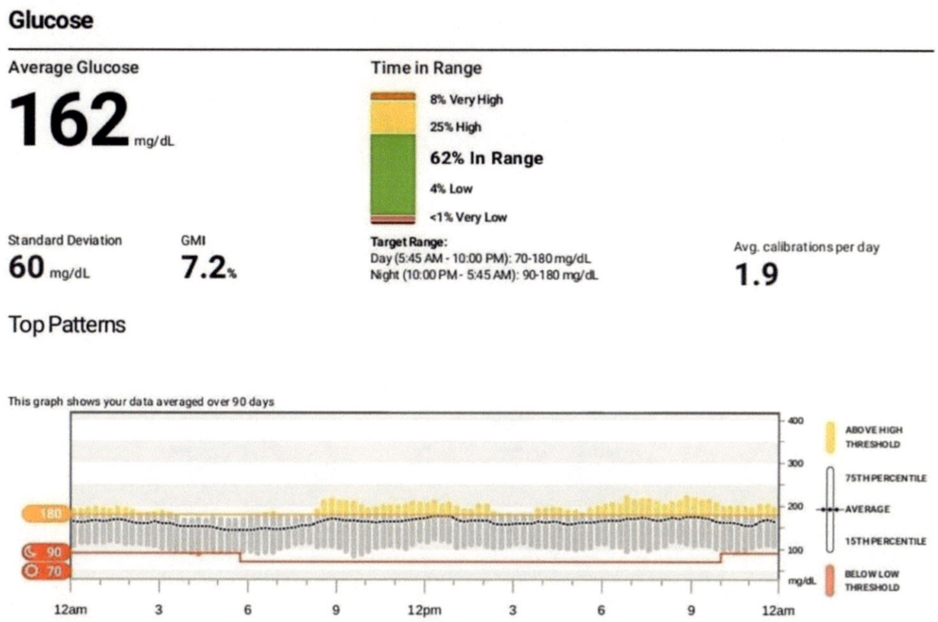

Figure 4.
90-day CGMS analytical report.

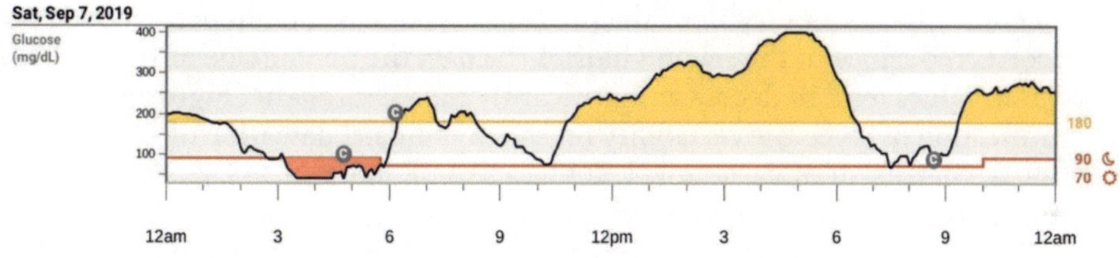

Figure 5.
Daily CGMS report (Sep 7, 2019).

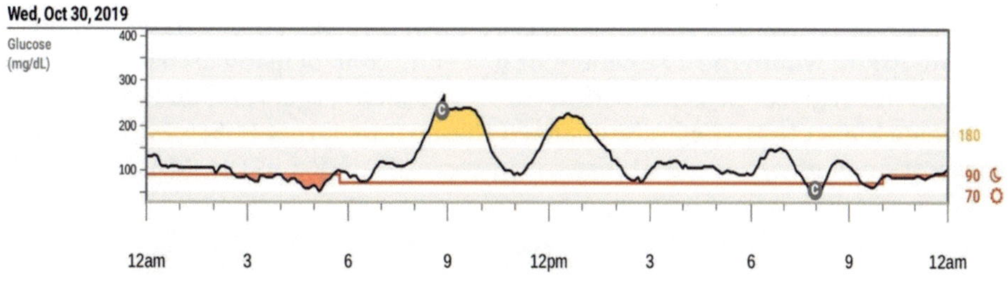

Figure 6.
Daily CGMS report (Oct 30, 2019).

Based on the hourly statistics, it is found that the patient presents in the time interval 02:00 a.m.–05:00 a.m., the highest percentage of time in which the glycemic values are below 70 mg/dl (3.9 mmol/l) (9–13% of the time), this being the period with the highest risk of hypoglycemia since cortisol secretion is low. Most likely,

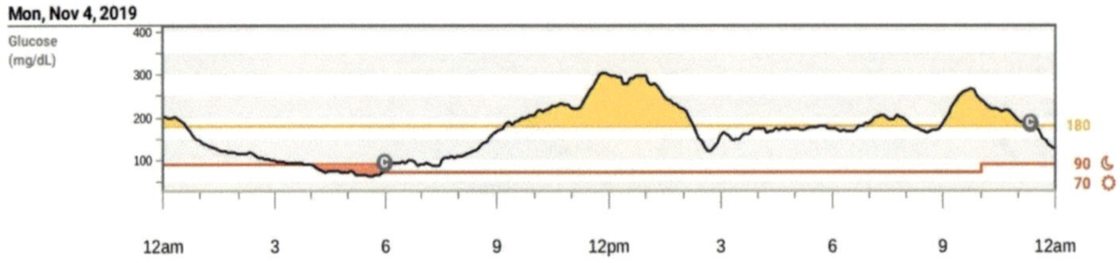

Figure 7.
Daily CGMS report (Nov 4, 2019).

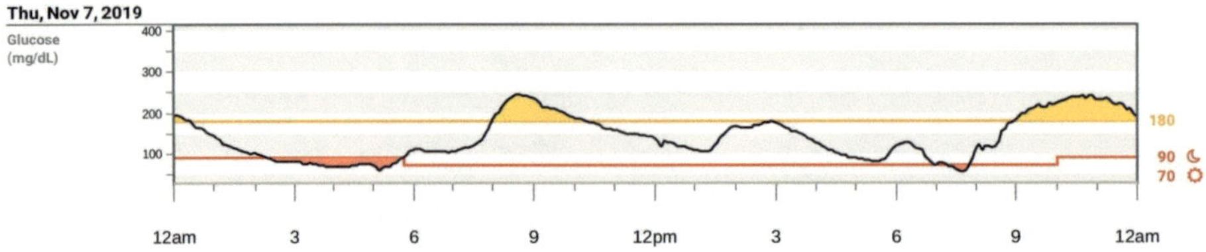

Figure 8.
Daily CGMS report (Nov 7, 2019).

taking into account the reproducibility of the profile, hypoglycemia not being an isolated one, a possible cause of its occurrence is represented by the increased basal rates compared to the insulin requirement. Later, during the morning, the tendency to hyperglycemia appears as a result of the previous hypoglycemia, hyperglycemia possibly overcorrected, since in the second half of the day, the percentage of time in which the glycemic values tend to decrease significantly increases again (**Figure 9**).

Quantification of glycemic variability revealed: standard deviation of 60 mg/dl (3.3 mmol/l), coefficient of variation of 37.3%, a MAGE index of 143.45, this value indicating major glycemic excursions within the same day, and a MODD index of 57.96, a value indicating a large variation in glycemic profiles from one day to the next, also highlighted by the overlay of CGMS graphs from seven consecutive days (**Figure 10**).

6.5 Case 5

We present the case of a patient with type 1 DM on sensor augmented insulin pump therapy, in whom the assessment of glycemic control using classical parameters indicated a mean glycemic value within the established targets and an HbA1c of 7.1%, a value higher than the individualized therapeutic target (6.5–6.7%) (**Table 1**). Quantification of glycemic variability parameters (SD, CV, J index, MAGE, MODD)

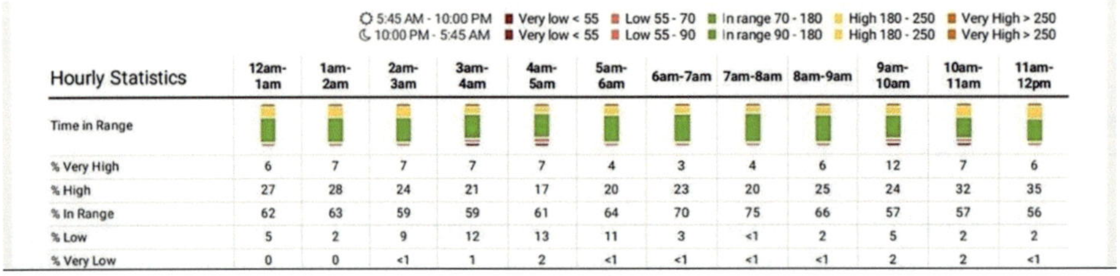

Hourly Statistics	12am-1am	1am-2am	2am-3am	3am-4am	4am-5am	5am-6am	6am-7am	7am-8am	8am-9am	9am-10am	10am-11am	11am-12pm
Time in Range												
% Very High	6	7	7	7	7	4	3	4	6	12	7	6
% High	27	28	24	21	17	20	23	20	25	24	32	35
% In Range	62	63	59	59	61	64	70	75	66	57	57	56
% Low	5	2	9	12	13	11	3	<1	2	5	2	2
% Very Low	0	0	<1	1	2	<1	<1	<1	<1	2	2	<1

Figure 9.
CGMS hourly statistics report.

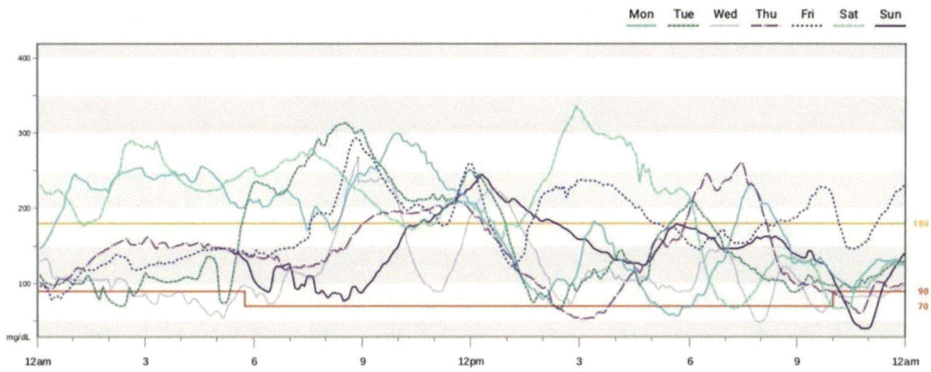

Figure 10.
Case 4 - CGMS weekly report.

	MAGE (mg/dl)	MODD (mg/dl)	HbA1c (%) (estimated)	MBG (mg/dl)	SD (mg/dl)	CV (%)	J Index (mg/dl)
Overall	102.1	29.7	5.9	123.6	50.4	40.7	30.2
Night time			5.8	121.1	30.7	25.4	23.1

Table 1.
Case 5 - Classical parameters of glycemic control.

on CGMS recordings indicated increased glycemic variability (CV >36%), poor glycemic control (J index > 30), with significant glycemic excursions within the same day (MAGE), but glycemic profiles are reproducible from one day to another (MODD) (**Table 1**). The difference between the dosed HbA1c value and the estimated HbA1c value is justified by the fact that the dosed HbA1c value indicates the average glycemic value in the last 3 months, while the HbA1c estimate is based on the glycemic values recorded during the 7 days of using the glycemic sensor. This difference suggests the predominance of hypoglycemia during the CGMS monitoring period and implies the identification of the precipitating factors of hypoglycemia during this period (the tendency to "force" the achievement of glycemic control during the CGMS monitoring period, more intense physical activity than usual, change in diet, etc.).

The CGMS graphs (**Figure 11**) and the data from **Table 2** suggest that the patient has frequent hypoglycemia, with both glucose values <70 mg/dl (3.9 mmol/l) being recorded in 8.2% of the total CGMS recording time, and <54 mg/dl (3.0 mmol/l) in 1.91% of the total CGMS recording time. Hypoglycemia predominates during the night, especially glucose values <54 mg/dl (3.0 mmol/l), which induces a high risk of asymptomatic and/or severe hypoglycemia.

Significant hyperglycemia (> 250 mg/dl (13.9 mmol/l)) was recorded in only 3.93% of the total CGMS recording time, occurring only during the day. Glucose values >180 mg/dl (10.0 mmol/l) were recorded in 9.49% of the time, also prevailing during the day. According to the CGMS graphs, hyperglycemia was generally the consequence of hypoglycemia, being due to counterregulatory hormones secreted during unrecognized hypoglycemia but also to the ingestion of carbohydrates to correct symptomatic hypoglycemia. Hyperglycemia can also be the consequence of the

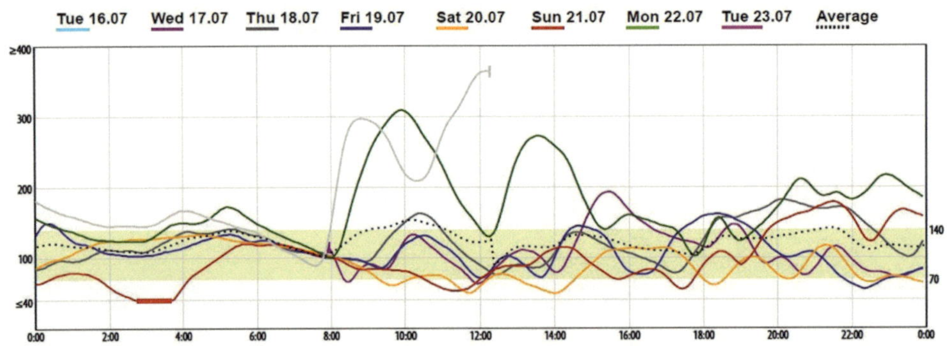

Figure 11.
Case 5 - CGMS weekly report.

	TBR (%)		TIR (%)	TAR (%)	
	< 70 mg/dl (3.9 mmol/l)	< 54 mg/dl (3.0 mmol/l)	70–180 mg/dl (3.9–10.0 mmol/l)	> 180 mg/dl (10.0 mmol/l)	> 250 mg/dl (13.9 mmol/l)
Overall	8.20	1.91	82.31	9.49	3.93
Night time	7.87	4.86	91.90	0.23	0.00

Table 2.
Case 5 - Percent of time spent below/above or in glycemic target.

imbalance between the amount of carbohydrates ingested at meals and the calculated insulin bolus, as a result of the incorrect estimation of the amount of carbohydrates.

Most of the time (82.31% of the total time of CGMS recording and 91.90% of the nighttime), the patient had glycemic values within the individualized therapeutic target.

Calculation of LBGI and HBGI, respectively, based on CGMS records indicated an increased risk of nocturnal hypoglycemia and an increased risk of daytime hyperglycemia (**Table 3**).

The consequence of glycemic variability, hypoglycemia, and hyperglycemia, respectively, was quantified using GRADE, indicating an increased risk attributable to nocturnal hypoglycemia and daytime hyperglycemia, respectively (**Table 3**).

CGMS records provided valuable data on the patient's glycemic control in the presence of asymptomatic nocturnal hypoglycemia. In this case, HbA1c and mean glycemic control do not accurately indicate glycemic control, making it impossible to identify glycemic variability and asymptomatic nocturnal hypoglycemia.

	LBGI	HBGI	GRADE total	GRADE hypoglycemia	GRADE hyperglycemia
Overall	2.14	2.80	4.99	18.25	63.50
Night time	2.31	1.23	5.21	33.48	38.03

Table 3.
Case 5 - Risk parameters associated with hypoglycemia/hyperglycemia.

6.6 Case 6

We present the case of a patient with type 1 DM on basal-bolus insulin therapy with HbA1c above the target (7.0%). The classic parameters of glycemic control highlight the HbA1c value higher than the therapeutic target, precarious glycemic control (J index > > 30), and important glycemic variability (CV >36%) (**Table 4**). The higher value of the estimated HbA1c (calculated based on the glycemic values of the 7 days of sensor operation) is observed compared to the dosed HbA1c (glycemic average of the last 3 months), the difference suggesting the presence of hyperglycemic episodes during CGMS monitoring. However, the HbA1c value estimated based only on CGMS recordings during the nights is much lower than the dosed HbA1c value, suggesting frequent nocturnal hypoglycemia.

The data presented in **Table 5** and the CGMS graphs in **Figure 12** indicate that blood glucose values <70 mg/dl (3.9 mmol/l) are present in 8.13% of the total recording time, and significant hypoglycemia values <54 mg/dl (3.0 mmol/l) are also recorded in 0.10% of the time, but hypoglycemic episodes are frequent and prolonged in duration during the night (28.97%). In contrast, the patient presented both blood glucose values >180 mg/dl (10.0 mmol/l) in 45.61% of the total time, and severe hyperglycemia values (> 250 mg/dl (13.9 mmol/l)) in 25.50% of the total time of CGMS recording. Hyperglycemias were recorded during the day (**Figure 12**).

Thus, hyperglycemia (predominantly diurnal) can be the consequence of hypoglycemia (predominantly nocturnal), justified by the ingestion of carbohydrates in order to correct the hypoglycemic episode, but also by the triggering of the secretion of counterregulatory hormones in the context of hypoglycemia.

Hypoglycemia can be explained by the administration of increased doses of insulin (prandial or basal), low carbohydrate intake, or lack of meals (especially dinner, because hypoglycemia is predominantly nocturnal).

The patient remained within glycemic targets in only 46.27% of the total time of CGMS recording.

	MAGE (mg/dl)	MODD (mg/dl)	HbA1c (%) (estimated)	MBG (mg/dl)	SD (mg/dl)	CV (%)	J Index (mg/dl)
Overall	139.76	69.76	8.35	192.83	95.6	49.60	83.22
Night time			5.96	124.47	67.8	54.51	36.99

Table 4.
Case 6 - Classical parameters of glycemic control.

	TBR (%)		TIR (%)	TAR (%)	
	<70 mg/dl (3.9 mmol/l)	<54 mg/dl (3.0 mmol/l)	70–180 mg/dl (3.9–10.0 mmol/l)	<70 mg/dl (3.9 mmol/l)	<54 mg/dl (3.0 mmol/l)
Overall	8.13	0.10	46.27	45.61	25.50
Night time	28.97	0.40	46.83	24.21	2.18

Table 5.
Case 6 - Percent of time spent below/above or in glycemic target.

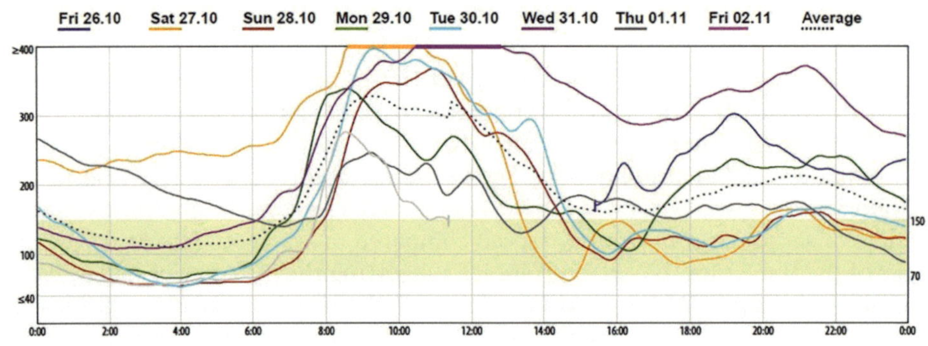

Figure 12.
Case 6 - CGMS weekly report.

The evaluation of LBGI/HBGI and GRADE hypo/hyperglycemia indicated an increased risk attributable to nocturnal hypoglycemia and, respectively, daytime hyperglycemia (**Table 6**).

6.7 Case 7

We present a patient with type 1 DM on sensor augmented insulin pump therapy, with poor glycemic control (HbA1c 7.2%, J index>30), with significant glycemic variability during the day, with significant glycemic excursions within the same day (MAGE), but also glycemic variation from one day to another (MODD), but with an estimated HbA1c value lower than the dosed one, explained by the difference between the period of evaluation of metabolic control with dosed HbA1c and the 7-day period over which HbA1c is estimated (**Table 7**).

The presence of hypoglycemia during the CGMS monitoring period further suggests this difference between the dosed and estimated HbA1c value and implies the identification and correction of the determining factors.

	LBGI	HBGI	GRADE total	GRADE hypoglycemia	GRADE hyperglycemia
Overall	1.38	14.43	13.11	4.14	91.86
Night time	4.79	4.85	7.36	27.13	66.58

Table 6.
Case 6 - Risk parameters associated with hypoglycemia/hyperglycemia.

	MAGE (mg/dl)	MODD (mg/dl)	HbA1c (%) (estimated)	MBG (mg/dl)	SD (mg/dl)	CV (%)	J Index (mg/dl)
Overall	143.45	57.96	6.49	139.6	56.8	40.7	38.6
Night time			6.48	139.5	47.2	33.8	34.8

Table 7.
Case 7 - Classical parameters of glycemic control.

The data in **Table 8** and **Figure 13** indicate that the patient presents hypoglycemia, with both glucose values <70 mg/dl (3.9 mmol/l) being recorded in 7.31% of the total time of CGMS recording, but also values <54 mg/dl (3.0 mmol/l) in 2.15% of the total time. Hypoglycemic episodes predominate during the evening and night, with glucose values <54 mg/dl (3.0 mmol/l) being frequent. According to the CGMS graphs, hypoglycemia occurs after the hyperglycemic episode, which can be explained by the administration of incorrectly calculated corrective boluses, in doses that are too high.

Significant hyperglycemia (> 250 mg/dl (13.9 mmol/l)) was recorded both during the day and at night, and glucose values >180 mg/dl (10.0 mmol/l) were recorded in 19.04% of the time, predominantly during the night. Hyperglycemia can be explained by the lack of concordance between the amount of carbohydrates ingested and the insulin bolus administered.

In 73.65% of the total time of CGMS recording and 78.95% of the nighttime, the patient had glycemic values within the individualized therapeutic target.

The evaluation of risk indices associated with hypo/hyperglycemia (**Table 9**) revealed an increased risk attributable to both daytime and nocturnal hyperglycemia and an increased risk attributable to hypoglycemia, especially in the second half of the day.

6.8 Case 8

Analysis of classic glycemic control parameters in a patient with type 1 DM on basal-bolus insulin therapy, highlights a measured HbA1c—6.90% and a good

	TBR (%)		TIR (%)	TAR (%)	
	<70 mg/dl (3.9 mmol/l)	<54 mg/dl (3.0 mmol/l)	70–180 mg/dl (3.9–10.0 mmol/l)	<70 mg/dl (3.9 mmol/l)	<54 mg/dl (3.0 mmol/l)
Overall	7.31	2.15	73.65	19.04	5.79
Night time	4.14	0.73	78.95	16.91	3.04

Table 8.
Case 7 - Percent of time spent below/above or in glycemic target.

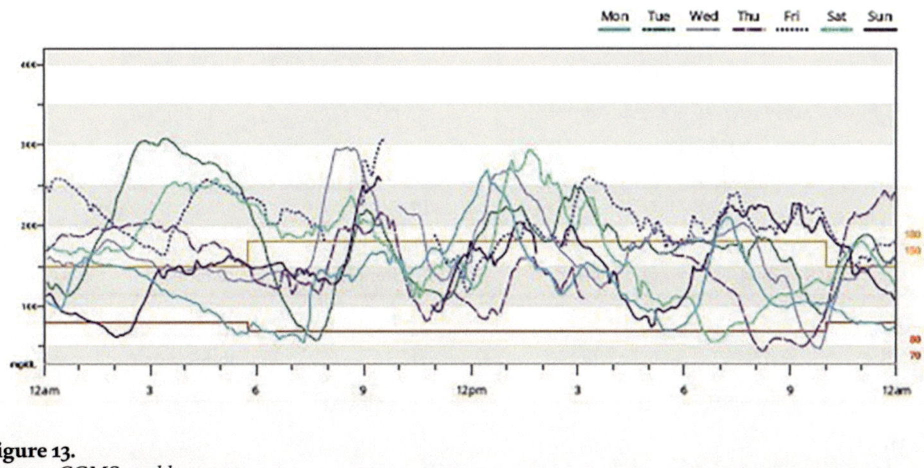

Figure 13.
Case 7 - CGMS weekly report.

glycemic control, with a coefficient of variation < 36%, but the MAGE and MODD values indicate significant glycemic excursions within the same day and reduced reproducibility of glycemic profiles from one day to the next (**Table 10**).

Despite the good glycemic control suggested by the values of the classic parameters, according to the data in **Table 11** and the CGMS graphs in **Figure 14**, the patient presents frequent hypoglycemia, especially during the night, spending 18.09% of the night with glycemic values < 70 mg/dl (3.9 mmol/l), half of this period presenting glycemic values < 54 mg/dl (3.0 mmol/l).

The consequence of glycemic variability, hypoglycemia, and hyperglycemia is determined using total GRADE, hypoglycemia GRADE, and hyperglycemia GRADE, and reveals an increased risk induced by nocturnal hypoglycemia (**Table 12**).

6.9 Case 9

Determination of glycemic control in a patient with type 1 DM on sensor augmented insulin pump therapy, using classical parameters indicated a measured HbA1c of 7.40% and an average glycemic level within the target range (100–180 mg/dl (5.6–10.0 mmol/l)), but the J index (**Table 13**) and HbA1c higher than the therapeutic target (6.5–6.7%) indicate poor metabolic control, characterized predominantly by hyperglycemia, as shown in **Table 14**. However, even in the presence of significant

	LBGI	HBGI	GRADE total	GRADE hypoglycemia	GRADE hyperglycemia
Overall	1.73	4.67	6.80	11.48	76.33
Night time	1.01	8.26	10.41	0.00	89.95

Table 9.
Case 7 - Risk parameters associated with hypoglycemia/hyperglycemia.

	MAGE (mg/dl)	MODD (mg/dl)	HbA1c (%) (estimated)	MBG (mg/dl)	SD (mg/dl)	CV (%)	J Index (mg/dl)
Overall	121.08	41.58	5.80	120.1	42.4	35.3	26.4
Night time			4.93	95.1	26.6	27.9	14.8

Table 10.
Case 8 - Classical parameters of glycemic control.

	TBR (%)		TIR (%)	TAR (%)	
	< 70 mg/dl (3.9 mmol/l)	< 54 mg/dl (3.0 mmol/l)	70–180 mg/dl (3.9–10.0 mmol/l)	< 70 mg/dl (3.9 mmol/l)	< 54 mg/dl (3.0 mmol/l)
Overall	6.81	2.25	81.46	11.74	0.89
Night time	18.09	8.75	81.91	0.00	0.00

Table 11.
Case 8 - Percent of time spent below/above or in glycemic target.

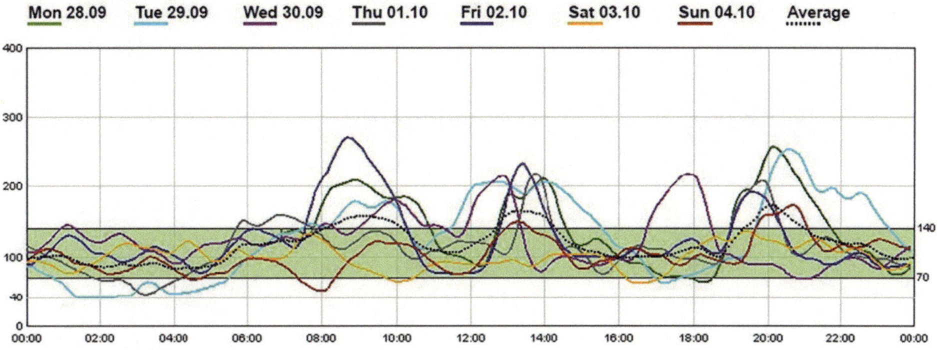

Figure 14.
Case 8 - CGMS weekly report.

	LBGI	HBGI	GRADE total	GRADE hypoglycemia	GRADE hyperglycemia
Overall	1.93	2.21	4.41	18.69	62.77
Night time	4.60	0.23	3.86	71.89	8.38

Table 12.
Case 8 - Risk parameters associated with hypoglycemia/hyperglycemia.

	MAGE (mg/dl)	MODD (mg/dl)	HbA1c (%) (estimated)	MBG (mg/dl)	SD (mg/dl)	CV (%)	J Index (mg/dl)
Overall	120.63	52.79	6.72	146.18	53.8	36.86	40.02
Night time			6.97	153.36	51.6	33.67	42.02

Table 13.
Case 9 - Classical parameters of glycemic control.

	TBR (%)		TIR (%)	TAR (%)	
	< 70 mg/dl (3.9 mmol/l)	< 54 mg/dl (3.0 mmol/l)	70–180 mg/dl (3.9–10.0 mmol/l)	< 70 mg/dl (3.9 mmol/l)	< 54 mg/dl (3.0 mmol/l)
Overall	5.36	1.22	70.20	24.44	3.93
Night time	2.59	0.00	68.66	28.74	2.79

Table 14.
Case 9 - Percent of time spent below/above or in glycemic target.

hyperglycemia, the patient spends a higher percentage of time than the therapeutic target with glycemic values < 70 mg/dl (3.9 mmol/l), which indicates that the presence of hyperglycemia does not exclude the existence of hypoglycemia.

Considering that hypoglycemia occurs during the day and after episodes of hyperglycemia, hypoglycemia is most likely precipitated by aggressive correction of hyperglycemia through corrective boluses or by reducing carbohydrate intake as a way to correct hyperglycemia (**Table 14**, **Figure 15**).

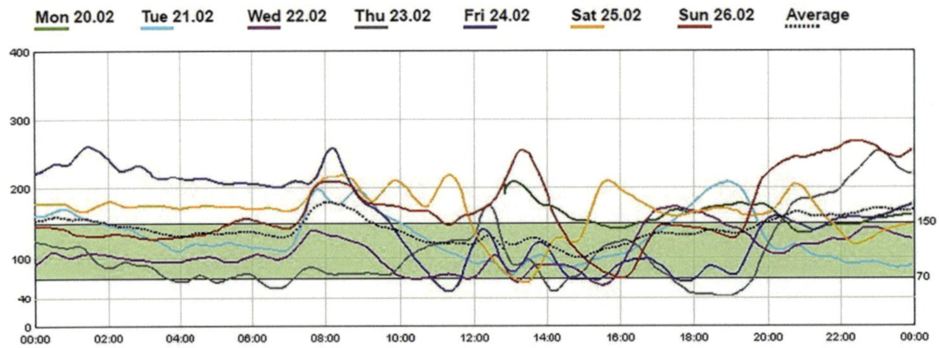

Figure 15.
Case 9 - CGMS weekly report.

	LBGI	HBGI	GRADE total	GRADE hypoglycemia	GRADE hyperglycemia
Overall	1.38	5.29	7.37	6.75	84.98
Night time	0.66	5.96	7.70	1.72	88.77

Table 15.
Case 9 - Risk parameters associated with hypoglycemia/hyperglycemia.

The LBGI and HBGI indices suggest the presence of the risk of hyperglycemia during the night and the risk of hypoglycemia during the day (**Table 15**).

The GRADE hypo/hyperglycemia indices indicate an increased risk attributable primarily to nocturnal hyperglycemia but also a risk attributable to daytime hypoglycemia (**Table 15**).

The presented cases indicated that the use of continuous glucose monitoring systems offers a more precise assessment of metabolic control and glycemic variability, but also of the presence of hypoglycemia, especially asymptomatic and/or nocturnal, and the quantification of the risk attributable to them, compared to classical methods such as HbA1c, glycemic mean, and even coefficient of variation.

For the metabolic control of these patients, the identification of glycemic variability indices using CGMS may be relevant.

As can be seen in **Figure 16**, in the cases presented, the dosed HbA1c values did not differ between patients, being generally within the therapeutic target range and the overall TIR values were within the therapeutic target, except for the case 6 in which the TIR was lower than the target due to prolonged nocturnal hypoglycemic episodes, with similar values being recorded in most patients, but the separate analysis of the parameters during the night highlighted in all patients significant hypoglycemic episodes that explain the lower estimated HbA1c values.

Regarding the consequences of hypoglycemia, as can be seen from **Figures 16** and **17**, the longer the time spent with glycemic values < 70 mg/dl (3.9 mmol/l), the higher the GRADE of hypoglycemia, especially in patients who experience hypoglycemia but otherwise do not exceed the glycemic threshold of 180 mg/dl (10.0 mmol/l).

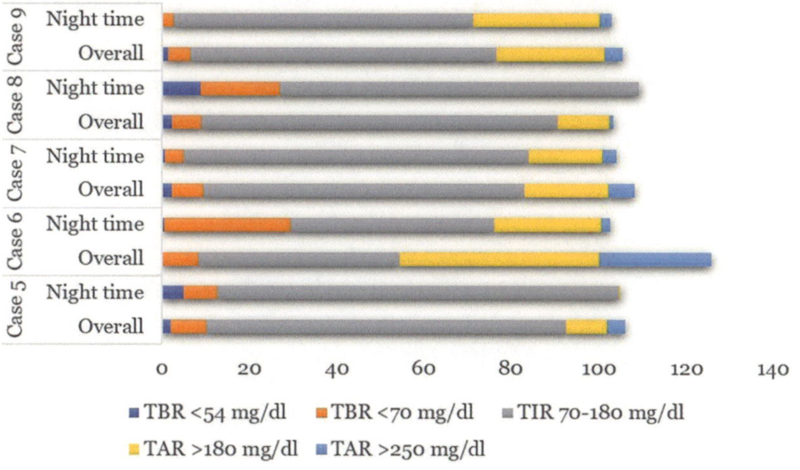

Figure 16.
Time in range (TIR), Time above the range (TAR), and Time below the range (TBR) in the presented cases 5–9.

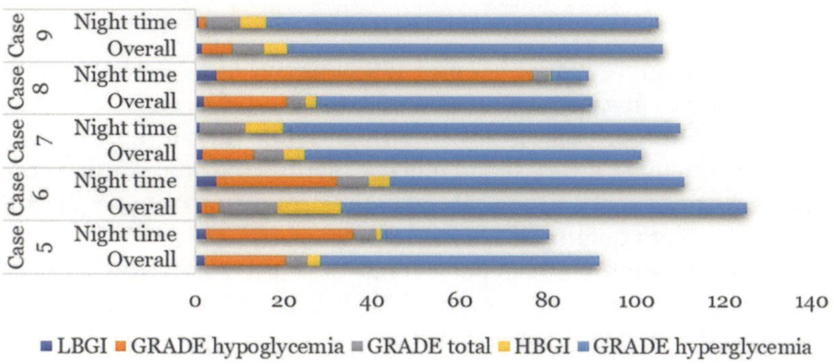

Figure 17.
Low Blood Glucose Index (LBGI), Blood Glucose Index (HBGI), Glycemic Risk Assessment in Diabetes Equation (GRADE) for hypoglycemia and hyperglycemia in the presented cases 5–9.

Also, in all patients, the hypoglycemic episodes were accompanied by hyperglycemia either prior to the hypoglycemia (these being the consequence of the correction of hyperglycemia) but also subsequent to the hypoglycemia as an effect of neurohormonal counterregulatory response, thus generating a significant glycemic variability suggested by the modified values of the glycemic variability parameters and a poor glycemic control detected in all patients (**Figure 18**).

These data suggest that the use of HbA1c but also of TIR alone to quantify glycemic control can be misleading, especially if only overall TIR is assessed and not separately during the night. It is necessary to include overall TBR and during the night as a parameter for assessing glycemic control and establishing optimal therapeutic measures.

Thus, the presented cases emphasize the fact that HbA1c is not sufficient for the exact evaluation of glycemic control, CGMS recordings bringing added accuracy in terms of glycemic variability parameters and awareness of asymptomatic and/or nocturnal hypoglycemia.

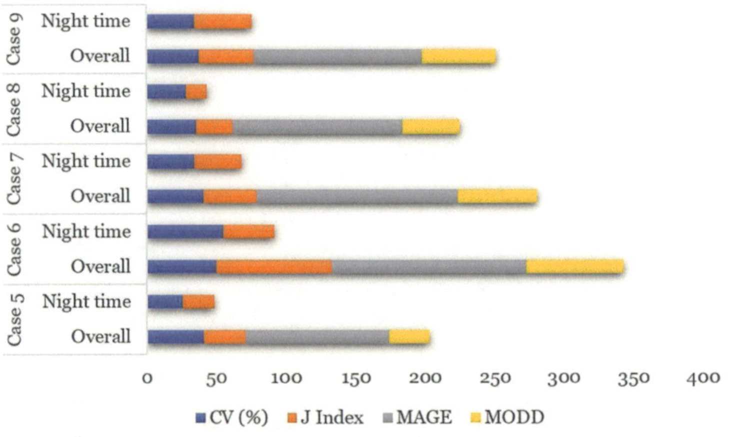

Figure 18.
Coefficient of variation (CV), J Index, Mean Amplitude of Glycemic Excursions (MAGE), Mean daily differences (MODD) in presented cases 5–9.

7. Prevention

Prevention of hypoglycemia is an important objective of DM management.

Individualization of glycemic goals, patient education, dietary intervention, physical effort management, periodic review of hypoglycemic therapy and adjustment of insulin and sulfonylurea doses, blood glucose monitoring, and routine clinical evaluation are measures that can contribute to the prevention of hypoglycemia and can improve the patient's quality of life [6].

In patients with asymptomatic hypoglycemia or those with frequent episodes of severe hypoglycemia, glycemic targets should be increased over a period of several weeks to improve the perception of hypoglycemia.

In the case of driving, patients with DM should determine their blood glucose before, or, if determination is not possible, have a snack. They should also have a snack every 2 hours of driving and always have a sufficient amount of sugar for one day.

8. Treatment of hypoglycemia in patients with diabetes

The management of hypoglycemia involves three goals: improving symptoms, restoring normal blood glucose levels, and correcting the causes of hypoglycemia [1, 14, 15, 16].

Treatment of hypoglycemia, if the patient is conscious, consists of ingesting 15-20 g of glucose from sugar, honey, candy, or rapidly absorbed carbohydrates (fruit, dairy). Patients should be instructed that hypoglycemia is a situation in which sugar is not only permitted, but even mandatory for people with diabetes.

Young children usually need less than 15 grams of carbohydrates to correct hypoglycemia: infants may need 6 grams, toddlers (1–3 years) may need 8 grams, and preschoolers (3–6 years) may need 10 grams. Patients on acarbose (α-glucosidase inhibitors - an enzyme that breaks down disaccharides) should only ingest glucose tablets or milk to correct hypoglycemia (lactase is not inhibited by acarbose).

15 g of ingested glucose causes an increase in blood glucose by approximately 40 mg/dl (2.2 mmol/l) in 20 minutes; therefore, 15 minutes after carbohydrate ingestion, blood glucose is repeated and if hypoglycemia persists, repeated carbohydrate ingestion is recommended (**Figure 19**). Chocolate should be avoided due to its lipid content, which can delay glucose absorption.

Once blood glucose returns to normal, the patient should eat a snack composed of foods with slow and fast absorption carbohydrates, to prevent the recurrence of hypoglycemia, possibly due to the continuation of the hypoglycemic effect of insulin or sulfonylureas already administered prior to hypoglycemia.

Parenteral administration of glucose should be avoided if the patient is conscious and able to swallow.

In severe hypoglycemia, in which the patient has lost consciousness or has convulsions or jaw contraction, 75–100 ml of 20% glucose, or 150–200 ml of 10% glucose, or 33% glucose will be administered intravenously. Glucose administration is performed slowly (in the case of rapid injection of hypertonic glucose solution, acute pulmonary edema may occur). The aim is to obtain persistent normal blood glucose or even mild hyperglycemia. Glucagon is, along with glucose, a very important therapeutic agent in severe hypoglycemia. Glucagon, at a dose of 1 mg, administered i.m. or s.c., causes a significant increase in blood glucose (by approx. 100 mg/dl) for 60 minutes, not being effective for more than 1–1.5 hours. Currently, glucagon is available for intranasal administration, in a single dose of 3 mg, which is passively absorbed through the nasal mucosa; inhalation or deep inspiration is not necessary after administration, and absorption is not influenced by nasal congestion. Administration of glucagon temporarily restores blood sugar levels, allowing the patient to have oral carbohydrate intake.

Immediately after regaining consciousness, 20 g of glucose and 40 g of slow-absorbing carbohydrates should be administered to prevent the recurrence of hypoglycemia. Glucagon is useful in patients with hepatic glycogen reserves (it is not effective in chronic ethanol users, in glycogenosis, and in hypoglycemia caused by long-acting sulfonylureas).

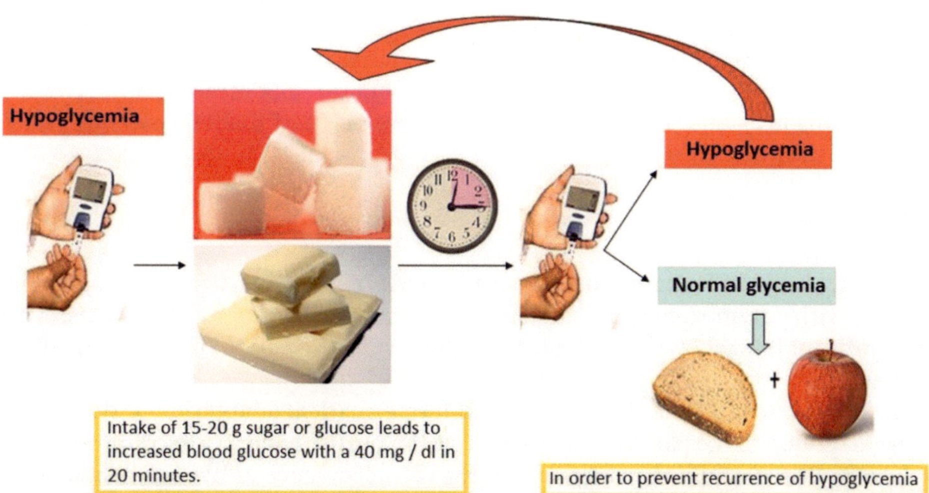

Figure 19.
Treatment of hypoglycemia when the patient is conscious.

If consciousness has not returned after the first 2–3 hours, coma should be considered very serious, making subsequent full recovery of cerebral disorders problematic. If prolonged for more than 6 hours, the complication of hypoglycemic coma with a meningeal hemorrhage or cerebral edema should be considered. In the presence of signs of cerebral edema, hydrocortisone hemisuccinate 500 mg in 500 ml glucose solution or 20% mannitol should be administered. In agitated patients or with convulsions, phenobarbital 2 ml/day or magnesium sulfate should be administered.

9. Prognosis

If the treatment of hypoglycemia is applied correctly and in time, the clinical manifestations can be completely reversible. If the carbohydrate intake necessary to balance blood sugar is delayed, irreversible lesions may occur in the central nervous system and the cardiovascular system, which can lead to death.

Regarding the immediate effects of hypoglycemia, several hypoglycemic clamp studies performed in patients with type 1 diabetes mellitus have shown the association of acute hypoglycemia, both significant (glycemia <2.5 mmol/l), moderate (2.5–2.9 mmol/l) and mild (glycemia <3.1 mmol/l) with impaired cognitive performance, increased cerebral blood flow (assessed by H215O-positron emission tomographies) in the striatum, which is involved in the regulation of memory, emotions, language and motor function, but also with reduced working memory performance evidenced by functional MRI and H215O-positron emission tomographies [26, 27]. In addition, the cognitive dysfunction associated with acute hypoglycemia can persist during the recovery period after hypoglycemia [26, 28]. Acute hypoglycemia also has deleterious effects on cognitive function in patients with type 2 diabetes [29].

The more pronounced the neurological manifestations, the worse the prognosis. Patients may be left with posthypoglycemic neuropsychiatric sequelae: posthypoglycemic encephalopathy, which consists of progressive personality changes, the appearance of memory disorders, psychoses, and progressive dementia [1].

Severe hypoglycemia, not properly corrected, can precipitate the occurrence of myocardial infarction in the context of increased heart contractility and vasospasm, but also serious cardiac arrhythmias by increasing heart rate and prolonging the QT interval, secondary to the catecholaminergic response induced by hypoglycemia, and also strokes precipitated by a hypoglycemic coma are not rare [14, 30]. Overall, hypoglycemia may negatively influence the quality of life of diabetic patients [29, 31].

10. Conclusions

Hypoglycemia is the main impediment to achieving optimal glycemic control in diabetes, with polymorphic clinical manifestations that vary from mild forms, without significant impact on the patient, to severe forms, the patient requiring medical intervention.

The cases presented emphasize the need for permanent adaptation of the insulin therapy regimen to the patient's status, one of the most frequently encountered impediments in diabetes management, being the occurrence of hypoglycemia secondary to inadequate titration of insulin doses after the remission of acute conditions/improvement of glucotoxicity or in the context of the appearance of associated pathologies.

DOI: http://dx.doi.org/10.5772/intechopen.1012541

Continuous glycemic monitoring allows the recording of a large number of glycemic values, the detection of asymptomatic hypoglycemia, the assessment of their severity and duration, the assessment of the risk, but also of the consequences of hypoglycemia, and addresses many of the limitations of HbA1c and capillary blood glycemic self-monitoring, being a critical aspect in the effective management of diabetes mellitus.

Therapeutic medical education and patient-clinician communication are essential in effectively preventing, identifying, and correcting hypoglycemic episodes and their consequences by ensuring the most effective treatment.

Author details

Simona Georgiana Popa[1*] and Andreea Loredana Golli[2]

1 Department of Diabetes, Nutrition and Metabolic Diseases, University of Medicine and Pharmacy, Craiova, Romania

2 Department of Public Health, University of Medicine and Pharmacy, Craiova, Romania

*Address all correspondence to: simona.popa@umfcv.ro

References

[1] American Diabetes Association Professional Practice Committee. 6. Glycemic goals and hypoglycemia: Standards of care in diabetes-2025. Diabetes Care. 2025;**48**(1):S128-S145. DOI: 10.2337/dc25-S006

[2] Yale JF, Paty B, Senior PA. Diabetes Canada clinical practice guidelines expert committee. Hypoglycemia. Canadian Journal of Diabetes. 2018;**42**(1):S104-S108

[3] MacDonald PE, Joseph JW, Rorsman P. Glucose-sensing mechanisms in pancreatic beta-cells. Philosophical Transactions of the Royal Society of London. Series B, Biological Sciences. 2005;**29**(1464):2211-2225

[4] Borg MA, Borg WP, Tamborlane WV, et al. Chronic hypoglycemia and diabetes impair counterregulation induced by localized 2-deoxy-glucose perfusion of the ventromedial hypothalamus in rats. Diabetes. 1999;**48**(3):584-587

[5] Borg WP, Sherwin RS, During MJ, et al. Local ventromedial hypothalamus glucopenia triggers counterregulatory hormone release. Diabetes. 1995;**44**:180-184

[6] Oyer DS. The science of hypoglycemia in patients with diabetes. Current Diabetes Reviews. 2013;**9**(3):195-208. DOI: 10.2174/15733998113099990059

[7] Cryer PE. Hypoglycemia in diabetes: Pathophysiological mechanisms and diurnal variation. Progress in Brain Research. 2006;**153**:361-365

[8] McCrimmon RJ, Sherwin RS. Hypoglycemia in type 1 diabetes. Diabetes. 2010;**59**(10):2333-2339. DOI: 10.2337/db10-0103

[9] Cryer PE. Minireview: Glucagon in the pathogenesis of hypoglycemia and hyperglycemia in diabetes. Endocrinology. 2012;**153**(3):1039-1048. DOI: 10.1210/en.2011-1499

[10] Amiel SA. Joslin's diabetes mellitus. ed. In: Kahn CR et al., editors. Chapter 40. Latrogenic Hypoglycemia. Philadelphia: Lippincott Williams & Willkins; 2005. pp. 671-686. ISBN-10: 0781727960

[11] Ryder RE, Owens DR, Hayes DM, et al. Unawareness of hypoglycaemia and inadequate counterregulation: No causal relationship to diabetic autonomic neuropathy. BMJ. 1990;**301**:783-787

[12] Cryer PE, Davis SN, Shamoon H. Hypoglycemia in diabetes. Diabetes Care. 2003;**26**(6):1902-1912. DOI: 10.2337/diacare.26.6.1902

[13] Abraham MB, Jones TW, Naranjo D, et al. ISPAD clinical practice consensus guidelines 2018: Assessment and management of hypoglycemia in children and adolescents with diabetes. Pediatric Diabetes. 2018;**19**(27):178-192

[14] Diabetes Canada Clinical Practice Guidelines Expert Committee, Yale JF, Paty B, Senior PA. Hypoglycemia. Canadian Journal of Diabetes. 2018;**42**(Suppl. 1):S104-S108. DOI: 10.1016/j.jcjd.2017.10.010

[15] Anderbro T, Amsberg S, Adamson U, Bolinder J, Lins PE, Wredling R, et al. Fear of hypoglycaemia in adults with type 1 diabetes. Diabetic Medicine. 2010;**27**(10):1151-1158. DOI: 10.1111/j.1464-5491.2010.03078.x

[16] American Diabetes Association Professional Practice Committee. 16.

Diabetes care in the hospital: Standards of care in diabetes—2025. Diabetes Care. 2025;**48**(Supplement_1):S321-S334. DOI: 10.2337/dc25-S016

[17] Casey A, Mann R, Banister K, et al. Effect of carbohydrate ingestion on glycogen resynthesis in human liver and skeletal muscle, measured by (13) C MRS. American Journal of Physiology. Endocrinology and Metabolism. 2000;**278**:E65-E75

[18] Krssak M, Petersen KF, Bergeron R, et al. Intramuscular glycogen and intramyocellular lipid utilization during prolonged exercise and recovery in man: A 13C and 1H nuclear magnetic resonance spectroscopy study. The Journal of Clinical Endocrinology and Metabolism. 2000;**85**:748-754

[19] Lin YK, Fisher SJ, Pop-Busui R. Hypoglycemia unawareness and autonomic dysfunction in diabetes: Lessons learned and roles of diabetes technologies. Journal of Diabetes Investigation. 2020;**11**(6):1388-1402. DOI: 10.1111/jdi.13290. Epub 2020 Jul 7

[20] Duelli R, Staudt R, Duembgen L, et al. Increase in glucose transporter densities of Glut3 and decrease of glucose utilization in rat brain after one week of hypoglycemia. Brain Research. 1999;**831**:254-262

[21] Davis SN, Tate D, Hedrington MS. Mechanisms of hypoglycemia and exercise-associated autonomic dysfunction. Transactions of the American Clinical and Climatological Association. 2014;**125**:281-291

[22] American Diabetes Association Professional Practice Committee. 6. Glycemic goals and hypoglycemia: Standards of care in diabetes-2024. Diabetes Care. 2024;**47**(1):S111-S125. DOI: 10.2337/dc24-S006

[23] Hill NR, Oliver NS, Choudhary P, Levy JC, Hindmarsh P, Matthews DR. Normal reference range for mean tissue glucose and glycemic variability derived from continuous glucose monitoring for subjects without diabetes in different ethnic groups. Diabetes Technology & Therapeutics. 2011;**13**(9):921-928. DOI: 10.1089/dia.2010.0247

[24] Kovatchev BP, Cox DJ, Kumar A, Gonder-Frederick L, Clarke WL. Algorithmic evaluation of metabolic control and risk of severe hypoglycemia in type 1 and type 2 diabetes using self-monitoring blood glucose data. Diabetes Technology & Therapeutics. 2003;**5**:817-828

[25] Leelarathna L, Thabit H, Wilinska ME, Bally L, Mader JK, Pieber TR, et al. Evaluating glucose control with a novel composite continuous glucose monitoring index. Journal of Diabetes Science and Technology. 2020;**14**(2):277-283. DOI: 10.1177/1932296819838525

[26] Gejl M, Gjedde A, Brock B, Møller A, van Duinkerken E, Haahr HL, et al. Effects of hypoglycaemia on working memory and regional cerebral blood flow in type 1 diabetes: A randomised, crossover trial. Diabetologia. 2018;**61**(3):551-561. DOI: 10.1007/s00125-017-4502-1

[27] Allen KV, Pickering MJ, Zammitt NN, Hartsuiker RJ, Traxler MJ, Frier BM, et al. Effects of acute hypoglycemia on working memory and language processing in adults with and without type 1 diabetes. Diabetes Care. 2015;**38**(6):1108-1115. DOI: 10.2337/dc14-1657

[28] Zammitt NN, Warren RE, Deary IJ, Frier BM. Delayed recovery of cognitive function following hypoglycemia in adults with type 1 diabetes: Effect of impaired awareness of hypoglycemia.

Diabetes. 2008;**57**(3):732-736. DOI: 10.2337/db07-0695

[29] Nilsson M, Jensen N, Gejl M, Bergmann ML, Storgaard H, Zander M, et al. Experimental non-severe hypoglycaemia substantially impairs cognitive function in type 2 diabetes: A randomised crossover trial. Diabetologia. 2019;**62**(10):1948-1958. DOI: 10.1007/s00125-019-4964-4

[30] International Hypoglycaemia Study Group. Glucose concentrations of less than 3.0 mmol/L (54 mg/dL) should Be reported in clinical trials: A joint position statement of the American Diabetes Association and the European Association for the Study of diabetes. Diabetes Care. 2017;**40**(1):155-157. DOI: 10.2337/dc16-2215

[31] Davis RE, Morrissey M, Peters JR, Wittrup-Jensen K, Kennedy-Martin T, Currie CJ. Impact of hypoglycaemia on quality of life and productivity in type 1 and type 2 diabetes. Current Medical Research and Opinion. 2005;**21**(9):1477-1483. DOI: 10.1185/030079905X61929

Chapter 10

Surgical Management of Hypoglycemia in Non-Diabetic Patients

Bonifacio García Ramos, Elías Guillermo Valdéz Montoya, Daena Judith Andrés Martínez, Victor García Ramos, Alvaro Alejandro Sánchez Ruiz, Jorge Luis Gordillo Magallanes and Patricio Alan Villarreal Aguirre

Abstract

Hypoglycemia predominantly occurs in adults with diabetes mellitus; however, all patients with hypoglycemia without diabetes mellitus who present Whipple's triad should undergo evaluation and targeted treatment. Depending on its etiology, non-diabetic hypoglycemia can be normoinsulinemic or hyperinsulinemic (insulinoma and hyperplasia of the islet cells, such as nesidioblastosis). To perform timely treatment, an accurate diagnosis is required, as it is crucial to understand the etiology in this group of patients. The basis for management is surgical resection when possible, which is curative in most cases.

Keywords: non-diabetic hypoglycemia, hyperinsulinemic hypoglycemia, normoinsulinemic hypoglycemia, tumors of the islet cells, surgical resection

1. Introduction

Hypoglycemia is a metabolic disorder characterized by low blood glucose levels, causing adrenergic and neuroglycopenic symptoms, significantly affecting patients' quality of life. It is common in patients with type 2 diabetes mellitus; however, it can also occur in patients without this condition. In some cases, hypoglycemia can be caused by certain conditions that require surgical treatment.

Hypoglycemia is a metabolic disorder characterized by low blood glucose levels, which causes adrenergic and neuroglycopenic symptoms, significantly affecting patients' quality of life. It is common in patients with type 2 diabetes mellitus; however, it can also occur in patients without this condition. In some cases, hypoglycemia may be due to certain conditions that require surgical treatment.

This chapter focuses on these conditions and the decision-making process for choosing the best surgical option available for their treatment, depending on the etiology of these patients. Although these are rare etiologies, it is important to be aware of their main clinical characteristics to make a timely diagnosis and provide surgical treatment that enhances the quality of life of patients.

It is important to mention that insulinoma is the most common functional pancreatic neuroendocrine tumor and one of the leading causes of hypoglycemia in non-diabetic patients. However, its clinical presentation is non-specific, so it should be suspected when adrenergic and neuroglycopenic symptoms are present, allowing for a timely diagnosis and subsequent surgical approach, improving the patients' quality of life. It is important to remember that there are multiple causes, which will be studied later; although they are less frequent, they can cause hypoglycemia and have differential diagnoses.

2. Tumor of pancreatic cells (insulinoma)

Pancreatic neoplasms can be divided based on their ability to secrete hormones into two categories: functioning and non-functioning. Among the functioning tumors, insulinomas are the most common type of pancreatic neuroendocrine tumor, making up 70–80% of all such tumors. They occur at a rate of 1–4 cases per million people. Most cases occur in adults, with the highest number between the ages of 40 and 60 [1, 2].

These cells are responsible for making insulin; but in some cases, these tumors can also release other hormones, such as gastrin, adrenocorticotropic hormone, glucagon, human chorionic gonadotropin, and somatostatin. Most of these tumors are small, measuring less than 2 cm in size [2].

About 90% of insulinomas occur on their own, while 10% are linked to a condition called multiple endocrine neoplasia type 1 (MEN-1).

Roughly, 10% of insulinomas are present in more than one part of the pancreas, 10% are cancerous, and 16% are related to MEN-1. However, only 21% of people with MEN-1 will develop an insulinoma in their lifetime. The 10-year survival rate for benign insulinomas is 91%, while it drops to 40% for those with the disease spreading locally and to 29% if the cancer has spread to other parts of the body [1, 2].

The exact reasons why insulinomas produce too much insulin are not completely understood.

However, research shows that these tumors often have a special form of insulin mRNA that is more efficient at making insulin compared to normal beta cells. This special form is present in up to 90% of insulinomas, whereas in normal cells, it is less than 1% [3]. Additionally, there is abnormal processing of proinsulin, a precursor to insulin. This leads to the presence of both insulin and proinsulin in the tumor cells, which results in a higher ratio of proinsulin to insulin in the blood [4].

It is very important to get a full medical history for a person who is not diabetic but has had episodes of low blood sugar. This should start with checking for the Whipple's triad, which includes: 1) signs that match low blood sugar, 2) actually low blood glucose levels, and 3) the symptoms going away after eating something with sugar. Symptoms of low blood sugar can be classified into two groups. The first group includes physical symptoms, such as sweating, feeling anxious, a fast heartbeat, feeling weak, hunger, nausea, and feeling warm. The second group includes brain-related symptoms, such as irritability, problems with thinking, temporary issues with movement or vision, seizures, confusion, double vision, and memory loss [5].

These symptoms should match up with actual blood sugar test results, usually below 2.5 mmol/L or 45 mg/dL, to suggest a need for more testing.

A helpful sign is recent weight gain, which is found in more than half of these patients, as they may eat often to prevent symptoms. It is also key to look at when the symptoms happen (like during fasting, at night, or after eating), any medications the person or family members are taking (to check for fake low blood sugar), and if there is a history of autoimmune diseases or previous weight loss surgery [1, 5–7].

In healthy beta cells, insulin and proinsulin do not increase during low blood sugar, and they are not much affected by calcium in the blood.

This lets healthy people go without food for up to 3 days without getting low blood sugar. When doctors do a test called arterial stimulation and hepatic venous sampling (ASVS), they do not see much insulin increase when calcium is given to normal pancreatic areas [4]. However, in insulinoma cells, insulin and proinsulin levels do not go down during low blood sugar and can actually rise when calcium is given. This means that insulinoma often causes high insulin and proinsulin levels when fasting and higher insulin levels in the liver after giving calcium near the tumor. These findings help doctors diagnose and find the tumor [4].

Patients with insulinoma might not respond properly to the body's normal reactions to low blood sugar, which can make them tolerate low glucose levels better than usual. This can cause their symptoms to be very mild or not clear, which can lead to delayed diagnosis that might take many years. In cases where the insulinoma has spread to the liver, other signs may include stomach pain from the tumor pressing on nearby tissues and higher levels of a protein called alpha-fetoprotein.

In people who show signs of low blood sugar, such as neurological symptoms or those related to the body's stress response, and who experience low blood sugar without an obvious cause (below 2.5 mmol/L), it is important to check for certain chemicals in the blood [7].

These tests should be done when the blood sugar is low, such as during a fast or after using a medication like glucagon. The tests usually include insulin, C-peptide, proinsulin, and ketones. Finding high levels of proinsulin can help diagnose insulinoma, especially in tricky cases.

The 72-hour fasting test is the best way to confirm insulinoma, with a 99% chance of detecting it [7].

During this test, blood is drawn every 6 hours to check the levels of glucose, insulin, C peptide, and proinsulin until the blood sugar drops to 60 mg/dL or lower. The testing continues more frequently once the glucose level is at 45 mg/dL or lower, and the test stops when the person starts showing symptoms of low blood sugar.

The diagnosis is confirmed if all six criteria are met:

1. Glucose level $\leq$ 2.5 mmol/L ($\leq$ 45 mg/dL).

2. Insulin level $\geq$ 6 μU/mL.

3. C-peptide level $\geq$ 200 pmol/L.

4. Proinsulin level $\geq$ 5 pmol/L.

5. β-hydroxybutyrate level $\leq$ 2.7 mmol/L.

6. Absence of sulfonylureas in plasma or urine.

Factitious hypoglycemia caused by using insulin from outside the body leads to low levels of C-peptide. In insulinoma, which is a tumor that makes insulin, proinsulin levels are high and not low, unlike in hypoglycemia that is not caused by a tumor. People who use insulin or oral medicines to lower blood sugar usually have normal or low proinsulin levels. If insulin does not go down during hypoglycemia, it shows there is a tumor making insulin on its own.

The European Neuroendocrine Tumor Society suggests using a mixed-meal test for people with symptoms after eating.

This test checks for Î^{2}-hydroxybutyrate, which goes down when insulin is present. Sometimes, glucose levels can be checked every 10 minutes after giving IV glucagon. In insulinoma, glucose levels go up because the body still has stored glycogen.

If someone does not have symptoms during a 72-hour fast, it is unlikely they have insulinoma.

Normal insulin levels during testing do not always rule out insulinoma, since not everyone has higher insulin levels. Proinsulin is a better marker because the tumor releases a lot of it. Measuring Î^{2}-hydroxybutyrate is helpful for people with kidney or liver issues, as insulin or C-peptide might not be cleared properly, which could affect results.

Most patients (90–95%) start having symptoms within 48 hours, but a full 72-hour fast is needed to avoid missing the condition.

Finding the tumor can be hard because of its size and location. About 30% of insulinomas are smaller than 1 cm, so there is debate about the best way to find and assess them. Non-invasive methods include ultrasound, CT scans, and MRI. MRI is currently the best option for diagnosis.

Somatostatin receptor scintigraphy uses a substance called octreotide to find tumors that have a lot of somatostatin receptors.

However, insulinomas have low receptor density, making this test less reliable—about 50% for benign and 70% for malignant tumors.

PET/CT scans are useful for managing pancreatic neuroendocrine tumors. Using C-5-hydroxytryptophan (C-5-HTP) in PET/CT has shown over 90% sensitivity for finding insulinomas because these tumors are more active in making serotonin. PET/CT using GLP-1R agonists such as Ga-exendin-4 helps find benign insulinomas. But it is not as accurate for malignant ones, since only 36% of patients with spread cancer have high GLP-1R expression.

F-DOPA PET, which uses dihydroxyphenylalanine, works because neuroendocrine cells like to take in amino acid precursors. It helps guide surgery in about 91% of cases. Gallium-labeled somatostatin analogs, which target SSTRs, are good for understanding pNETs in terms of their expression and metabolism. They are highly sensitive and useful for PET/CT scans and for thinking about peptide receptor radionuclide therapy (PRRT). There are three Ga-labeled radiopharmaceuticals available: Ga-DOTATATE, Ga DOTANOC, and Ga-DOTATOC. Each one has a different level of binding to various SSTR subtypes. For non-progressive or slow-growing insulinomas, 68Ga-DOTA PET is not very helpful because the SSTR2 expression is low. Instead, PET/CT with Ga-exendin-4 is better, as it targets GLP-1R.

Among invasive methods, selective arterial calcium stimulation with hepatic venous sampling (ASVS) used to be the standard for finding tumors before surgery, and it had a success rate of 90%.

Another method is percutaneous transhepatic portal venous sampling (PTPVS), where a catheter is placed into the portal vein to measure insulin levels in the veins that drain the pancreas. The area with the most insulin shows where the tumor is, and this method has a sensitivity between 77% and 100%.

Endoscopic ultrasound (EUS) can find tumors smaller than 5 mm in the pancreatic head, with a success rate of 82–92%, but only 40% for tumors in the pancreatic tail.

It also helps to see the edges of the tumor. Performing a fine-needle aspiration (FNA) during EUS can increase the chance of getting a correct diagnosis up to 98%, and it can help to test for certain proteins and hormones in the tumor. EUS-FNA is only recommended in unclear cases, non-functional tumors, and for people with MEN-1. It is especially helpful if surgery is needed.

During surgery, smaller tumors can be found by feeling the pancreas and using intraoperative ultrasound.

This method has a sensitivity of 75–95% and can show the exact location, the blood vessels around the tumor, and help guide the best way to perform the surgery.

In 2017, the 8th edition of the American Joint Committee on Cancer (AJCC) staging manual updated the TNM/AJCC system for pNETs.

This system is important for predicting how well a patient might do. To determine the tumor grade, a biopsy and precise measurement of the proliferation index (Ki-67) are needed. Grading is based on the ENETS and WHO classification for gastroentero-pancreatic neuroendocrine neoplasms [1].

Treatment for insulinoma depends on the size and location of the tumor, as well as whether it has spread to other parts of the body. The options for the treatment include surgery, medical treatment to manage symptoms in cases where the tumor cannot be removed or has spread, and targeted therapy that can be helpful when the tumor has specific genetic features.

Surgical removal is the best option for insulinomas that are localized.

The preferred surgical method is a parenchyma-sparing resection, which is recommended first when it is possible to do so. This choice depends on the tumor's characteristics, such as whether it functions, its grade, and stage. The goal of treatment is to relieve symptoms caused by low blood sugar and any physical pressure from the tumor, prevent it from becoming cancerous or spreading, and, if it is not curable, to reduce the tumor size and the impact of the symptoms.

Since the risk of cancer spreading to nearby lymph nodes is low, it is not typical to remove them during surgery.

The ENETS guidelines suggest that for insulinomas smaller than 2 cm at the main pancreatic duct, a parenchyma-sparing technique such as enucleation should be considered.

If the insulinoma is in the middle part of the pancreas and cannot be removed by enucleation, a central pancreatectomy might be a good option, as long as the remaining part of the pancreas can still work properly. These methods have better long-term results in terms of preserving pancreatic function compared to more extensive surgery. However, one major challenge is the high risk of complications after surgery, especially related to fluid leakage from the pancreas.

When it comes to the type of surgery, research has shown that laparoscopic procedures are safe and effective for insulinoma patients.

So, if the tumor is clearly located before surgery and it is possible to do so, a minimally invasive approach should be considered. On the other hand, if the tumor is not clearly located, an open surgery with the use of intraoperative ultrasound may be needed.

If the insulinoma has spread, which is linked to a worse outcome, it is important to remove the nearby lymph nodes around the pancreas and any accessible liver lymph nodes.

Removing the primary tumor can also help manage symptoms, slow the progression of the disease, and may improve survival. However, if the tumor is too advanced and involves major blood vessels or has spread widely, surgery may not be an option.

Recently, doctors have started combining endoscopic and imaging methods to treat insulinomas. A new method called EUS-guided radiofrequency ablation (EUS-RFA) has been explored. This technique uses heat to destroy small tumors in the pancreas. EUSRFA seems to be a safe and good option for treating small insulinomas (less than 2 cm), especially for people who cannot have surgery. Studies looking back at patient records and recent reviews show that this treatment works well, with success rates between 86% and 96%, and only minor side effects. However, more information is needed about long-term results, such as survival and whether the tumors come back, before it can be used widely. These procedures should be done only in specialized centers.

During surgery, the anesthesiologist must keep the patient's blood sugar levels normal, avoiding both low and high blood sugar. Hourly monitoring of blood glucose levels is recommended [4].

Most insulinomas can be cured with surgery [1].

3. Hyperinsulinemic hypoglycemia—Islet cell hyperplasia (nesidioblastosis)

Nesidioblastosis is a rare condition that typically occurs in infants and, in some cases (0.5–7%), [8] in adults. It is characterized by abnormal (non-neoplastic) proliferation of the islet cells of the pancreas, leading to persistent episodes of hyperinsulinemic hypoglycemia. Laidlaw coined the term "nesidioblastosis" in 1938 to describe the condition, in which endocrine cells differentiate and bud from the pancreatic ductal epithelium to form new islet tissue. It also encompasses a broad category of pathological overgrowth of pancreatic islet cells [9, 10].

Some authors suggest a genetic component, as mutations have been identified in the ABCC8 (SUR1) and KCNJ11 (Kir6.2) genes, which encode subunits of the ATP-sensitive potassium channels in the β-cell membrane. These mutations result in continuous insulin secretion, causing hypoglycemic episodes [11] diagnosed by Whipple's triad.

However, adult-onset nesidioblastosis has been reported following gastric bypass surgery for morbid obesity, particularly Roux-en-Y gastric bypass. Some studies suggest a link to glucagon-like peptide-1 (GLP-1), an incretin hormone secreted after such surgical procedures, which may induce neogenesis of islet cells from the pancreatic ductal epithelium [12].

There are three forms of presentation: [13, 14].

- Diffuse form: involving the entire pancreas (60–70%)
- Focal form: characterized by nodular hyperplasia (30–40%)
- Atypical form: rare (<1%), associated with morphological mosaicism.

Symptomatology is generally postprandial, and there are two types of symptoms: neuroglycopenic (loss of consciousness, dizziness, confusion, and seizures) and adrenergic (diaphoresis, tremor, and hunger) [13].

Endogenous hyperinsulinemia is diagnosed based on plasma glucose levels (≤55 mg/dL or < 3 mmol/L), insulin (≥18 pmol/L), and C-peptide (≥0.20 nmol/L) [9].

Conventional radiological tests are not useful, with a sensitivity of 50–80%. However, the selective arterial calcium stimulation test with hepatic venous sampling, a minimally invasive procedure, is useful in patients with negative or inconclusive non-invasive imaging, and it allows for tumor localization within the pancreas to guide surgical planning [14, 15]. This test involves cannulating the arteries supplying the pancreas (gastroduodenal, superior mesenteric, splenic, and hepatic) and the subsequent intraarterial injection of calcium gluconate (a pancreatic secretagogue) that stimulates insulin release from hyperfunctioning (abnormal) β-cells but not from normal ones. Blood samples are collected from the right hepatic vein to measure insulin levels at 0, 30, 60, 90, 120, and 180 seconds. A positive result is defined as a twofold or greater increase in insulin concentration from baseline and is considered a diagnostic criterion for localizing an occult insulinoma, with a sensitivity of 67–100%. The tumor's location corresponds to the artery where the response is noted: an increase in the gastroduodenal artery suggests a tumor in the pancreatic head; an increase in the superior mesenteric artery indicates a lesion in the uncinate process; and an increase in the splenic artery suggests localization in the body or tail of the pancreas [16].

In patients in whom no focal lesion is found and insulin secretion is stimulated by calcium in two or more arteries, a diagnosis of nesidioblastosis should be strongly considered [8]. When the test is positive in more than one artery, up to 75% of cases are nesidioblastosis and 25% insulinoma [15].

The definitive diagnosis is histological. There are four main criteria for the diagnosis of diffuse nesidioblastosis: exclusion of insulinoma (macroscopic, microscopic, and immunohistochemical examination); presence of multiple β-cells with enlarged, hyperchromatic nuclei, and abundant clear cytoplasm; and islets with normal spatial distribution and no proliferative activity of endocrine cells. Another characteristic is the presence of ductuloinsular complexes.

Other tools that can aid diagnosis include neuroendocrine markers (chromogranin, enolase, synaptophysin, and hematoxylin-eosin).

Medical treatment includes a low-carbohydrate diet combined with various medications, such as diazoxide (which inhibits insulin secretion by acting on sulfonylurea receptors), octreotide (which inhibits β-cell calcium channels), glucocorticoids, and calcium channel blockers (verapamil and nifedipine).

Definitive treatment is surgical resection. Partial pancreatectomy (60–80% resection of pancreatic tissue) has been shown to control nesidioblastosis in 50% of patients without additional medication, generally in focal forms [9]. However, the gold standard is subtotal pancreatectomy (90–95%), since more extensive resections result in exocrine pancreatic insufficiency and insulin-dependent diabetes [9, 10]. Nonetheless, according to Whitteles et al., approximately 40% of patients undergoing near-total (subtotal) pancreatectomy developed insulin-dependent diabetes mellitus [17].

Treatment is considered successful when symptoms resolve, serum glucose levels normalize, and histopathological confirmation of a lesion is obtained.

4. Non-islet cell tumor hypoglycemia (NICTH)

Non-islet cell tumor-induced hypoglycemia (NICTH) is a rare condition that happens when a tumor, not from the pancreas, causes severe low blood sugar levels without the body making too much insulin. This usually happens with large tumors that are either mesenchymal or epithelial, and these tumors make insulin-like growth factors, especially IGF-2 or its earlier forms. Diagnosing and treating this condition can be hard, especially if the tumor has spread or cannot be removed, so it often needs a team of doctors working together [18, 19].

Non-islet cell tumor hypoglycemia (NICTH) is a type of syndrome linked to tumors that are not in the pancreas.

It causes repeated episodes of low blood sugar. It is different from insulinomas because during these episodes, the levels of insulin, C-peptide, and proinsulin are low. It is a less common cause of low blood sugar compared to insulinomas, occurring about four times less often. However, the real number could be higher because it is often missed, especially in patients with widespread disease [19].

The idea that low blood sugar can be linked to cancer was first noticed in the middle of the last century. At first, there was confusion about why this happened, with theories such as tumors using up too much glucose or making extra insulin. Later, improved laboratory tests helped find out that insulin-like growth factors, especially IGF-2, are the main reason behind this condition [20, 21].

The predominant pathophysiological mechanism in non-islet cell tumor hypoglycemia (NICTH) involves the tumoral production of aberrant forms of insulin-like growth factor type 2 (IGF-2), primarily high-molecular weight precursor forms known as "big IGF-2." Under normal conditions, IGF-2 circulates in plasma bound to carrier proteins, mainly insulin-like growth factor binding protein 3 (IGFBP-3), along with an acid-labile subunit (ALS), which limits its bioavailability. However, the precursor forms of IGF-2 produced by these tumors have reduced affinity for these carrier proteins, resulting in an increased free fraction with biological activity [21, 22].

The hypoglycemic effect of IGF-2 occurs through several complementary mechanisms: activation of insulin receptors (promoting peripheral glucose uptake), inhibition of hepatic glucose production (suppressing gluconeogenesis and glycogenolysis), inhibition of lipolysis in adipocytes (limiting the availability of alternative energy substrates), and suppression of counter-regulatory hormones (glucagon and growth hormone), enhancing susceptibility to hypoglycemia [23].

A characteristic finding in patients with non-islet cell tumor hypoglycemia (NICTH) is the suppression of circulating IGF-1 and growth hormone (GH), which contributes to the pathophysiology of the condition and has diagnostic significance [21]. Tumoral overproduction of IGF-2 exerts negative feedback on pituitary GH secretion, leading to reduced levels of both GH and IGF-1. This imbalance is reflected in an elevated IGF-2/IGF-1 ratio (typically >3:1, often >10:1), which serves as a characteristic biochemical marker of this entity.

Although tumoral production of IGF-2 is the predominant mechanism, there are documented cases of tumor-induced hypoglycemia mediated by other mechanisms [18]: ectopic insulin production by non-pancreatic tumors (bronchial, ovarian, and small cell cervical carcinomas), tumoral secretion of IGF-1 (metastatic large cell lung carcinoma), and secretion of GLP-1 (glucagon-like peptide 1) by tumors, which may induce hypoglycemia by stimulating insulin secretion from normal pancreatic beta cells.

Although less common, these alternative mechanisms should be considered in patients with a compatible clinical presentation, but an atypical biochemical profile for IGF-2-mediated hypoglycemia [24].

Types of Tumors Associated with NICTH

- Mesenchymal Tumors: approximately 60% of NICTH cases.
    - o Solitary fibrous tumor:
    - o This is the prototypical tumor associated with NICTH, characterized by its origin in mesenchymal tissue with fibroblastic differentiation.
    - o It may arise in the pleura, pericardium, peritoneum, or soft tissues.
    - o Fibrosarcomas and fibrohistiocytic tumors
    - o Leiomyosarcomas and rhabdomyosarcomas
    - o Liposarcomas (particularly the myxoid and well-differentiated variants)
    - o Malignant mesotheliomas (especially the fibrous subtype).

These mesenchymal tumors associated with NICTH often share characteristics, such as slow growth, favorable histological differentiation, and substantial size at diagnosis [25].

- Epithelial Tumors: Epithelial-origin tumors account for approximately 40% of NICTH cases.
    - o Hepatocellular carcinoma (one of the most frequently associated epithelial tumors)
    - o Adrenal carcinoma
    - o Gastrointestinal carcinomas (gastric, colorectal, and pancreatic adenocarcinomas).
    - o Renal and adrenal carcinomas (predominantly of the clear cell variant)
    - o Pulmonary carcinomas (particularly non-small cell subtypes)

These epithelial tumors associated with NICTH tend to present in locally advanced or metastatic stages, with hypoglycemia potentially serving as a marker of tumor progression.

- Other Tumor Types
    - o Hematologic malignancies (mainly non-Hodgkin lymphomas and multiple myeloma)
    - o Extra pancreatic neuroendocrine tumors
    - o Pheochromocytomas
    - o Carcinoid tumors
    - o Germ cell tumors

NICTH typically presents with recurrent episodes of hypoglycemia, most often occurring when a person has not eaten or during exercise.

The symptoms can be grouped into two main types: neuroglycopenic and autonomic symptoms. Neuroglycopenic symptoms are typically the most common in NICTH.

This is because the tumor produces IGF-2, which lowers the levels of hormones such as adrenaline and glucagon that normally help raise blood sugar [26–28].

Hypoglycemia can happen at different stages of the tumor's growth.

It might be the first sign that leads to finding the tumor, it can appear as the disease progresses with tumor growth or comes back, or it can happen in later stages when the disease is advanced or has spread [26].

Diagnosing NICTH relies on three main things: finding evidence of low blood sugar without high insulin levels, finding the tumor that is causing it, and ruling out other possible causes [26].

Biochemical Diagnostic Criteria

1. Documented hypoglycemia (blood glucose <45 mg/dL or < 2.5 mmol/L) with compatible symptoms.

2. Suppressed insulin, C-peptide, and proinsulin levels during the hypoglycemic episode (insulin ≥6 μU/mL, C-peptide ≥200 pmol/L, and proinsulin ≥5 pmol/L).

3. Absence of anti-insulin antibodies and negative screening for oral hypoglycemic agents.

4. Decreased IGF-1 levels (<100 ng/mL) and GH.

5. Normal or elevated IGF-2 levels (>275 ng/mL).

6. Elevated IGF-2/IGF-1 ratio (>3:1, often >10:1).

7. Low beta-hydroxybutyrate, reflecting inhibition of lipolysis.

Depending on the laboratory assays used, IGF-2 levels may appear "normal" quantitatively, as standard techniques may not detect higher molecular weight precursor forms ("big IGF-2"). In these cases, an elevated IGF-2/IGF-1 ratio is a more reliable diagnostic marker [27].

Complementary Studies

- Imaging studies for tumor localization: CT, MRI, and PET-CT as appropriate

- Biopsy and histopathological examination when technically feasible.

- Additional hormonal assessments: cortisol, glucagon, and epinephrine/norepinephrine.

- Liver and kidney function tests to rule out other causes of hypoglycemia.

The differential diagnosis for hypoinsulinemic hypoglycemia should include other possible causes, such as severe liver failure, kidney failure, adrenal insufficiency, lack of counterregulatory hormones, post-meal reactive hypoglycemia, hypoglycemia caused by taking external insulin or secretagogues, and hypoglycemia due to anti-insulin antibodies.

When hypoglycemia occurs along with low levels of insulin, C-peptide, and pro-insulin, and there is an increased ratio of IGF-2 to IGF-1 in the presence of a tumor that fits the clinical picture, it strongly suggests a diagnosis of non-islet cell tumor hypoglycemia (NICTH) [28].

The treatment for NICTH includes managing hypoglycemia immediately and addressing the underlying tumor.

The most effective and potentially curative treatment is complete surgical removal of the tumor, which can quickly restore normal blood sugar levels if the tumor is fully removed.

However, surgery may not always be possible due to the tumor's characteristics, such as its position or how much it has spread, or due to the patient's condition [29].

For patients with tumors that cannot be removed or have spread, treatment options may include chemotherapy based on the tumor type, targeted therapies such as pazopanib for mesenchymal tumors, and local treatments such as arterial embolization, radiofrequency ablation, and selective intra-arterial radiotherapy (SIRT).

These treatments can help control hypoglycemia by lowering the amount of tumor producing IGF-2.

If surgery is not an option or is not enough, there are other medications that can be used, such as corticosteroids, diazoxide, somatostatin analogs, and growth hormone.

Continuous glucose monitoring is helpful in managing these patients, allowing for better adjustments in treatment and early warning of severe hypoglycemia.

Along with this, general strategies such as eating small, frequent meals, following a diet high in complex carbohydrates, and avoiding long fasting periods can help manage symptoms (see **Table 1**).

Characteristics	Insulinoma	Nesidioblastosis	NICTH
Definition	Neuroendocrine pancreatic tumor secreting insulin (70–80% of pNET).	Focal or diffuse beta cell hyperplasia of the pancreas (non-neoplastic).	Paraneoplastic hypoglycemia by non-pancreatic tumors (production of "Big IGF-2" or related peptides).
Epidemiology	Most common in 40–60 years; 1–4 cases/million/year. Associated with MEN-1 (10%).	Predominant in infants; rare in adults (0.5–7%). Associated with bariatric surgery.	Much less frequent than insulinoma (4–1). Associated with mesenchymal (60%) and epithelial tumors.
Clinical manifestations	Fasting or nocturnal hypoglycemia symptoms >50%, weight gain, possible neuroglycopenic or neurogenic signs.	Mostly postprandial. Neuroglycopenic and neurogenic symptoms (sweating, tremor, palpitations, hunger, weight loss, sometimes increased appetite).	Mostly fasting hypoglycemia, neuroglycopenic symptoms over adrenergic symptoms. Symptoms due to underlying tumor.
Biochemical diagnostic criteria	Glucose ≤45 mg/dL, insulin ≥6 μU/mL, C-peptide ≥200 pmol/L, proinsulin ≥5 pmol/L, low β-hydroxybutyrate.	Glucose ≤55 mg/dL, insulin ≥18 mU/L, C-peptide ≥0.20 nmol/L, indistinguishable from insulinoma by laboratory.	Glucose ≤45 mg/dL with low insulin, C-peptide, and proinsulin; elevated IGF-2, IGF-2:IGF-1 ratio > 10:1.

Characteristics	Insulinoma	Nesidioblastosis	NICTH
Gold standard diagnostic test	72-h fasting (99% sensitivity), confirmation with biochemical criteria 6 hours.	Pancreatic stimulation test with selective arterial calcium. Diagnosis is histological (ductuloinsular complexes).	IGF-2 and IGF-2:IGF-1 ratio high. Imaging to localize the tumor (CT, MRI, and PET).
Imaging	CT/MRI sensitivity (33–90%). PET with GLP-1R (Ga-exendin-4) in benign insulinoma. EUSFNA.	Conventional images not very useful (50–80% sens.). Selective arterial calcium stimulation test assists diagnosis.	Tumor extension studies (CT, MRI, and PET-CT). Pancreatic lesion not found.
Surgical treatment	Curative resection: enucleation if <2 cm >3 mm from main pancreatic duct. Central or formal pancreatectomy as indicated.	Subtotal (90–95%) in diffuse cases or distal pancreatectomy (60–80%) for focal cases. High risk of postsurgical diabetes.	Complete resection of the primary tumor (only curative treatment).
Other treatments	EUSRFA in non-surgical candidates.	Low-carbohydrate diet, diazoxide, octreotide, and verapamil.	If not resectable: chemotherapy, embolization radiotherapy, somatostatin analogs, GH, and glucocorticoids.
Prognosis	Benign (90%) curable with surgery. Malignant (10–30%).	Frequent recurrence (>40% with subtotal pancreatectomy) may become insulin-dependent.	Depends on tumor type. Malignant advanced tumors: poor prognosis.

Source: Prepared by the authors (2025).

Table 1.
Comparative diagnostic insulinoma, nesidioblastosis, and NICTH.

5. Case 1: Hypoglycemia associated with hepatocellular carcinoma

A 72-year-old woman from Mexico with a past medical history of hypertension managed with candesartan/hydrochlorothiazide 16/12.5 mg, with no other medications.

She reports an 11-month history of episodes involving fine tremor in the upper limbs, profuse sweating, dizziness, and skin pallor, which resolve with sugary drinks. Capillary glucometer readings during episodes have shown glucose levels as low as 38 mg/dL or < 2.1 mmol/L. She attributes symptoms to poor food intake and reports intermittent early satiety. She was referred to an endocrinology outpatient clinic, where a fractionated diet, self-monitoring, and laboratory workup were recommended.

On initial physical examination, she was neurologically intact, no skin changes, normocephalic skull, normal neck, chest with adequate respiratory dynamics, rhythmic and unremarkable precordium, normal breath sounds, distended abdomen due to abundant adipose tissue, non-tender on palpation, and extremities without compromise.

At her next visit, self-monitoring data showed fasting 46 mg/dL, pre-breakfast 79 mg/dL, pre-lunch 83 mg/dL, pre-dinner 68 mg/dL, and 3 a.m. 70 mg/dL. Despite 100% adherence to the diet, five hypoglycemic readings were reported in previous days (35, 38, 42, 36, and 35 mg/dL).

Initial laboratory results:

- Hemoglobin: 14 g/dL, hematocrit: 38%, platelets: 122,000, leukocytes: 3.4 × 10^3/µL, glucose: 59 mg/dL, creatinine: 0.6 mg/dL, sodium: 139 mEq/L, potassium: 4.2 mEq/L, chloride: 104 mEq/L, total 10 bilirubin: 3.1 mg/dL, direct bilirubin: 2.6 mg/dL, indirect bilirubin: 0.5 mg/dL, albumin: 2.9 mg/dL, AST: 87 U/L, ALT: 89 U/L, LDH: 347, TSH: 3.2 µIU/mL, viral serologies: Negative for Hepatitis B, C, and HIV.

Due to persistent hypoglycemia of unclear cause, additional specialized laboratories were requested, showing:

- Insulin: 2.1 µU/mL, C-peptide: 0.2 ng/mL, proinsulin: 3.4 pmol/L, beta-hydroxybutyrate: 3.2 mmol/L, sulfonylurea and glinide levels: pending/not available, endocrine panel: basal and stimulated, cortisol: 18.2 µg/dL, ACTH: 19.1 pg./mL, LH: 17 mIU/mL, prolactin: 18.9 ng/mL, and IGF-I: 25 ng/mL.

The markedly suppressed IGF-I levels, along with low insulin, C-peptide, proinsulin, and beta-hydroxybutyrate, combined with abnormal liver function tests, prompted hospitalization for observation, supportive care, and further diagnostic evaluation.

Given the suspicion of paraneoplastic hypoglycemia and the patient's clinical course, alpha-fetoprotein (AFP) levels and a liver CT scan were ordered.

- AFP (<10 ng/ml): 1280 ng/mL, CT findings: A lesion involving a large portion of liver tissue with a heterogeneous appearance and contrast enhancement (**Figure 1**).

IGF-II or big IGF-II levels were not available in the unit. However, based on the clinical-laboratory correlation and imaging findings, the diagnosis of hypoglycemia secondary to a non-islet cell tumor was made. The patient died a few months later due to tumor progression.

Hypoglycemia secondary to hepatocellular carcinoma is a well-recognized, albeit rare, clinical syndrome. It is generally accepted that both impaired hepatic endocrine function from local tumor effects and overproduction of IGF-II/Big IGF-II can result in recurrent hypoglycemia. Elevated IGF-II levels cause supraphysiological glucose uptake by skeletal muscle, along with suppression of gluconeogenesis, glycogenolysis, ketogenesis, and glucose-6-phosphate dehydrogenase activity [26, 30].

Increased IGF-II production also reduces circulating IGF-I levels, as observed in this case. While the tumor volume itself alters hepatic architecture and function, the glycemic profile—marked by low insulin, C-peptide, beta-hydroxybutyrate, and IGF-I levels—is particularly indicative. Despite the absence of IGF-II assays, the clinical, biochemical, and imaging context allows for a reliable diagnosis of tumor-induced hypoglycemia [26].

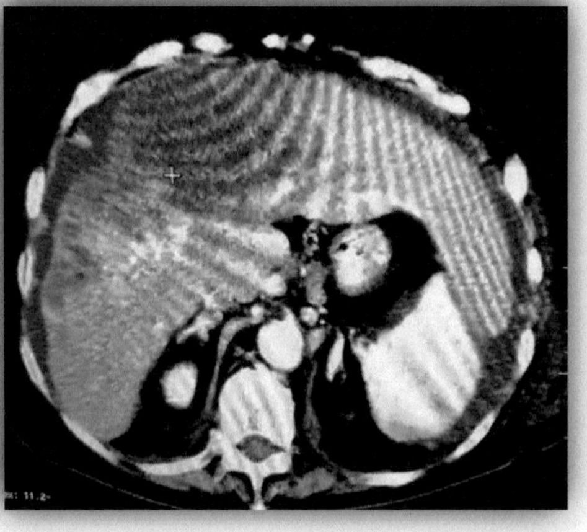

Figure 1.
Axial section computed tomography shows a heterogeneous mass with irregular contours. Predominantly hypodense relative to the adjacent liver parenchyma, containing internal areas suggestive of necrosis. It demonstrates heterogeneous, predominantly peripheral, and irregular enhancement.

6. Case 2: Paraneoplastic hypoglycemia in metastatic adrenal cortical carcinoma (ACC)

A 53-year-old female was admitted to the Affiliated Hospital of Ningxia Medical University (Yinchuan, China) in May 2024 due to abdominal pain and recurrent hypoglycemic coma episodes. During hospitalization, she continued to experience hypoglycemic coma episodes, which improved with active symptomatic glucose supplementation treatment. However, the cause of these episodes remained unidentified. Even after discharge, the patient experienced hypoglycemic coma episodes while resting at home. On further evaluation at Hexi University Affiliated Zhangye People's Hospital (Zhangye, China) in July 2024, the patient's vital signs were within normal ranges. Physical examination revealed right upper abdominal tenderness, a palpable mass, facial acne, and obesity, with a body weight increase from 54 to 69 kg over the past 2 months. The patient exhibited mental distress and general fatigue, with weight gain and redistribution of body fat, resulting in the characteristic appearance of a moon face and buffalo hump [31].

Endocrine evaluation revealed low insulin and C-peptide levels during hypoglycemic episodes, with an elevated IGF-2/IGF-1 ratio exceeding 10, suggesting hypoglycemia mediated by IGF-2. Abdominal computed tomography (CT) scan revealed a right-sided adrenal mass. The patient underwent surgical resection of the adrenal tumor [31].

Postoperative recovery was uneventful, and follow-up evaluations showed resolution of hypoglycemic episodes (**Figure 2**) [31].

This case underscores the rarity of hypoglycemia as a manifestation of metastatic adrenal cortical carcinoma and emphasizes the importance of considering paraneoplastic syndromes in the differential diagnosis of unexplained hypoglycemia [31].

The prognosis of patients with NICTH is closely linked to that of the underlying neoplasm. In benign or completely resectable malignant tumors, surgical removal is curative for hypoglycemia, resulting in immediate normalization of glycemic profile

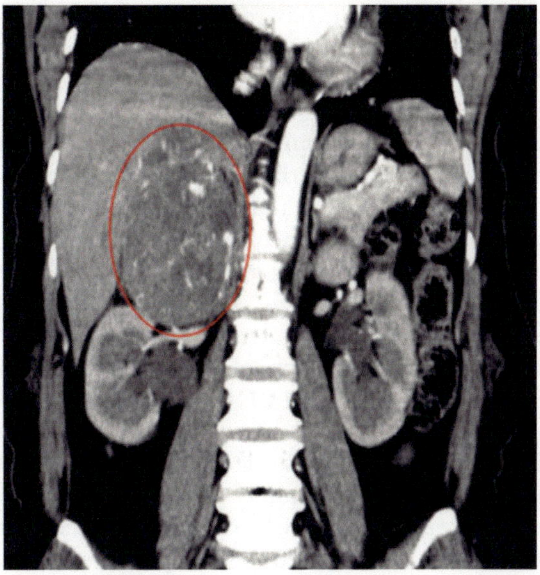

Figure 2.
Imaging manifestation of right adrenal cortical carcinoma. Contrast-enhanced computed tomography coronal section, where the right adrenal tumor can be seen. Obtained from the work by Li et al. [31].

and symptom resolution. However, in advanced or metastatic malignant tumors, paraneoplastic hypoglycemia often represents a marker of poor prognosis, associated with increased tumor burden and biological aggressiveness.

Follow-up of these patients should include both oncologic and metabolic aspects, including periodic blood glucose monitoring (especially during therapeutic changes), regular tumor response assessment using appropriate imaging techniques, serial measurements of the IGF-2/IGF-1 ratio as a marker of tumor activity, and surveillance for adverse effects related to prolonged treatment, particularly corticosteroids.

Recurrence of previously controlled hypoglycemia should raise suspicion of possible tumor progression or recurrence, warranting a thorough oncologic reevaluation.

7. Discussion

Hypoglycemia in non-diabetic patients represents a complex clinical challenge, given the heterogeneity of its etiologies and the potential severity of its manifestations. The present chapter emphasizes the need for a structured diagnostic approach guided by Whipple's triad, as timely recognition and differentiation among insulinoma, nesidioblastosis, and non-islet cell tumor hypoglycemia (NICTH) are essential to avoid delays that may compromise patient outcomes.

Insulinoma remains the most frequent surgically correctable cause of hypoglycemia in non-diabetic adults. Although most are benign and localized, their nonspecific presentation often results in prolonged diagnostic intervals. Advances in functional imaging, particularly GLP-1 receptor, PET/CT, and endoscopic ultrasound-guided fine-needle aspiration, have significantly improved preoperative localization, facilitating minimally invasive surgical strategies. Nevertheless, postoperative morbidity, especially pancreatic fistula formation, continues to be a relevant concern. From a therapeutic standpoint, enucleation and parenchyma-sparing resections should be prioritized whenever feasible, as they preserve pancreatic function while providing high cure rates.

Adult-onset nesidioblastosis, although rare, underscores the diagnostic difficulties in distinguishing diffuse islet cell hyperplasia from insulinoma. The condition's association with bariatric surgery highlights the interplay between incretin physiology and pancreatic adaptation, suggesting that metabolic interventions may precipitate pathological insulin secretion. Surgical treatment through subtotal pancreatectomy remains the gold standard, yet carries substantial risks, including the development of insulin-dependent diabetes. For this reason, patient selection must balance the likelihood of surgical benefit against the long-term metabolic burden.

In contrast, NICTH represents a paraneoplastic syndrome with entirely different pathophysiology and prognosis. Unlike insulinoma or nesidioblastosis, these patients exhibit hypoinsulinemic hypoglycemia driven predominantly by tumoral production of aberrant IGF-2. The clinical predominance of neuroglycopenic symptoms and the correlation with advanced malignancy underline the need for a multidisciplinary approach. Complete tumor resection, when feasible, remains the only curative option. In unresectable or metastatic cases, palliation through systemic therapy, selective embolization, or radiotherapy must be complemented with pharmacological agents, such as glucocorticoids or somatostatin analogs, to mitigate hypoglycemia. Case series consistently demonstrate that the recurrence of hypoglycemia is a harbinger of tumor progression, reinforcing the importance of integrated oncologic and metabolic surveillance.

The illustrative cases presented in this chapter highlight the clinical spectrum of hypoglycemia in non-diabetic patients—from the potentially curable insulinoma to the devastating paraneoplastic hypoglycemia of hepatocellular carcinoma and adrenal carcinoma. These cases underscore the critical role of a systematic evaluation, beginning with biochemical confirmation and extending to advanced imaging and histopathology, to guide therapeutic decisions.

Overall, surgical intervention remains the cornerstone of treatment when feasible, offering definitive management and, in most cases, resolution of hypoglycemia. However, the complexity of these conditions requires individualized management plans that consider tumor biology, patient comorbidities, and long-term quality of life. The integration of endocrinology, oncology, radiology, and surgery is paramount in optimizing outcomes. Future directions will likely focus on molecular-targeted therapies and novel minimally invasive interventions, which may provide additional options for patients with otherwise limited prognoses.

8. Conclusions

This chapter explores some of the main causes of hypoglycemia that affect insulin production in the pancreas in non-diabetic patients. Through a discussion of its main clinical characteristics, diagnosis, and treatment, the importance of early detection for appropriate management and the goal of preventing serious complications have been highlighted.

Insulinoma is the most common neuroendocrine tumor of the pancreas; however, diagnosis is often inopportune due to its nonspecific symptoms. Despite being generally benign, it is associated with high morbidity.

It is crucial to keep in mind that episodes of low blood sugar are characterized by a well-established set of symptoms known as Whipple's triad.

Signs of low blood sugar encompass autonomic (adrenergic) symptoms, including sweating, nervousness, heart palpitations, lack of strength, rapid heartbeat, intense hunger, nausea, and a feeling of heat. Symptoms related to neuroglucopenia may consist of mood swings, mental impairments, brief neurological deficits, seizures, unconsciousness, double vision, and memory loss.

The management of insulin-producing tumors varies based on the tumor's size and position, along with whether it has spread to other areas. Treatment options involve surgery (removal of the tumor), medical management (relief of symptoms for tumors that cannot be surgically removed or have metastasized), and targeted treatments (effective for tumors with particular molecular profiles).

Surgical intervention is considered the best option for insulinomas, and in the majority of instances, removing the tumor can effectively resolve this condition.

Nesidioblastosis is an uncommon disorder marked by an increase in pancreatic beta cell count, resulting in too much insulin being made. The symptoms typically occur after eating, which include fainting, lightheadedness, confusion, convulsions, sweating, shaking, and intense hunger. Diagnosing and treating this condition can be difficult, often necessitating a mix of medications and surgical options. The definitive method of treatment is the surgical removal of tissue. A partial pancreatectomy, involving the removal of 60–80% of the pancreas, has been effective in managing nesidioblastosis in about half of the cases without the need for further medication, usually when the condition is focal. However, the most accepted procedure is a subtotal pancreatectomy, which entails removing 90–95% of the pancreas. Severe hypoglycemia that occurs alongside liver cancer, metastatic adrenal cancer, and metastatic solitary fibrous tumors requires a comprehensive approach to both diagnosis and treatment. Its actual frequency might be higher than reported due to underdiagnosis, especially in those with widespread disease.

Initially, there was some uncertainty about the underlying mechanisms, with different theories suggested, including high glucose utilization by large tumors or abnormal insulin production in other sites.

The treatment method for NICTH includes not only the immediate handling of low blood sugar but also a targeted approach to address the tumor responsible for it. It is vital to grasp these issues, as timely identification and suitable intervention can enhance the well-being and outlook of patients.

Conflict of interest

The authors declare no conflict of interest.

Author details

Bonifacio García Ramos[1*], Elías Guillermo Valdéz Montoya[2],
Daena Judith Andrés Martínez[3], Victor García Ramos[4],
Alvaro Alejandro Sánchez Ruiz[1], Jorge Luis Gordillo Magallanes[1]
and Patricio Alan Villarreal Aguirre[5]

1 High Specialty Medical Unit (UMAE) Manuel Ávila Camacho Traumatology and Orthopedics Hospital, Puebla, México

2 General Hospital of Zone N°. 1 Dr. Demetrio Mayoral Pardo, Oaxaca, México

3 Oaxacan Children's Hospital, Oaxaca, México

4 High Specialty Medical Unit (UMAE) Adolfo Ruiz Cortines, Veracruz, México

5 General Hospital of Monclova, Coahuila, México

*Address all correspondence to: bonifacio_bonice@hotmail.com

References

[1] Castro, Gomez KG, Contreras Romero JA, Afanador Jaimes DV, Álvarez Herrera LV, Gaitán Díaz NL, Saavedra López HF. Abordaje del insulinoma: revisión actualizada de la literatura. Revista Colombiana de Endocrinología, Diabetes & Metabolismo. 2024;**11**(1):1-23. DOI: 10.53853/encr.11.1.822

[2] Medina-Zamora P, Lucio-Figueroa JO. Insulinoma: revisión actual de manejo y tratamiento. Revista médica MD. 2016;7(2):83-90

[3] Minn AH, Kayton M, Lorang D, Hoffmann SC, et al. Insulinomas and expression of insulin splice variant. Lancet. 2004;**363**(9406):363-367. DOI: 10.1016/S0140-6736(04)15438-X

[4] Wiesli P, Perren A, Saremaslani P, Pfammatter T, Spinas GA, Schmid C. Abnormalities of proinsulin processing in functioning insulinomas: Clinical implications. Clinical Endocrinology (Oxford). 2004;**61**(4):424-430. DOI: 10.1111/j.1365-2265.2004.02095.x

[5] Shin JJ, Gorden P, Libutti SK. Insulinoma: Pathophysiology, localization and management. Future Oncology. 2010;**6**(2):229-237. DOI: 10.2217/fon.09.165

[6] Hofland J, Falconi M, Christ E, Castaño JP, Faggiano A, Lamarca A, et al. European neuroendocrine tumor society 2023 guidance paper for functioning pancreatic neuroendocrine tumour syndromes. Journal of Neuroendocrinology. 2023;**35**(8):e13318. DOI: 10.1111/jne.13318

[7] De Herder WW, Niederle B, Scoazec JY, Pauwels S, Klöppel G, Falconi M, et al. Well-differentiated pancreatic tumor/carcinoma: Insulinoma. Neuroendocrinology. 2006;**84**(3):183-188. DOI: 10.1159/000098010

[8] Witteles RM, Straus FH 2nd, Sugg SL, Koka MR, Costa EA, Kaplan EL. Adult-onset nesidioblastosis causing hypoglycemia: An important clinical entity and continuing treatment dilemma. Archives of Surgery. 2001;**136**(6):656-663. DOI: 10.1001/archsurg.136.6.656

[9] Dravecka I, Lazurova I. Nesidioblastosis in adults. Neoplasma. 2014;**61**(3):252-256. DOI: 10.4149/neo_2014_047

[10] Raffel A, Krausch MM, Anlauf M, Wieben D, Braunstein S, Klöppel G, et al. Diffuse nesidioblastosis as a cause of hyperinsulinemic hypoglycemia in adults: A diagnostic and therapeutic challenge. Surgery. 2007;**141**(2):179-184. DOI: 10.1016/j.surg.2006.04.015

[11] Palladino AA, Stanley CA. Nesidioblastosis no longer! It's all about genetics. The Journal of Clinical Endocrinology and Metabolism. 2011;**96**(3):617-619. DOI: 10.1210/jc.2011-0164

[12] Service GJ, Thompson GB, Service FJ, Andrews JC, Collazo-Clavell ML, Lloyd RV. Hyperinsulinemic hypoglycemia with nesidioblastosis after gastric-bypass surgery. The New England Journal of Medicine. 2005;**353**(3):249-254. DOI: 10.1056/NEJMoa043690

[13] García B, Álamo MV, Gonzalez EA. Nesidioblastosis focal y difusa que simula un insulinoma. Medicina Clínica (Barcelona). 2023;**162**(9):457-459. DOI: 10.1016/j.medcli.2023.11.034

[14] Fajardo D, Aguirre DAU, Chaviano AR. Hipoglucemia

hiperinsulínica en un adulto con nesidioblastosis. Revista Cubana de Cirugía. 2020;**59**(4):1-8

[15] Thompson SM, Vella A, Thompson GB, Rumilla KM, Service FJ, Grant CS, et al. Selective arterial calcium stimulation with hepatic venous sampling differentiates insulinoma from nesidioblastosis. The Journal of Clinical Endocrinology and Metabolism. 2015;**100**(11):4189-4197. DOI: 10.1210/jc.2015-2404

[16] Torres-Arano SE, Fernández-Baez N, Torres-González MG, González-Cabrera IG, López-Rosales F. Hipoglucemia hiperinsulinémica en el adulto. Reporte de un caso de nesidioblastosis y revisión de la literatura. Cirugia y Cirujanos. 2021;**89**(S1):70-75

[17] Demartin S, Goffette P, Christ E, Freitag MT, Maiter D, Furnica RM. Adult onset nesidioblastosis: A challenging diagnosis revealed by glucagon like peptide 1 receptor imaging. Endocrinology, Diabetes & Metabolism Case Reports. 2022;**2022**(1):edm220325. DOI: 10.1530/EDM-22-0325

[18] Stivaros S, Hynes SO, Cremeens CR, et al. Management of non-islet-cell tumor hypoglycemia: A clinical case and review of the literature. The Journal of Clinical Endocrinology and Metabolism. 2014;**99**(3):713-719. DOI: 10.1210/jc.2013-2959

[19] Bodnar TW, Acevedo MJ, Pietropaolo M. Management of non-islet-cell tumor hypoglycemia: A clinical review. The Journal of Clinical Endocrinology and Metabolism. 2014;**99**(3):713-722. DOI: 10.1210/jc.2013-3382

[20] Takahashi H, Masuda T, Tadokoro M, Matsumoto S, Iwasaki Y, Kubo T, et al. Hypoglycemia mediated by paraneoplastic production of insulin-like growth factor-2 (IGF-2). Endocrine Journal. 2014;**61**(6):537-544. DOI: 10.1186/1472-6823-14-49

[21] De Groot JW, Rikhof B, van Doorn J, Bilo HJ, Alleman MA, Honkoop AH, et al. Paraneoplastic hypoglycemia: An overview for optimal clinical management. Endocrine-Related Cancer. 2024;**31**(7):R125-R137. DOI: 10.1016/j.metop.2024.100305

[22] Igaz P, Paszt A, Stefanova D, et al. Non-islet cell tumor hypoglycemia: Pathophysiology and clinical implications. Frontiers in Endocrinology (Lausanne). 2022;**13**:968077. DOI: 10.3389/fsurg.2022.968077

[23] Hojfeldt G, Mørup M, Kristensen JM, Sandberg M, Jørgensen JO, Nielsen S, et al. Non-islet cell hypoglycemia: Case series and review of the molecular mechanisms with emphasis on IGF-2 mediated insulin receptor activation. Frontiers in Endocrinology (Lausanne). 2019;**10**:316. DOI: 10.3389/fendo.2019.00316

[24] Abdulhadi B, Anastasopoulou C, Lekprasert P. Tumor-induced hypoglycemia: An unusual case report and review of literature. Cureus. 2020;**12**(12):e12345. DOI: 10.1016/j.aace.2020.11.002

[25] Ata F, Choudry H, Khan AA, et al. A systematic review of literature on insulin-like growth factor-2-mediated hypoglycaemia in non-islet cell tumours. Endocrinology, Diabetes & Metabolism. 2024;**7**(2):e00471. DOI: 10.1002/edm2.471

[26] Karamanolis N, Kounatidis D, Vallianou NG, et al. Paraneoplastic hypoglycemia: An overview for optimal clinical guidance. Metabolism Open. 2024;**23**(1):1-9. DOI: 10.1016/j.metop.2024.100305

[27] Crowley MT, McDonald JR, McDonald JR, et al. IGF-2 mediated hypoglycemia and the paradox of an insulin-like growth factor II-producing tumor. BMC Endocrine Disorders. 2022;**22**(1):175. DOI: 10.1186/s12902-022-01175-4

[28] Dizon AM, O'Dorisio MS, O'Dorisio TM, et al. Neuroglycopenic and other symptoms in patients with non-islet cell tumor hypoglycemia. The Journal of Clinical Endocrinology and Metabolism. 1999;**84**(3):1055-1060. DOI: 10.1210/jcem.84.3.5534

[29] Kurihara T, Nakano Y, Iwasaki Y, et al. Non-islet cell tumor hypoglycemia that required immediate surgery after a long-term asymptomatic state: recommendation for early intervention. Endocrinology, Diabetes & Metabolism Case Reports. 2024;**3**(1):e00250. DOI: 10.1002/edm2.250

[30] Sanchez L, Delgado-Cruz DA, Basurco V. Reporte de caso. Hipoglucemia asociada a hepatocarcinoma. Rev Soc Peru Med Interna; 2014;**27**(1):1-4

[31] Li Y, Yang R, Zhang L, et al. Adrenal cortical carcinoma with non-islet cell tumor hypoglycemia: A case report. Oncology Letters. 2025;**29**:225. DOI: 10.3892/ol.2025.14971